T0237278

Family Poverty in Diverse Contexts

Family Poverty in Diverse Contexts addresses the context of poverty in the United States and focuses on poverty issues that family members must confront as they move through the life course.

This edited collection provides a unique perspective that draws together macro and micro research about how poverty affects families throughout their lives, increasing risks and reducing opportunities at every stage. Individual chapters emphasize the context of poverty in the United States, then go on to examine specific life cycle stages and what happens when poverty intersects with family concerns. Contributing authors are respected experts in their fields and represent a broad range of disciplines and perspectives including child development, community health, education, family studies, gerontology, disability, public policy, social work and sociology.

Family Poverty in Diverse Contexts includes a range of pedagogical features to enhance learning, such as exercises and discussions relating to each chapter, which will encourage readers to think critically and apply the knowledge to their own lives. It will interest students, academics and researchers of sociology, family studies, social work and health, as well as other related disciplines.

C. Anne Broussard is a sociologist and Associate Professor of Social Work at the University of New Hampshire, USA.

Alfred L. Joseph is Associate Professor in the Department of Family Studies and Social Work at Miami University, USA.

Family Poverty in Diverse Contexts

Edited by
C. Anne Broussard
and
Alfred L. Joseph

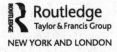

Routledge
Taylor & Francis Group

NEW YORK AND LONDON

First published 2009
by Routledge
711 Third Avenue, New York, NY 10017, USA

Simultaneously published in the UK
by Routledge
2 Park Square, Milton Park, Abingdon, Oxon OX14 4RN

Routledge is an imprint of the Taylor & Francis Group, an informa business

© 2009 Routledge

Typeset in Goudy by
Book Now Ltd, London

All rights reserved. No part of this book may be reprinted or reproduced
or utilized in any form or by any electronic, mechanical, or other means,
now known or hereafter invented, including photocopying and recording,
or in any information storage or retrieval system, without permission in
writing from the publishers.

Trademark Notice: Product or corporate names may be trademarks or
registered trademarks, and are used only for identification and
explanation without intent to infringe.

Library of Congress Cataloging-in-Publication Data
Family poverty in diverse contexts / edited by C. Anne Broussard and
Alfred L. Joseph.
    p. cm.
1. Poverty—United States. 2. Poor—United States. 3. Poor families—
United States. 4. Family—United States. 5. United States—Economic
conditions. I. Broussard, C. Anne. II. Joseph, Alfred L.
HC110.P6F36 2008
362.50973—dc22   2008012662

ISBN10: 0–7890–3740–8 (hbk)
ISBN10: 0–7890–3741–6 (pbk)
ISBN10: 0–203–89067–1 (ebk)

ISBN13: 978–0–7890–3740–4 (hbk)
ISBN13: 978–0–7890–3741–1 (pbk)
ISBN13: 978–0–203–89067–7 (ebk)

Contents

Illustrations

Contributors

C. Anne Broussard holds a PhD in Sociology from Washington State University. Currently, she is Associate Professor in the Department of Social Work at the University of New Hampshire. Her work has appeared in a variety of scholarly journals, including *Children and Schools, Equity and Excellence in Education, Health and Social Work* and *Sociological Perspectives*. Professor Broussard serves on the editorial review boards of the *Journal of Poverty*, the *Journal of Social Work Values and Ethics* and *Marriage and Family Review*. She can be reached at anne.broussard@unh.edu.

Alfred L. Joseph holds a PhD in Social Work from the Ohio State University and is currently Associate Professor in the Department of Family Studies and Social Work at Miami University. He is co-editor of the *Journal of Poverty* and has published in *Children and Schools, Social Work in Education* and *School Social Work Journal*. Professor Joseph has also authored and co-authored a number of book chapters. He can be reached at josephal@muohio.edu.

Mimi Abramovitz, DSW, Hunter College School of Social Work and the Graduate Center, City University of New York, 129 East 79th St, New York, NY 10021, iabramov@hunter.cuny.edu.

Robert Aponte, PhD, IUPUI—Sociology (CA303), 425 University Blvd., Indianapolis, IN 46202, raponte@iupui.edu.

Sandra Austin, EdD, School of Social Welfare, 203 Richardson Hall, University of Albany, 135 Western Ave. Albany, NY 12222, saustin@albany.edu.

L. Rene Bergeron, PhD, Department of Social Work, 55 College Road, University of New Hampshire, Durham, NH 03824, lb@cisunix.unh.edu.

Katharine Briar-Lawson, PhD, Dean, School of Social Welfare, 101 Richardson Hall, University of Albany, 135 Western Ave., Albany, NY 12222, kbriar lawson@uamail.albany.edu.

Karen Carlson, PhD, Department of Social Work, Ohio University Zanesville, 1425 Newark Rd, Zanesville, OH 43701, carlsonk@ohio.edu.

Carrie E. Foote, PhD, IUPUI—Sociology (CA303), 425 University Blvd., Indianapolis, IN 46202, foote@iupui.edu.

Charles B. Hennon, PhD, Department of Family Studies and Social Work, Miami University, Room 101D McGuffey Hall, Oxford, OH 45056, hennoncb@muohio.edu.

Bruno Hildenbrand, PhD, Institut für Soziologie, Friedrich-Schiller Universität Jena, D 07740 Jena, Germany, bruno.hildenbrand@uni-jena.de.

Keith M. Kilty, Professor Emeritus, OSU College of Social Work, 225E Stillman Hall, 1947 College Road, Columbus, OH 43210, kilty.1@osu.edu.

W. Sean Newsome, PhD, Department of Family Studies and Social Work, Miami University, Room 101J McGuffey Hall, Oxford, OH 45056, new somws@muohio.edu.

Michael D. Niles, PhD, School of Social Work, Arizona State University, Office of American Indian Projects, College of Public Programs, 411 N. Central Ave, Ste 880M, Phoenix, AZ 85004-0689, michael.niles@asu.edu.

Gary W. Peterson, PhD, Department of Family Studies and Social Work, Miami University, Room 101C McGuffey Hall, Oxford, OH 45056, petersgw@muohio.edu.

M. Elise Radina, PhD, Department of Family Studies and Social Work, Miami University, Room 101E McGuffey Hall, Oxford, OH 45056, radiname@muohio.edu.

Tammy Anne Schwartz, EdD, Department of Teacher Education, Miami University, Room 401 McGuffey Hall, Oxford, OH 45056, schwarta@muohio.edu.

Karen Seccombe, PhD, School of Community Health, Portland State University, PO Box 751, Portland, OR 97207-0751, seccombek@pdx.edu.

Elizabeth A. Segal, PhD, School of Social Work, Arizona State University, Mail Code 3920, 411 N. Central Ave, Ste 800, Phoenix, AZ 85004-0689, esegal@asu.edu.

Patrick Shannon, PhD, School of Social Work, University at Buffalo, 658 Baldy Hall, Buffalo, NY 14260-1050, pshannon@buffalo.edu.

Karen Slovak, PhD, Department of Social Work, Ohio University Zanesville, 1425 Newark Rd, Zanesville, OH 43701, slovak@ohio.edu.

Carrie Jefferson Smith, DSW, Syracuse University College of Human Services and Health Professions, School of Social Work, 307 Sims Hall, Syracuse, NY 13244, cjsmit04@syr.edu.

Stephan W. Wilson, PhD, Human Development and Family Sciences, 106 HES, Stillwater, OK 74078, stephen.wilson@okstate.edu.

Acknowledgments

We want to begin by acknowledging the significant contributions made by our distinguished group of authors, without whom this book would not have become a reality. We want to thank our Haworth editor—Suzanne Steinmetz—who helped at every step of the process. Thank you for sharing your expertise with us. Thank you to Gary Peterson, who kick-started the book by putting us in touch with Suzanne, and to Keith Kilty for his valuable advice throughout the process. Many thanks to Ruth Edmonds, Anne's graduate assistant, who searched the literature for hours on end. We also want to thank Grace McInnis, Eloise Cook, and the other fine people at Routledge for pulling us through the final rabbit hole. Finally, we want to thank our own families who have been there through reams of electronic "paper" and who have spent many evenings and weekends without us as we wrote and edited this book.

I would like to thank my husband, Bob Kennedy, and children, Forrest and Reeve, for being my constant source of support as I worked on this book. I could not have done it without you. CAB

I would like to thank my family—wife Dorothy and sons, Shane, Paul and Jonathan. Thank you for allowing me time to work. I apologize for missing too many dinners. ALJ

1 Introduction
The Poverty Context

C. Anne Broussard and Alfred L. Joseph

The United States (U.S.) boasts one of the highest per capita incomes in the world. Yet it leads other industrialized nations with the highest poverty rate. In 2000, Smeeding, Rainwater, and Burtless compared poverty rates across 18 developed nations using three different poverty measures. Their results showed that the U.S. poverty rate was considerably higher than all 17 of the other nations. More recently, Smeeding (2006) ranked 11 wealthy nations and again the United States scored first or second on nearly all poverty measures. In addition to noting that poverty among the elderly was particularly high in comparison to other wealthy nations, Smeeding (2006, p. 86) expressed special concern over U.S. child and family poverty:

> In most rich countries, the relative child poverty rate is 10 percent or less; in the United States, it is 21.9 percent. What seems most distinctive about the American poor, especially poor American single parents, is that they work more hours than do the resident parents of other nations while also receiving less in transfer benefits than in other countries.

Closer to home, the U.S. Census Bureau (2007a) recorded the U.S. poverty rate at 22.2% in 1960. Throughout the 1960s and into the early 1970s, the rate declined dramatically, reaching a low of 11.1% in 1973. It has changed little since then, fluctuating between 11.2% and 15.2%, tending to decrease with economic expansion and increase with economic recession (Rank, 2001, p. 883). The 2006 poverty rate was 12.3, which represented about 36.5 million people. When we add those who were near poverty—living at 125% of poverty level— the rate increases to 16.8% or more than 49 million Americans. That year, more than 15 million of these individuals (5.2%) lived in extreme poverty (below 50% of poverty level).

While the overall rates are high, these numbers vary substantially by context within the United States: They are much higher for some groups than for others. For example, the 12.3% poverty rate listed above represented all races. Breaking this rate down by racial and ethnic status reveals wide variation in the numbers: For Whites, the 2006 poverty rate was 8.2%, for Blacks it was 24.3% and for all Hispanics, the rate was 20.6% (U.S. Census Bureau, 2007a). If we break down Hispanic poverty by national origin, we would find that some Hispanic populations experience considerably higher poverty than others.

The results are similar if we examine poverty by gender (U.S. Census Bureau, 2007a). For people of all races in families with a female householder and no husband present, 30.5% were below poverty level in 2006, but the rate ranged from 22.5% (Whites alone) to 39.1% (Blacks alone). In contrast, the poverty rate for all married couple families was a significantly lower 4.9%.

How can such wide variations be explained? The simple answer is context. The family life course is situated within a broadbased structural context that provides opportunities and constraints for individuals and families living in a given culture. Sewell, (1992, p. 862) explained that, "social structures intersect in complex ways such that structures of the life course will interact with broader structures of a gendered, racialized, and class-based society." Sewell pointed to sociohistorical context and stratification as two important dimensions that dictate opportunities and constraints across the life course (p. 862).

This book examines family poverty across a number of important contexts, highlighting family characteristics that result in disadvantages for broad cross-sections of people. First, though, it is important to define poverty in the United States and to discuss how our history has unfolded to place some people at greater disadvantage than others.

What Is Poverty?

Two common poverty measures are absolute and relative poverty. Absolute poverty refers to the least amount of money needed to meet basic human survival needs, such as food and shelter, while relative poverty is where people fall relative to other members of the society in which they live. Poverty was first measured officially in the United States in the mid-1960s after President Lyndon Johnson launched his War on Poverty. In response to the President's plan, the President's Council of Economic Advisors (CEA) and the Office of Economic Opportunity (OEO) began to actively seek a poverty measure that would avoid an inequality focus (i.e. relative poverty), and focus instead on the specific level of income needed to subsist at a minimal level (i.e. absolute poverty). At the same time, and apart from OEO and CEA, a Social Security Administration economist and statistician named Mollie Orshansky developed a poverty measure (see Orshansky, 1965).

Orshansky's measure determined the minimum income (using 1963 dollars) required for families of various sizes to purchase a minimally adequate diet according to the U.S. Department of Agriculture (USDA) Economy Food Plan (Fisher, 1997). Since individuals need more than a minimal diet (for example, minimal clothing and minimal shelter), she multiplied each of the calculated amounts by three. This multiple of three was not arbitrary; rather it was based on 1955 Household Food Consumption Survey data, which found that families with three or more members spent approximately one-third of their after-tax income on food (Fisher, 1997). Orshansky's measure defined poor families as those whose

Table 1.1 U.S. Department of Health & Human Services (DHHS) Poverty Guidelines by Size of Family, 2008

Size of family unit	Poverty threshold
One person	$10,400
Two people	$14,000
Three people	$17,600
Four people	$21,200
Five people	$24,800
Six people	$28,400
Seven people	$32,000
Eight people	$35,600
For each additional person, add	$3,600

U.S. DHHS (2008).

pre-tax income fell below the calculated threshold for families of given sizes. While Orshansky's approach is still used today, her original measure, which took into account the relative wealth of the United States, has evolved into a measure of absolute poverty (Fisher, 1997; Iceland, 2003). If the U.S. government had recalculated the cost of a minimal diet in the United States each year, the poverty rate would to some extent take into account both absolute and relative poverty; however, in 1969, officials began to adjust poverty thresholds for inflation using the Consumer Price Index (CPI). In order to adjust for growth in U.S. incomes, which have increased faster than the CPI, the proportion of income spent on food would have to be recalculated each year. As it is, poverty threshold buying power has not changed since the 1960s. Take a look at the 2008 poverty guidelines in Table 1.1. The income information in this table represents weighted average thresholds. The actual thresholds vary by several characteristics, including whether the family lives in the 48 contiguous states, Alaska or Hawaii and whether individuals in the household are over or under age 65 (the complete 2008 guidelines table is available at: http://aspe.hhs.gov/poverty/08poverty.shtml). In order to be considered officially poor, a family of four could not have made a penny over $21,200. Families that live above the official threshold may not be able to afford basic necessities; nevertheless, they are not included in the determination of the official poverty rate. Neither are the millions of poor who move frequently, or many of those who live in places like nursing homes, mental hospitals, and prisons (Rodgers, 2006). Rodgers points to a number of other flaws with the official poverty measure, including lack of regional cost adjustments for shelter, health care, and food (pp. 18–19).

Who Are the Poor?

The poor are all around us if we would only bother to look. They are invisible. It takes extraordinary people, movements or catastrophes to "remind" us that we need to (re)discover poverty in the "land of plenty."

Hurricane Katrina, a category-four storm, hit the southeast United States before dawn on 29 August 2005 with unforgiving ferocity. It destroyed millions of dollars worth of residential and commercial property. It disrupted the lives of hundreds of thousands of people in Mississippi and Louisiana. In New Orleans alone, over 1000 men, women, and children lost their lives. The rest of America watched in horror as the extent of the devastation became clear. We all watched stunned as our fellow citizens gathered on rooftops, waded chest-deep in flood-waters, and crammed into public buildings in an effort to survive the storm and the subsequent flooding. A tragedy like this can expose the weaknesses and contradictions of any society. In times of crisis, fault lines that go unnoticed in "normal" times make their presence known in ways that are difficult, if not impossible, to ignore. The Hurricane Katrina catastrophe taught us a great deal about American society, though the lessons can be uncomfortable. Lessons like these require that we reassess much of our conventional wisdom about the fundamental inequality that permeates all aspects of the American social order. Hurricane Katrina laid bare the deep racial and class divisions in the United States that many of our leaders desperately try to ignore and pretend do not exist. Those who go out on a limb and talk about what is obvious if we would only look are often derided and labeled as proponents of "class warfare."

Imagine yourself in New Orleans just before, during, and immediately after Hurricane Katrina made contact. Your chances of getting out of New Orleans and other threatened areas increases as your class position edges up the socioeconomic ladder. Access to a car or cars, and access to cash or credit cards, greatly increases your chances of being able to escape to a more hospitable place. Being middle-class or wealthier increases your chances of having others in your immediate circle of friends or family who can help you. They can use their resources to assist you in your hour of need. You need not wait on the authorities.

The storm taught us that an individual's chances of living or dying could depend on whether or not they live in poverty. These are not facts that are easy to confront or to accept. Of course, we all realize, on some level, that there are poor people in our midst. But our political leaders and the media, almost to a person, focus on the "great middle class" to the exclusion of the more than 35 million people living in poverty in the United States. The impoverished were and are largely ignored. Indeed, a Brookings Institution analysis (Berube & Katz, 2005) reported that the areas most affected by Hurricane Katrina housed 80% of New Orleans minority residents. In contrast, 54% of the residents in the flooded areas were White.

Another lesson Hurricane Katrina taught us is equally important. Katrina showed us that we hold the poor in contempt. The contempt is based on the fact that many people blame the poor for their own predicament. Writing in 1976, scholar William Ryan defined blaming the victim as, "justifying inequality by finding defects in the victims of inequality" (p. xiii). Think back to Hurricane Katrina: The feelings of pity for those left behind faded quickly as "stories" of various types of criminality began to fill the airwaves. Stories of selflessness and sacrifice that could have been broadcast were pushed aside for stories about criminality, whether verifiable or not. These news stories confirmed what many people already believed about the poor. Pity turned to anger and then to scorn. The storm victims were seen as responsible for their own situation. The message was clear, even in the midst of a grave natural disaster: Poor people behave in ways that exacerbate their already unfortunate situation. This lesson—that poor people continue to behave in ways that further their own degradation, even in the midst of a natural disaster—was powerful.

Even though it took extraordinary circumstances to expose both the vulnerability of the poor and the contempt with which they are held, we must remind ourselves that this is a normal part of the daily lives of poor people. We must also be aware that this is not unique to adults; it is applicable to children as well. The lives of poor children and adults are distorted by their vulnerability to both the vagaries of life and the political reality that many of their fellow citizens hold them accountable for their own poverty. There is no refuge from this reality.

Who Should Be Interested in this Book?

Family Poverty in Diverse Contexts is designed for students, scholars, practitioners, policymakers, and other stakeholders invested in alleviating family poverty. There is a great deal of high-quality research about poverty outcomes at various stages throughout the life cycle. There is also abundant research that addresses individual, neighborhood, and structural contexts. However, poverty research cuts across disciplines, which fragments the information and makes it difficult to synthesize. This book pulls together some of the latest family poverty knowledge across the life cycle addressed by scholars from diverse disciplines, including economics, education, family studies, psychology, public health, medical fields, social work, and sociology. Because the contributors and the research they address cuts across a variety of disciplines, this book could serve as a text for a broad range of graduate- and advanced undergraduate-level courses that deal with poverty, structural inequality, the family, and individual life cycles, women and children, and public policy.

The book is organized into three sections. The first section sketches the structural context of family poverty in the United States. Rank (2001) defines three structural sources of poverty—economic, social/political and structural vulnerability—all of which are touched upon in this first section. Kilty (Chapter 2) addresses the way ideology has helped to shape policies that greatly impact the lives of those with little power and influence in society. In Chapter 3, Abramovitz examines the historical relationship between women and the state that has resulted in policies that place women at far greater risk of experiencing poverty throughout the life cycle. Seccombe (Chapter 4) examines the consequences of the Personal Responsibility and Work Opportunity Reconciliation Act (PRWORA; PL 104-193) and Temporary Assistance for Needy Families (TANF) for poor families in the United States. The final two chapters in this section address specific family poverty contexts: Chapter 5 juxtaposes rural against urban family poverty, while Aponte and Foote (Chapter 6) examine family poverty among Hispanics, the fastest-growing minority population in the United States (U.S. Census Bureau, 2007b).

The second section addresses individual and family contexts of poverty at a range of stages across the life cycle from childhood through old age. A key theme throughout the chapters in this section is that poverty and associated policy affect the lives of all generations, from infants through the elderly. Another key theme is that poverty-related problems multiply and continue in the lives of individuals and families; they come not just in threes, but in fours, sixes, and eights, causing stress, lost income, transportation difficulties, compromised physical and mental health, and family conflict and breakup, among other things, and can result in lifelong disadvantage. This section addresses poverty outcomes that change normal development for small children (Segal & Niles, Chapter 7) as well as special problems faced by poor families with children who have disabilities (Shannon, Chapter 8). In Chapter 9, Smith addresses the U.S. foster care system and what it means for poor families in various contexts, while Joseph and Schwartz (Chapter 10) examine the many ways children in poverty experience our nation's schools. The last two chapters in this section examine family poverty during adulthood in depth: mental health and other outcomes for single mothers (Broussard, Chapter 11) and special problems facing the elderly poor (Bergeron, Chapter 12). Certainly this book does not address all aspects of family poverty across the life cycle. That would take many volumes, as there is enough information in the literature, even using research conducted just since the millennium, to devote multiple books to each chapter topic. Neither do we have solutions for creating equitable and family-friendly policy. Rather, this book provides a cross-section of information about contexts in which poverty exists and a call to begin to think about family poverty research differently as we move forward.

The final two chapters look to the future of family research and policy. Chapter 13 (Hennon, Newsome, Peterson, Wilson, Radina, & Hildenbrand) presents a multidimensional family action and intervention model that suggests new research avenues, in addition to providing guidelines for reducing resource-related stressors caused by poverty. Finally, Briar-Lawson and Austin (Chapter 14) return to U.S. structures that promote poverty by addressing values and belief systems that drive the continued development of policy that fosters the persistence of family poverty. They point to antipoverty agendas in other nations as models to developing pathways out of poverty in the United States and reversing the U.S. "race to the bottom."

As you will see, poverty statistics are disturbing. And they confirm that poor families are all around us. If we look closely, we will see that the primary difference between poor families and other families in the United States is that poor families lack opportunity on many fronts, including adequate housing, food, health care and education. Ehrenreich (2001, p. 214) has declared that poverty in America is in a "state of emergency." Others ask what has become of the American Dream and urge policymakers to stop blaming and start developing antipoverty public policy that can restore this dream (Edwards, Crain & Kalleberg, 2007).

References

Berube, A. & Katz, B. (2005). *Katrina's window: Confronting concentrated poverty across America, special analysis in metropolitan policy.* Washington, DC: Brookings Institution, Metropolitan Policy Program. Available HTML: www.brookings.edu/~/media/Files/rc/reports/2005/10poverty_berube/20051012_Concentratedpoverty.pdf.

Edwards, J., Crain, M., & Kalleberg, A. (2007). *Ending poverty in America: How to restore the American Dream.* New York: New Press.

Ehrenreich, B. (2001). *Nickel and dimed: On (not) getting by in America.* New York: Henry Holt.

Federal Register (2008, 23 January). The 2008 HHS poverty guidelines. *Federal Register, 73.* Available HTML: http://aspe.hhs.gov/poverty/08poverty.shtml (accessed 27 June 2008).

Fisher, G. (1997). The development and history of the poverty thresholds. *Newsletter of the Government Statistics Section and the Social Statistics Section of the American Statistical Association,* Winter, 6–7. Available: http://aspe.hhs.gov/poverty/papers/hptgssiv.htm (accessed 12 December 2007).

Iceland, J. (2003). *Poverty in America: A handbook.* Berkeley: University of California Press.

Orshansky, M. (1965). Counting the poor: Another look at the poverty profile. *Social Security Bulletin, 28,* 3–29.

Rank, M. (2001). The effect of poverty on America's families: Assessing our research knowledge. *Journal of Family Issues, 22,* 882–903.

Rodgers, H. (2006). *American poverty in a new era of reform* (2nd ed.). Armonk, NY: M. E. Sharpe.

Ryan, W. (1976). *Blaming the victim.* New York: Vintage.

Sewell, W., Jr. (1992). A theory of structure: Duality, agency, and transformation. *American Journal of Sociology, 98,* 1–29.

Smeeding, T. (2006). Poor people in rich nations: The United States in comparative perspective. *Journal of Economic Perspectives, 20,* 60–90.

Smeeding, T., Rainwater, L., & Burtless, G. (2000). *United States poverty in a cross-national context* (Luxembourg Income Study, Working Paper Series No. 244). Syracuse, NY: Maxwell School of Citizenship and Public Affairs, Syracuse University.

U.S. Census Bureau. (2007a). Table 2—Poverty Status of People by Family Relationship, Race, and Hispanic; Table 6—People Below 125 Percent of Poverty Level and the Near Poor: 1959 to 2006 (Numbers in Thousands) Origin: 1959 to 2006; Table 22—Number and Percent of People Below 50 Percent of Poverty Level: 1975 to 2006. Current Population Survey, Annual Social and Economic Supplements. Washington, DC: Author. Available HTML: www.census.gov/hhes/www/poverty/histpov/perindex.html (accessed 9 December 2007).

U.S. Census Bureau. (2007b, 17 May). Minority population tops 100 million. *U.S. Census Bureau News.* Washington, DC: Author.

Critical Thinking Questions

1 The authors assert that social class and race played a large part in the aftermath of Hurricane Katrina. Think about the constraints related to race and class (also called institutionalized racism and institutionalized classism). What are their effect on individuals and families? How is your own cultural background demonstrated in your family life? Does it mean different things to be White, Black, or Hispanic, for example? What does it mean to be a poor White person or a wealthy Black person in U.S. society?

2 Evaluate the U.S. official federal poverty measure, and then search the Internet to see if you can find reference to other types of poverty measures (two sites to start with are: www.cbpp.org/11-15-99wel.htm and www.npc.umich.edu/poverty/). Are there better measures available? How would you improve on the official U.S. measure?

3 Choose a social issue such as health care, civil rights, gender, or mental health and plot historical events through the twentieth century (use Internet sources) indicating how cultural shifts, societal attitudes, or social policies have changed the ways in which families have experienced these social issues over time.

Part I

Cross-Sections of Oppression and Poverty

2 "Greed Is Good"

The Idle Rich, the Working Poor, and Personal Responsibility[1]

Keith M. Kilty

When Hurricane Katrina came ashore on the morning of 29 August 2005, it left behind horrific images of people trapped throughout the city of New Orleans. Other parts of the southeastern Gulf coast were also devastated, but it was the pictures of the suffering in a flooded New Orleans that captured the hearts of many people in this country—at least for a few short hours. Suddenly poverty and desperation, especially among minorities, were all too visible. That is unusual in America. For the most part, Americans have long suffered from "historical amnesia" when it comes to poverty (Kilty, 2006). But every now and then, poverty becomes visible, even if for just a little while.

Some 40 years ago was another time when poverty and its connection to race and ethnicity became strikingly visible in America. In many ways, this era—"the sixties"—is unique in U.S. history. Largely as a result of being the only major industrial state not devastated by the ravages of World War II, the United States was then in the midst of an amazing period of affluence (Blau, 2006). For the generation that grew up during the Great Depression, achieving the American Dream—a "hopeful, more prosperous future" (Peck & Gershon, 2006, p. 98)—seemed finally within reach.

There was another side to the 1960s. This was also a time of social activism, especially focused on civil rights. While opportunities were available for many, poverty was still common, especially for older people, minorities of color and Appalachians (Ehrenreich, 1985). However, it was not only poverty that touched the lives of far too many, but also continuing blatant discrimination in who got hired or fired, in where some could go to school or live and in being allowed to vote. Civil rights demonstrations and rallies brought nightly images of poverty and race to the public through national television news coverage. Seminal books like Michael Harrington's *The Other America* (1962) challenged the widespread belief that poverty had been eradicated. Many people worked hard, trying to make a better life for their families, but remained mired deep in poverty—contrary to the American ethos that hard work will bring prosperity.

The nation's historic amnesia about poverty, inequality, and race and ethnicity could not prevail, especially when anticolonial movements throughout what was then called the Third World were focusing greater and greater attention on the racist and imperialist histories of the United States and its western European allies

(Ehrenreich, 1985). The very public images of racism and poverty challenged the freedom and equality rhetoric championed by the leaders of this country. This combination of social forces culminated in efforts by the Lyndon B. Johnson administration to deal with a growing public perception that poverty and racism were deeply entrenched in the lives of Americans. On the economic front came the War on Poverty and Great Society programs, particularly the Economic Opportunity Act of 1964. On the racism and discrimination front came major legislative initiatives, including the Civil Rights Act of 1964 and the Voting Rights Act of 1965.

While debate continues as to which factors provoked which political responses, the 1960s were an era where broad policies emerged. As Katz (1989, p. 81) points out, "Histories of the War on Poverty disagree about the relative influence of ideas, bureaucratic politics and political strategy." It was, in fact, all three factors at work: efforts to understand poverty and inequality, conflicts between different national bureaucracies, and attempts to create new constituencies and a degree of compassion for the poor and oppressed.

Unfortunately, the 1960s did not last long. Poverty turned out to be more intractable than modestly funded social programs could counteract, especially with the growing war in Vietnam consuming a larger and larger share of the national wealth (Blau, 2004). Civil rights gains were met with increasing hostility from Whites, and conservative politicians soon learned to exploit those sentiments in their election campaigns (Neubeck & Cazenave, 2001). Little by little, a perception emerged that War on Poverty programs were failures, allowing an explanation of poverty and inequality that focused on the individual as responsible for his or her situation to surface: the notion of a "culture of poverty." As Ehrenreich (1985, p. 164) describes, "In its simplest form, it was nothing more than the observation that prolonged poverty leads to poor health, inadequate education, high rates of marital instability, aberrant subcultural value systems and behaviors and ultimately to individual and community apathy, lack of self-esteem and powerlessness; and that all of these characteristics handicap people in their efforts to improve their situation."

While this conception does not necessarily place the blame for poverty and inequality on the victim, it was interpreted by some exclusively in individualistic terms. This process started with one of the more controversial versions of the "culture of poverty" thesis, Daniel Patrick Moynihan's (1965) report titled simply *The Negro Family*. He argued that the problems Blacks experienced were due to a dysfunctional family structure that had its roots in slavery when Blacks were not allowed stable marital patterns. Those traditions led to female-headed households where male children lacked adequate role models. However, as Ehrenreich (1985) pointed out, Moynihan ignored the simple fact that poor White families were also likely to be female-headed, in favor of a racialized version of the culture of poverty thesis. Later writers, such as George Gilder (1981) and Charles Murray (1984) individualized this framework even more, by taking race out of the equation and focusing instead on gender roles, where they proposed that women ended up in poverty because of their inability to achieve economically on their own and to their poor choices of fathers for their children. Whether the focus was on race or gender, these proposals were nothing new, just contemporary Malthusian versions of biological determinism or "blaming the victim" (Kilty & Segal, 1996). That is, individuals were responsible for their own life circumstances. A revitalized version of "personal responsibility" was being born, one that became the catchphrase for "understanding" poverty and creating poverty policy for the next three decades. It also provided a mechanism for making poverty invisible again.

How deeply embedded "personal responsibility" has become as an explanation for why the poor are poor can be seen in the aftermath of Hurricane Katrina. At first, the country was shocked by TV images of poor Blacks stranded at the Superdome and the Convention Center in New Orleans. Within hours, though, those same desperate people came to be identified as "looters" and "thieves," as gun-toting and dangerous, as gang members shooting at potential rescuers, as people who had failed in their responsibility to take care of themselves and to evacuate in the first place (Dyson, 2006). No longer were they victims, but rather victimizers and failures.

Sentiments toward the working class have historically been relatively negative (Coontz, 1992). But, since the days of the Reagan presidency, a mean-spiritedness toward those at the bottom of American society has been especially rampant. "Greed is good," a line memorialized in the movie Wall Street, became the mantra for achieving success in this society. The market takes care of those who take care of themselves, and the spirit of the entrepreneur is the key to rising out of poverty. Those that do not rise up have just not worked hard enough or persevered. As we have heard repeatedly from conservatives for some 30 years now, discrimination—whether due to race and ethnicity, gender, or class—is a thing of the past, and the playing field is level for those willing to roll up their sleeves and get to work.

The reality of life in America is much different. Most adults participate in the labor force. Yet what many receive for the long hours they labor is far from fair. For 2005, median household income in the United States was $46,344 (DeNavas-Walt et al., 2006), a value that reflects virtually no increase during the six years of the George W. Bush administration. But the median tells only part of the story. The full distribution of household income explains just how inequitably it is distributed. As Table 2.1 shows, the upper limit of the bottom quintile of the household income distribution was $19,178. Fully one of every five households had an income of $19,178 or less. With an average household size of 2.6 in 2005, that puts households at the upper limit of the quintile at about 120% of the poverty threshold. In fact, the mean of $10,655 indicates that the typical household in the bottom 20% of the household income distribution fell well below the poverty threshold. In 2005, the official family poverty rate was 9.9%, while the individual rate was 12.6%—a rate that had finally leveled off after five years of increases (DeNavas-Walt et al., 2006). As Table 2.1 also shows, the share of total aggregate income that year for the bottom quintile was only 3.4%.

Those in the second quintile were somewhat better off, with an upper limit of $36,000. That quintile averaged $27,357. Keep in mind, though, that this represents gross (or pre-tax) income, amounting to about $2,280 a month. In most

Table 2.1 Household Income for the United States by Quintile for 2005

Quintile	Upper limit ($)	Mean ($)	Share (%)
Top	—	159,583	50.4
Fourth	91,705	72,825	23.0
Third	57,660	46,301	14.6
Second	36,000	27,357	8.6
Bottom	19,178	10,655	3.4

Source: DeNavas-Walt et al. (2006).

urban areas, close to half of that income would be consumed by rent alone. This quintile's share of aggregate income is only 8.6%. For the bottom two quintiles combined, the share of aggregate income amounts to a meager 12.0% of the total of all earned income in the United States. The 2005 poverty threshold for a family of four with two children was $19,806. Some safety net programs, like food stamps or reduced-fee school lunches, allow up to 130% of the poverty guidelines in order for households to quality. For a family of four in 2005, that threshold was $25,748—significantly lower than the mean household income for the second quintile. Most of the households that fall in the bottom 40% of the income distribution are struggling working families. The official household poverty rate of 9.9% falls far short of reflecting the true life situations for these families.

If we look at the top of the income distribution, we see a very different picture—one of affluence and ease. The top quintile's share of aggregate income amounted to 50.4%—four times that of the bottom two quintiles combined. Would anyone seriously argue that the bottom 40% of American households deserve only a quarter of the aggregate income that poured into the pockets of the top 20%? That those at the top really work that much harder than those at the bottom? This is not just a ludicrous notion, but also a slap in the face of all hard-working individuals in households below the median income.

How critical race and ethnicity remain as factors in income inequality can be seen in Table 2.2, which presents median household and per capita income by race and ethnicity for 2005. The median for Asian Americans was probably an overstatement of their situation, since they are clustered in five large metropolitan areas (Los Angeles, San Francisco, Seattle, Chicago, and New York), while the median for non-Hispanic Whites includes that entire population group, which is much more geographically dispersed. Per capita income for Asian Americans reflects that fact. For Blacks and Latinos, both median and per capita household income show the depth of disadvantage that continues to prevail in the United States. Once again, it seems ludicrous to suggest that what these groups earn reflects their efforts, relative to the efforts of the dominant racial and ethnic group in America. Why do we see those at the bottom as irresponsible and lazy and to blame for their poverty? Why do we see those at the top as having earned what they have, when the reality is that most were born with a silver spoon (Tabb, 2006; Mishel et al., 2005).

Table 2.2 Household Income for the United States by Race and Ethnicity for 2005

Race/Ethnicity	Median	Per capita
White, non-Hispanic	50,784	28,946
Black	30,858	16,874
Asian	61,094	27,331
Hispanic/Latino	35,967	14,483

Source: DeNavas-Walt et al. (2006).

Responsibility: Personal and Collective

Why has there been this emphasis on "personal responsibility" when it comes to the poor and poverty in the United States? Responsibility is not just individual. It is also collective, and we often hear statements from political leaders about the "common good" or the "general welfare." In fact, one of the guiding principles underlying human relations is that the needs of the many outweigh the needs of the few. Yet the preamble for the Personal Responsibility and Work Opportunity Reconciliation Act of 1996 (PRWORA)—popularly known as "welfare reform"—tells us that the poor are poor simply because of their own lack of personal responsibility. As Segal (2006, p. 207–8) points out:

> Although Aid for Families with Dependent Children (AFDC) was typi-cally included as a major part of the arsenal of the War on Poverty, the cri-sis that prompted the shift to create Temporary Assistance for Needy Families (TANF) was not poverty (Segal & Kilty, 2003). Thus, all the needs associated with poverty, such as low wages, lack of health care, disappearing jobs, inadequate education, lack of affordable housing, hunger, homelessness, lack of child care, sexism and racism—the corollaries of poverty—were not on the table when welfare reform was discussed. Because poverty was not the national crisis, addressing poverty was not important to leading lawmakers. Instead, what was on the table were the issues of marriage and out-of-wedlock births.

If only poor people would quit being lazy and give up their immoral ways and accept their personal guilt for their plight, then the problem of poverty would be eliminated. In other words, a "tough love" approach was needed to help the poor shape up. Social conditions are not responsible for poverty—a classic Malthusian principle.

Personal responsibility is a sentiment that is compatible with this country's core values and beliefs: hard work, rugged individualism, self-sufficiency, and reliance on the family. Marriage has been a particularly significant institution, especially in determining who is "deserving" of help and who is not. Widows and children have often been exempt from culpability for their circum-stances, at least if they were White. Most others, especially "able-bodied" men and minority women and children, were not, which made early federal programs for public assistance (e.g. Aid for Dependent Children) open to hostility and challenge, particularly after World War II (Blau, 2004).

These core values and beliefs are deeply entrenched in American social ideology. They also connect to deeply held religious convictions. For many Americans, the United States has long been a "Christian" nation, which is illustrated by the way that Puritan settlers in New England have been revered as a group that was forced to flee religious persecution in their homeland in search of a safe haven in the "New World." According to Hughes (2003, p. 28):

> Every schoolchild learns that the Puritans settled America for the sake of freedom. To a degree, that is true. The freedom the Puritans envisioned, however, was a far cry from the freedom Americans prize today. The Puritans sought freedom for themselves but for no one else.

At the core of Puritan beliefs was the Calvinist notion of predestination: that God has already decided what is going to happen and that nothing can change that fate. Because of hard work and perseverance, some individuals and families will do well, and their success serves as a sign that they are righteous and among God's chosen. Hard work and self-reliance combined with religious values to create a special version of the Protestant work ethic here. Hughes (2003) argues that a "gospel of wealth" developed in the United States, flourishing from the end of the Civil War through the end of the nineteenth century. This was a gospel of wealth that would serve as a justification for why the rich are rich and the poor are poor:

> Many, therefore, came to view the wealth of the barons of industry as God's reward for individual righteousness. Likewise, if many viewed southern poverty as God's curse on the South for the institution of slavery, they also came to view the poverty of the masses in northern cities as God's curse for laziness and immorality.
>
> (Hughes, 2003, p. 128)

Wealth is righteousness and poverty is sinfulness. Those were powerful ideas, especially at a time when Social Darwinism and eugenics dominated supposedly scientific conceptions of human nature. Perhaps what was developing here was not a commitment to "the needs of the many outweighing the needs of the few" but rather one to "the needs of the few outweighing the needs of the many."

At the same time, we need to recognize that there are other values and beliefs that are deeply ingrained in the American worldview, including freedom, equality, and justice—principles that are more collective in nature. Throughout our history, social movements have arisen in response to struggles in the names of those principles, including abolitionism and the early women's rights movements in the nineteenth century. Further, not all those who identify themselves as

Christians incorporate Calvinist traditions in their religious beliefs. Many believers are devoted to social justice and peace, and religiously affiliated individuals as well as congregations have pursued social change, as exemplified in the civil rights and the peace and antinuclear movements of the past 50 years.

Yet many in this society have a narrow vision of religion, especially Christianity. Religion is important to most Americans, probably more so than in any other industrialized society, and for many that includes the notion that the United States was founded as a Christian nation (Hughes, 2003). Since the Reagan era, religion has been an increasingly powerful force in national elections, especially the religious rightwing (Phillips, 2006). It is important to keep in mind, though, that one of the divisions among Christians involves those identifying as "evangelicals" or fundamentalists and those identifying as "progressives." Some have described this as a "culture war," where conservative, fundamentalist Christians who reject many scientific ideas, including Darwinian theory, have moved increasingly to the right, supporting social policies such as welfare reform that are ever more punitive and harmful. These are people who see themselves as on a mission to resurrect the Christian nature of this country, one that has supposedly been taken away by "secular humanists" and "atheists" (Goldberg, 2006). Even the statements of some political leaders reflect notions of "sin" in the provision of public assistance, when seen as being provided to those who supposedly do *not* need it (Segal & Kilty, 2003). Individuals with these attitudes have been among the core supporters of political leaders devoted to what they see as reforming public welfare policies.

Whether connected to religious sentiments or not, the nucleus of the American Dream lies in certain values: "hard work, individual responsibility for failure, and unlimited possibility for success" (Peck & Gershon, 2006, p. 99). Even President Ronald Reagan remarked in 1983 that this is still a country where anyone can get rich (Peck & Gershon, 2006). Being successful continues to be seen largely in materialistic terms. Cultural values and beliefs are not monolithic, but some are central and broadly accepted.

Americans see themselves as caring people. After the 9/11 attacks and Hurricane Katrina, donations flowed in to private charities. When a child falls down a well, people are glued to their TV sets and offer up prayers and donations for medical expenses. But they seem to have no qualms about taking food out of children's mouths or taking away their wheelchairs by supporting welfare reform. After all, parents have to learn to be responsible for their children. Nor do there seem to be qualms about refusing to support tax levies that are necessary for providing adequate public education for many other children. The government spends too much money, anyway, and the tax burden is too great. In sum, do the needs of the many outweigh the needs of the few, or is it the needs of the few that are paramount?

Personal Responsibility: Who Has It and Who Does Not?

One of the great American myths is the belief that this is a classless society. That conviction should come as no surprise: If this is truly a land of unlimited possibilities for success, how could it be otherwise? This may be a land of opportunity, but the real issue is for whom. According to Tabb (2006, p. 11), "When Ronald Reagan said, 'What I want to see above all is that this remains a country where someone can always get rich,' his base understood him to say, 'where those already rich can get vastly richer'."

While the gap between rich and poor has widened dramatically in recent decades, this wealth gap is not really anything new. Phillips (2002) shows how, even at the founding of the United States, wealth was vastly unequally distributed. After independence, the colonial era inequality grew rapidly, especially during the nineteenth century—"The largest fortune in the U.S. had grown from an ambiguous $1 million to somewhere in the $300 to $400 million range" (Phillips, 2002, p. 4)–a period of about 125 years. Much of that growth was due to federal policies on taxation, banking regulations, and tariffs and trade. For the most part, governmental policies throughout U.S. history have favored the wealthy (Tabb, 2006).

In recent times, the impact of such policies has been striking in extending the gap between rich and poor, to the point that the U.S. media have even publicly acknowledged it—a rare occurrence on their part. The concentration of wealth closes doors of opportunity for those without it, and there is now an abundance of statistical evidence showing, "that the U.S. is a more class-bound society than its major Western European counterparts, with the exception of Britain" (Foster, 2006, p. 1). In other words, class is an increasingly serious factor influencing the opportunity to "get rich." According to Tabb (2006, pp. 7–8):

> The specifics of the way the Bush administration and the Republican Congress are changing tax laws—such as who is favored and who is hurt—carry echoes which have been heard down through our nation's history and have taken on resonance analogous to the Gilded Age and the Roaring Twenties, other periods when conservative ideology and politics held sway and rapid increases in inequalities were produced by deregulation and variants of laissez faire policy and Social Darwinist thinking. But in all periods, we have had a government of the rich that has acted in the interests of the rich.

That appears unlikely to change in the near future. If anything, we will probably see only an increasing concentration of wealth in the hands of the already wealthy.

While the poor are often looked upon as lacking a sense of personal responsibility, it is actually the rich who have the least sense of personal responsibility in America. No doubt there are some poor individuals who take advantage of social welfare programs and public resources, but it is in fact the rich who have the most opportunities to take advantage of scarce social resources. We will look at two examples of how the rich use wealth irresponsibly: through excess and extravagance and through U.S. tax codes.

Excess and Extravagance

One of the leading organizations that has helped to document the growth of excess and extravagance among the wealthy is the Council on International and Public Affairs (CIPA), which publishes a weekly online magazine titled *Too Much*. According to CIPA, *Too Much* provides "a weekly commentary on excess and inequality." In their 17 July 2006 issue were the following examples of what *Too Much* editors (www.cipaapex.org/toomuch/index.html) identified as "Greed at a Glance":

> Public service pays—at least for House of Representatives Speaker Dennis Hastert. The Illinois Republican entered Congress, in 1987, with a $77,400 salary and a $290,000 family net worth, about six times the net worth of 1987's typical American family. Hastert's net worth, the *Chicago Tribune* reports, currently totals over $6.2 million, over 65 times the net worth of today's typical U.S. family. How amazing has Hastert's climb been? He picked up nearly $6 million in net worth over a 20-year period that saw him put two kids through college—and Hastert has never made more, in annual salary, than the $212,100 he's now making as House speaker . . .

> The world's most discriminating motorists have a brand-new option: the just-released Bentley Azure, a hi-tech convertible that will retail, with tax, near $400,000. Over the next year, Bentley expects to move 150 of these 18-foot-long gas guzzlers worldwide, with most of the sales in the U.S. But the company insists the new Azure won't add much at all to global warming. The average Azure buyer, Bentley officials point out, will already own eight other cars, a reality that means that the typical 10-mile-per-gallon 2007 Azure won't see terribly much time on the roads . . .

The *Too Much* archives include many other instances of excess. Stories about the lavish lives of the rich are commonplace, providing material for gossip columns and tabloid newspapers and television shows. Other time periods in the United States have been notable for extravagance, including the Gilded Age and the Roaring Twenties (Tabb, 2006). Obviously, that is true not only in this country but in other places and times as well.

What is important to understand is that a rationale commonly used to justify greed and avarice is that it is necessary—that without it all of society will suffer. According to this logic, it is only through wealth accumulation by the few that the many will benefit. Those who are wealthy will use some of their affluence to invest, creating jobs, as well as to donate to philanthropic organizations, including the arts, education, health, and more. According to Pizzigati (2004), that is rarely the case. What tends to happen, in fact, is just the opposite: The wealth that is accumulated by those at the top stays right there or is invested in possessions such as homes, boats, vehicles, and personal art collections. Typically, the outcome of a period such as the one that started during the Reagan era is an economic downturn, leading to progressive reforms (e.g. the Progressive Era and the

New Deal policies) where wealth is somewhat deconcentrated, and benefits flow from the top to the bottom (Phillips, 1990)—at least for a time, until those at the top find new ways to siphon society's wealth back into their hands.

Tax Policy

Tax policy is another way in which the wealthy use their vast riches to benefit themselves. Politics in the United States, especially at the national level, revolves around money. Politicians need large amounts to get themselves elected, and it is, of course, the affluent who can provide the most. The theory goes that money merely provides access to political leaders—and does not necessarily influence how they will actually vote on particular legislation (Palast, 2004). Of course, the real world does not always reflect the ideal, and wealth produces not merely access but great influence. As Johnston (2003) puts it in the subtitle to his book *Perfectly Legal*, what we actually have is a "covert campaign to rig our tax system to benefit the super rich—and cheat everybody else." Yet, as noted earlier, this is nothing new. Virtually since the founding of this country, tax policy has been used to benefit the rich (Phillips, 2002; Tabb, 2006). Let us look at a few examples of how tax policy benefits those at the top—especially the very top.

We should start by noting that the U.S. tax burden is among the lowest of OECD (Organization for Economic Cooperation and Development) nations, which includes the G7 and other major industrialized states. That is true whether the focus is on personal income, corporate income, Social Security contributions, property, or goods and services taxes (Hoo & Todor, 2006).

Income Taxes

Since Ronald Reagan was elected president, the federal income tax burden for those at the top has declined sharply. Depending on what kinds of statistics are presented, though, it can appear that the income tax is heaviest on those at the very top. According to Riskind and Torry (2006, p. B1), the highest earners pay the bulk of income taxes: The top 1% alone paid 34.3% of the total, while the top 5% paid 54.4% of the total, and the top 10% paid 65.8% of the total. Of course, the aggregate share of income is greatest for precisely these groups. Yet, as we saw in Table 2.1, the top quintile of the income distribution alone accounted for 50.4% of total aggregate income in the United States, with the bottom of this quintile starting at $91,765 (DeNavas-Walt et al., 2006).

When we are talking about the top 1, 5 or 10% of earners, we are dealing with people with very high incomes. For example, the lower limit for the top 5% for household income was $166,000 in 2005—when the *personal* incomes of U.S. senators and representatives was $162,100. And it is precisely those individuals who are getting the bulk of the latest round of tax cuts: The highest 1% had an average benefit of $39,020 and the top quintile averaged $5,400. The middle quintile averaged $748, while the bottom quintile had an average of $23 (Riskind & Torry, 2006). Those with incomes over $1 million dollars received a benefit of $111,549 (Friedman *et al.*, 2006). In fact, between 1979 and 2003, the middle quintile had an after-tax increase in income of $5,900 (an increase of 15.2%), while the top 1% saw an after-tax increase of $395,700 (an increase of 129.4%) (Friedman *et al.*, 2006).

The income tax was originally designed as a progressive tax, where high earners would pay increasing levels of tax as their earnings got higher. It was not intended to be a flat tax, which would in effect be regressive and put a greater burden on those at the bottom. Thus, the fact that high earners pay a high relative share of the total of income taxes paid simply reflects the original design of this tax plan—the idea of fairness. Those at the top should assume a higher proportion of the tax burden while still having more than adequate after-tax incomes on which to live.

Typically, depictions of the U.S. budget include all federal spending, from military to infrastructure to human resources. Financing that spending is generally presented as coming largely from income taxes. However, not all federal programs rely specifically on those taxes. Human resources spending—particularly the Old Age, Survivors and Disability program (OASDI)—has its own payroll tax—one that is regressive in nature and puts a much greater burden on working families. The Social Security payroll tax, collected under the authority of the Federal Insurance Contributions Act (FICA), is another "income tax," but one that is not included in reports like Riskind and Torry (2006). This tax is a flat tax of 7.65% of wages (matched by the same amount from employers)—but actually not on all wages. In 2005, it was capped at $90,000. Those with earnings over that amount, which includes everyone in the top 20% of the income distribution, only pay 7.65% of their first $90,000 of earnings and nothing on any further earnings. That actually reduces their effective tax rate, if the percentage is based on what they paid out of the total earned. So a large part of the federal budget is actually paid out of taxes specifically earmarked to cover those costs, but surplus funds (the Social Security "trust funds") can be "borrowed" to supplement general revenues, including the income tax—thus reducing the federal deficit. Analysts like Riskind and Torry (2006), then, are providing inaccurate figures on the supposed tax burden of those at the top, since their figures do not include this second income tax—the Social Security payroll tax. These taxes are a heavy burden on low-income workers, and the Earned Income Tax Credit (EITC) was originally created in part to offset the regressive nature of the payroll tax. Unfortunately, far too few low-wage workers make use of the EITC (Mendenhall, 2006).

Estate Taxes

The estate tax—or the "death tax" as its opponents often refer to it—is another type of tax that has benefited the wealthy greatly in recent years. According to Citizens for Tax Justice, there were a total of 30,276 estates large enough to be taxable in 2003—representing only 1.24% of all the people who died that year (McIntyre, 2006). A total of $21.6 billion dollars was collected by the federal government that year, but that mainly came from the very largest estates. In fact, estates under $1 million were not even required to file tax returns, and no fed-eral estate tax was collected on any. For estates between $1 and $2.5 million, the average estate tax was $80,000, while it was $427,600 for estates worth between $2.5 and $5 million, $1,148,600 for estates worth between $5 and $10 million, $2,466,800 for estates worth between $10 and 20 million and $7,715,100 for estates worth $20 million or more. Most of the total tax, then, was paid by only a very small number of extremely large estates (McIntyre, 2006). Even that will be gone in a few years, since the estate tax is supposed to be completely phased out by 2010. But it has never been the family farm or the small family business that were taxed to any significant extent—the motif used by opponents of the estate tax to garner support for eliminating it. Even those who do pay estate taxes pay only a small proportion of the total value of their estates. That helps to main-tain relatively rigid class strata.

Taxes and Housing Subsidies

One last example involves deductions that can be used to reduce federal income taxes, and this is a clear example of public welfare for the affluent (Kilty, 2006). The major type of housing subsidy available in the United States is a tax deduction for interest payments on mortgages—a tax deduction that mainly benefits income tax payers at the top of the income distribution. In 2004, some $68 billion was lost to the federal treasury because of this deduc-tion, with about 60% of that savings going directly into the pockets of house-holds with incomes in excess of $100,000. According to Zepezauer (2004, p. 20), "One study found that in 1997, the total amount of tax subsidies to homeowners was more than seven *times* what the Department of Housing and Urban Development (HUD) spent on its housing programs for the poor". In fact, households with incomes under $40,000 were generally unable to make use of this potential deduction.

There are many other examples throughout the U.S. tax codes, whether at the federal, state, or local levels, where the affluent are privileged compared to the rest of Americans. So who is showing personal responsibility, and who is not?

Conclusion

During the past 25 years, the code of personal responsibility has been used as a powerful tool for changing public opinion about poverty and the poor. It has been repeated endlessly, becoming virtually a mantra. Many political leaders and aca-demics have questioned the virtue of the poor, transforming the war on poverty into a war on the poor. Yet it is important to realize that blaming the victim is nothing new, but rather a recurrent theme in American history. If it is recurrent, though, that means that there have been times when a different image of the poor captured the public imagination.

Block (2006, p. 16) identifies the currently dominant economic principle in the United States as "market fundamentalism"—what he describes as, "a dogmatic belief in the power of Adam Smith's 'invisible hand' to create prosperity." This is not a new idea, either, and it has been used repeatedly since the early days of the country to justify the growth of capitalism and the vast increase of wealth concentrated in the hands of a few. It certainly fits well with the Protestant work ethic, the "gospel of wealth" and Social Darwinism. It is simply a matter of personal responsibility; those who work hard get their just rewards.

There are times when this Market Fundamentalism falters. During the Great Depression of the 1930s, almost a quarter of the labor force was unemployed, and many people who had worked hard lost their homes, businesses, farms, and possessions, not through any failure on their own part but rather through the failure of an economic system oriented around greed and speculation. Out of that social disaster emerged a different political agenda—one focused on collective responsibility. Out of that era came a more humane view of the poor. A moral argument for social change emerged around the perspective that it was the avarice of business that had brought about catastrophe. That language was essential in the creation of a social welfare state in the United States, particularly through the Social Security Act of 1935.

Advocates of market fundamentalism never give up. Challenges were made from the beginning of the Social Security Administration to its provisions, but it would be some 40 years before those efforts would gradually lead to a retrenchment in the social welfare state. This retrenchment is not just in terms of public assistance but also in other areas, including the Old Age pensions and Medicare provisions of Social Security. Since the Reagan administration, calls for privatizing Old Age pensions have been made, and the current Bush administration recently tried to make such changes again. After all, individuals should have the right to invest their own money as they wish, and they can then have the opportunity to see a greater return than public pensions can possibly provide—or so goes the argument. This is just another version of personal responsibility, with the argument phrased now in terms of individuals being able to make better decisions personally than can be made collectively. Public bureaucracies supposedly constrain and interfere with the actions of rational, hard-working individuals (Block, 2006). Government cannot do for people what they need to do for themselves. Personal responsibility provides the opportunity to advance on one's own, while it ensures that those who do not work hard enough will not become dependent on government largesse.

What else should we expect in a society that reveres wealth, whatever the means necessary to acquire it? The excesses of corporate leaders in the past two decades do not seem to have led to a crisis of faith in private institutions. Even those convicted of corporate crime, such as Ken Lay of Enron, are typically treated with sympathy rather than with disgrace. If those at the top of this society can openly display avarice and larceny and get away with it, why should we expect anything different from the rest?

The reality of daily life for many Americans is one of constant struggle (Mishel *et al.*, 2005). All those families that fall below the median household income work hard just trying to pay the rent, feed, clothe, and educate their children, keep their cars running. Yet they are forgotten—put out of sight and out of mind.

The notion of personal responsibility helps to maintain a belief that this is a country where anyone can still become rich. It implies that making lots of money is the most important aspiration any of us can have. It allows us to turn a blind eye to collective responsibility. It hides away the reality of just how highly stratified the United States is, of how limited mobility actually is. Problems such as poverty recede into invisibility. As Clarence Page (2006) recently pointed out, President Bush seems to have forgotten in less than a year that poverty still needs to be fought. Since he included it in two speeches shortly after Hurricane Katrina, he has brought it up only six more times.

Poverty will not remain invisible, no matter how much Bush and the other Market Fundamentalists might want it to. Many people are aware of its reality. Many know that collective responsibility is essential for the well-being of any society. As Block (2006: p. 18), notes, "Market ideology focuses only on competition, but a productive economy depends on cooperation." For those who cannot put themselves into someone else's shoes, it may be hard to be empathetic (Segal, 2006). But many people can put themselves into the shoes of strangers and understand that that person's life could be their life. It is time now to challenge the personal irresponsibility of the rich, to make their excesses as visible as possible, to make them accountable to the very society that has given them so much. It is also time once again to put a human face on poverty, to show the reality of being poor and working.

Note

1   An earlier version of this paper was presented at the Second Japan–U.S. Symposium on Poverty, Inequality and Social Justice held at Hosei University in Tokyo on 6 and 7 September 2006. I would like to thank Elizabeth Segal, Lisa Raiz, Alfred Joseph, and Anne Broussard for their helpful comments on previous drafts.

References

Blau, J. (2004). *The dynamics of social welfare policy*. New York: Oxford University Press.
Blau, J. (2006). Welfare reform in historical perspective. In K. Kilty & E. Segal (Eds.), The *promise of welfare reform* (pp. 49–56). Binghamton, NY: Haworth.
Block, F. (2006). A moral economy. *The Nation, 282*, 16–19.
Coontz, S. (1992). *The way we never were*. New York: Basic.
DeNavas-Walt, C., Proctor, B., & Lee, C. (2006). *Income, poverty and health insurance coverage in the United States: 2005* (Current Population Reports (P60–231). Washington, DC: U.S. Census Bureau.
Dyson, M. (2006). *Come hell or high water: Hurricane Katrina and the color of disaster*. New York: Basic Civitas.
Ehrenreich, J. (1985). *The altruistic imagination*. Ithaca, NY: Cornell University Press.
Foster, J. (2006). Aspects of class in the United States. *Monthly Review, 58*, 1–5.
Friedman, J., Shapiro, I., & Greenstein, R. (2006, 10 April). *Recent tax and income trends among high-income taxpayers*. Washington, DC: Center on Budget and Policy Priorities. Available HTML: http://www.cbpp.org.
Gilder, G. (1981). *Wealth and poverty*. New York: Basic.
Goldberg, M. (2006). *Kingdom coming: The rise of Christian nationalism*. New York: Norton.
Harrington, M. (1962). *The other America*. New York: Collier.

Hoo, S. & Todor, E. (2006). *The U.S. tax burden is low relative to other OECD countries.* Washington, DC: Urban-Brookings Tax Policy Center. Available HTML: http://taxpolicycenter.org/home/index.cfm.

Hughes, R. (2003). *Myths America lives by.* Chicago: University of Chicago Press.

Johnston, D. (2003). *Perfectly legal.* New York: Portfolio.

Katz, M. (1989). *The undeserving poor: From the war on poverty to the war on welfare.* New York: Pantheon.

Kilty, K. (2006). Welfare reform: What's poverty got to do with it? In K. Kilty & E. Segal (Eds.), *The promise of welfare reform* (pp. 109–20). Binghamton, NY: Haworth.

Kilty, K. & Segal, E. (1996). Genetics and biological determinism: Scientific breakthrough or blaming the victim revisited? *Humanity & Society, 20,* 90–110.

McIntyre, B. (2006, 4 April). *Who pays the federal estate tax.* Washington, DC: Citizens for Tax Justice. Available HTML: www.ctj.org.

Mendenhall, A. (2006). A guide to the earned income tax credit: What everyone should know about the EITC. *Journal of Poverty, 10,* 51–68.

Mishel, L., Bernstein, J., & Allegretto, S. (2005). *The state of working America 2004/2005.* Ithaca, NY: Cornell University Press.

Moynihan, D. (1965). *The Negro family.* Washington, DC: U.S. Government Printing Office.

Murray, C. (1984). *Losing ground: American social policy 1950–1980.* New York: Basic.

Neubeck, K. & Cazenave, N. (2001). *Welfare racism: Playing the race card against America's poor.* New York: Routledge.

Page, C. (2006, 25 July). Glaring omission: President avoided poverty issue in NAACP speech. *Columbus Dispatch,* p. A9.

Palast, G. (2004). *The best democracy money can buy.* New York: Plume.

Peck, L. & Gershon, S. (2006). Welfare reform and the American dream. In K. Kilty & E. Segal (Eds.), *The promise of welfare reform* (pp. 97–107). Binghamton, NY: Haworth.

Phillips, K. (1990). *The politics of rich and poor.* New York: Random House.

Phillips, K. (2002). *Wealth and democracy: A political history of the American rich.* New York: Broadway Books.

Phillips, K. (2006). *American theocracy.* New York: Viking.

Pizzigati, S. (2004). *Greed and good.* New York: Apex.

Riskind, J. & Torry, J. (2006, 16 July). On taxes, senate candidates differ sharply. *Columbus Dispatch,* pp. B1–B2.

Segal, E. (2006). Welfare as we should know it: Social empathy and welfare reform. In K. Kilty & E. Segal (Eds.), *The promise of welfare reform* (pp. 265–74). Binghamton, NY: Haworth.

Segal, E. & Kilty, K. (2003). Political promises for welfare reform. *Journal of Poverty, 7,* 51–67.

Tabb, W. (2006). The power of the rich. *Monthly Review, 58,* 6–17.

Zepezauer, M. (2004). *Take the rich off welfare.* Cambridge, MA: South End Press.

Critical Thinking Questions

1   This chapter asserts that poverty is a structural problem and not an individual problem. Yet in the United States, we value hard work, rugged individualism, and self-sufficiency. Are individuals personally responsible for "pulling themselves up by their bootstraps" or do the "needs of the many outweigh the needs of the few"? Which is it? Explain your answer. Can you think of examples from your own experience that address this issue?

2   Think about the community where you spent your childhood. Were neighborhoods in your community segregated by social class or were they mixed? Did children from different social class groups attend different schools? Did their parents tend to shop at certain stores or did families worship at different religious centers? Were there social clubs in your community? Was the membership at these clubs segregated along social class lines or did different groups mix at these clubs? Who held the power in local government?

3   Kilty mentions that upward social mobility is very limited in the United States, which implies that people are likely to live out their lives in the social class into which they were born. Why do you think this occurs? How might it be changed?

3   Women in a Bind

The Decline of Marriage, Market, and the State

Mimi Abramovitz

Poverty has long been a woman's issue. More than one in two poor adults in the United States is a women, more than one in four mother-only families live below the poverty line and one in two poor families is headed by a women (U.S. Census Bureau, n.d.). Limited by gender blindness or ideological views, most poverty explanations either fail to explain women's plight or blame it on the women themselves. Conservatives say that women are poor due to personal irresponsibility, such as failure to comply with prescribed wife and mother roles and other "family values." In contrast, liberals link women's poverty to the lack of labor market opportunity (sex discrimination, sexual harassment), lack of representation in public office, and difficulties balancing work and family roles. Feminists argue further that women's poverty reflects underlying structural forces like the gender division of labor, women's economic dependence on men, sex (and race) segregated occupations, and overall hierarchies of power including those based on class, race, and gender.

While poverty has many causes, this chapter assumes poverty is first and foremost the lack of money. Traditionally the two main sources of income for women have been marriage and the market. When these fail, many women turned to the state for help. However, the data suggest that all three institutions—marriage, the market, and the state—have become increasingly unreliable sources of economic support for women. From 1945 to the mid-1970s, fueled by peace, prosperity and a liberal political climate, all three institutions expanded. However, in the mid-1970s, deindustrialization, globalization, the rise of conservatism, and other changes in the domestic and international economies were accompanied by major reorganizations that reduced their capacity to protect women from poverty.

The Decline of Marriage

Traditional social expectations called upon men to provide for their families and women to marry and to depend on husbands for economic support. Access to male income historically both reduced women's autonomy and buttressed them against privation, especially if they were middle-class, heterosexual, and White. Although some women could not or chose not to marry, declining marriage rates, domestic violence, and stagnating male income means that contemporary marriage protects fewer and fewer women from poverty.

Falling Rates of Marriage

In 2005, married couples became a minority of all American households for the first time (Roberts, 2007). The declining rates make the institution of heterosexual marriage less available to women as a route out of poverty. With only minor fluctuations, marriage rates fell from 10.6 per 1000 population in 1970 to 7.4 per 1000 population in 2004 (U.S. Department of Health and Human Services, National Center for Health Statistics, n.d.). In 2004, 60.3% of all men and 57.1% of all women were married, down from 67.7% of men and 62.8% of women in 1970 (Statistical Abstract of the United States, 2006). While some men and women are widowed, separated, or divorced, nearly half of all adults currently live on their own because they have never married and growing numbers cohabit. From 1970 to 2003, the proportion of never-married men age 25–49 grew from 10.5% to 56.6%, and for women it grew from 19.1% to 40.8%. Both groups have also postponed marriage.

Heterosexual marriage as a route out of poverty is even less available to women of color, especially Black women. From 1960 to 2000, the percentage of Black women who married declined from 59.8% to 36.1%. The percentage of never-married Black women doubled, from 21.6 to 42.3% in that time period. Women of color seeking to marry face a shrinking pool of available men. Owing to racism, too many men of color are poor, jobless, or in jail or die prematurely. Indeed, the number of families with children under 18 headed by a women of color increased from 17.6% in 1970 to 22.4% in 2002 among Blacks, from 12.8 to 14.2% among Latina women and from 5.38 to 5.43% among Asians. For White women, the number rose from 4.65% (1970) to 5.46% (2002) (AmeriStat, 2003). Nor is heterosexual marriage a viable source of income for lesbians, bisexual, and transgender women, or other women who prefer to live on their own. In 2000, same-sex partners accounted for about 10% of all unmarried-partner households (Info Please, 2006).

Public policy touts single motherhood or marital breakup as a cause of poverty. In contrast researchers have found that poverty can both discourage and break up a marriage (Halle, 2002). While two incomes are better than one, low wages, unemployment, and poverty often keep people from marrying (Edin, 2000; Nakosteen & Zimmer, 1997). In 2001 one in three poor women living below 100% of the poverty line was married compared to a higher two in three women living at 300 or more% of the poverty line. From 1991–2001 the percentage of lower-income married women dropped from 37% to 33%, while the share of better-off married women stayed about the same (Halle, 2002).

Low-income can also erode family stability making it more likely that marriages will deteriorate (Edin, 2000; Nakosteen & Zimmer, 1997). Some 50% of all first marriages are expected to end in divorce (Ooms, 2002), yet a study of ever-married adults up to their early 30s found that low-income adults were more likely to marry than those with higher incomes. These poorer couples were also more prone to splitting up (Fein, 2004). That is, more women with less than a high school education and living in poorer neighborhoods were married than their better-off counterparts. However, their chance of splitting up in each year after the first marriage was consistently higher than for women with more education and living in better-off neighborhoods. The rates of marital disruption were highest for Black women and lower for Latinas (Fein, 2004).

The data led Fein (2004, p. 9) to observe that, "poverty brings a substantial array of stresses that spill over into marriages and create abundant marital distress." Coupled with domestic violence, the lack of access to education, well-paid jobs, affordable childcare, and other hardships associated with poverty can wreak havoc on relationships. Rather than a "haven-in-a-heartless land," for many women from all walks of life, the home is a site of physical and emotional violence. The data show that from 85 to 95% of all domestic violence victims are female and that domestic violence is the leading cause of injury to women. Each year 5.3 million women are abused, over 50,000 are stalked, and 1,232 are killed by an intimate partner (American Institute on Domestic Violence, n.d.).

These changes in family patterns since the mid-1970s posed a threat to the "traditional" family as did women's increased economic independence. Seeking to restore so-called "family values," during the last 25 years public policy has rewarded heterosexual marriage and stay-at-home moms while penalizing same-sex couples, single motherhood, and, in some cases, employed women. In the name of reducing poverty the government has directed recent marriage promotion and fatherhood initiatives to low-income households. Responding to this marriage mandate for women on welfare, Patricia Ireland (2001, as cited in Dorian & Miller, 2002, p. 3) former President of the National Organization of Women (NOW) concluded, "If marriage were a solution to poverty, it wouldn't take an act of Congress to promote it."

Falling Breadwinner Income

A second key reason why marriage has become a less solid guarantee against poverty for women is that in many households work does not pay—especially for men expected to be the prime, if not the only, breadwinner. From 1947 to 1973 wages and productivity (e.g. output per hour)—a key determinant of living standards—both doubled. In this period productivity and the median family income both grew by 103.7% (Mishel, Bernstein & Allegretto, 2006). The productivity gains made during the prosperous years following World War II spread broadly to the average family aided by strong unions, tight labor markets, adequate minimum wage, and balanced trade. Most shared the sustained increase in the quality of life—with unskilled workers and their families gaining proportionately more than most others.

The lockstep relationship between productivity and wages broke down in the mid-1970s as structural changes in the economy and public policy shifts pushed productivity and national income up and pressed wages down. Since then, with deindustrialization, the export of production abroad, the attack on organized labor, and the shredding of the safety net, productivity has continued to rise but the gains are barely shared. From 1973 to 2004, productivity rose by 75.7% compared to the much slower rate of 21.8% for median family income (Mishel *et al.*, 2006). The associated drop in wages weakened the breadwinning capacity of men and increased inequality.

Falling Wages

During the last three decades work has barely paid—despite an older, more experienced, better-educated, and therefore more productive, workforce. For one, the $5.15 federal minimum wage has not been raised since 1997. In 2006 it equaled only 31% of the average wage for private sector, nonsupervisory workers, the lowest share since 1949. Its purchasing power had dropped by 17%, reaching the second-lowest level since 1955 (Bernstein & Shapiro, 2006).

Second, from 1973 to 2005, the share of all male workers earning only poverty-level hourly wages rose from 17.5 to 19.9%. It increased from 14.9 to 15.9% for White men and from 31.7 to 35.0% for Latino men, but fell from 31.9 to 28.7% for Black men (Economic Policy Institute, 2006).

Finally, in 2005 dollars the real average (median) weekly income for men who worked full-time fell from $785 in 1979 to $722. (U.S. Department of Labor, Women's Bureau, 2006a). The *growth* in real median weekly earnings for all men also fell steadily from an increase of 1.3% (1995–2001) to an increase of only 0.2% (2001–2), to a drop of 1% (2003–5). The higher growth rate for Black men also fell from a 1.6% increase (1995–2001), to a 1.2% increase (2001–2), to a sharp 2% drop (2003–5) (Bernstein & Price, 2005). The 2001 recession and the subsequent "jobless recovery" erased the full employment conditions responsible for the healthy wage growth of the late 1990s. By mid-2006 the job market still could not generate the number and quality of jobs needed to support male breadwinning.

Greater Inequality

Most of the benefits of high worker productivity during the last 30 years flowed to the rich, marked by a decline in share of the GDP going to wages, greater consumption disparities, and reduced upward mobility.

In 2006, wages and salaries made up the smallest share of the nation's GDP (45%) since 1947, down from their historically high share of 53.5% in 1970 (Greenhouse & Leonhardt, 2006). In contrast, after-tax corporate profits soared to a record 10.1% of the GDP—the highest proportion in 87 years. Prior to 2005 profits never even reached 9% of the GDP. Somewhat ominously they came closest to the number in 1929—at 8.9% of the GDP (Fox, 2006). Likewise the share of national income going to wages fell from a high of 59.3% to 51.8% from 1970 to 2006 and the share going to profits jumped from 9% in 1970 to 13.6% (Aron-Dine & Shapiro, 2006). Reflecting these trends in 2005, 50.4% of the national income went to the top fifth of all households—their highest share since 1967. The 14.6% of national income received by the middle fifth and the 3.4% flowing to the bottom fifth are among the lowest shares on record (Bernstein & Gould, 2006).

Not surprisingly, from 2000 to 2005, the *growth* of consumer spending fell by 0.7% for low-income households and 0.4% for the middle class. It grew by 1.5% for the affluent. Fueled by tax cuts skewed to the rich, 2005 consumer spending disparities reached new highs. The top one-fifth of households made 39% of all consumer expenditures—the largest share on record. This compared to 8.2% for the bottom fifth, which tied with 2004 for the smallest share ever. Earlier, from 1984 (when data on consumption expenditures were first available) to 2000 consumption increases were distributed more broadly (Bernstein & Furman, 2006).

Finally, upward mobility came to a standstill for many families. Of those that started out in the bottom 20% of families in 1970, 49% were still there in 1980. From 1980 to 1990, 53% of families stayed put, with another 24% climbing only to the next fifth. That is, 77% of those who started out in the low end of the income scale in the 1980s were found there a decade later (Mishel, Bernstein, & Allegretto, 2005). Not surprisingly a 2006 Gallup poll found that 55% of Americans rate the economy as only "fair" or "poor," while 52% believe it is getting worse (Price, 2006).

In sum, since the mid-1970s three major trends—the decline of marriage, falling males wages, and increased economic inequality—have significantly eroded the capacity of the marriage institution to provide women a road out of poverty.

Markets: Work, Wages and Work Supports

The labor market was a main source of income for a record 66.6 million women who worked for wages outside the home in 2005. Economists predict that women will account for 51% of the *increase* in total labor force growth from 2004 to 2014, when they will represent 47% of all workers (U.S. Department of Labor, Women's Bureau, 2006a).

Although women comprise nearly half the workforce, the market is not a reliable source of income support for them for at least three reasons. Most fundamentally, the labor market has never offered the average women adequate protection against low wages and poor working conditions. Since the mid- to late 1970s, women have lost ground in the labor market marked by: (1) reduced labor force participation; (2) stagnating wages; (3) a wider gender wage gap; (4) sex-segregated occupations; (5) increased sexual harassment, and (6) ongoing difficulty balancing work and family responsibilities. The gender lens reveals that changes in the economy and the stubborn allocation of different tasks to women and men at home and at work have negatively affected women's labor force participation.

Lower Labor Force Participation Rates

The massive entry of women into the workforce since World War II is one of the most significant social trends in modern U.S. history. From 1948 to 2005, the fraction of all women age 20 and over working or looking for work (e.g. labor force participation) rose non-stop from 31.8 to 60.3% (U.S. Department of Labor, Bureau of Labor Statistics, n.d.). The influx accelerated in the mid-1970s due to: (1) the victories of the women's movement (the Equal Pay Act, the ban on sex discrimination in education and employment, etc.); (2) the increased demand for low-paid women workers in the expanding service sector; and (3) the greater availability of women for work because of fewer children, delayed mar-' riage, higher divorce rates, and improved household technology.

At the same time that more women entered the workforce, the growth rate slowed down. Women's labor force participation grew by 5.3 percentage points from 1975 to 1980, 3.4 percentage points from 1980 to 1985; and 3.3 percentage points from 1985 to 1990, after which it virtually halted until 1993. Women's labor force participation rates temporarily jumped from 58.8% in 1994 to an all-time high of 60.7% in 1999. However, by the end of the economic upswing of the late 1990s, the rate returned to its downward spiral, falling to 60.3% in 2005 (U.S. Department of Labor, Bureau of Labor Statistics, n.d.).

Many factors shaped the decline. The failure of economic growth to produce enough jobs—nearly unprecedented in postwar economic experience—played a key role. Since 1960, five years after the end of each of four recessions (1961, 1982, 1991, 2001), job growth became less and less robust. It rose by 17.3% after the 1961 recession, 16.4% after the 1982 recession, 9.5% after the 1991 downturn and only 4.5% since 2001 (Bernstein, 2006). From the end of the 2001 downturn to 2006 the economy grew but continued to shed jobs as if it were still in recession, leading to the term "a jobless recovery" (Stettner & Allegretto, 2005).

Historically recessions have hit the jobs filled by women (e.g. health care, education, and others) less hard than the jobs filled by men (manufacturing). But the recession in the early 1990s was different. Languid employment expansion did not provide those who lost their jobs during this downturn with opportunities to become reemployed (Stettner & Allegretto, 2005). Instead, the 2001 recession inaugurated the only period of sustained job losses for women in the past 40 years (Hartmann, Lovell, & Wershckul, 2004). Of the lost jobs 55% came from industries that had hired low-income women during the 1990s. A noticeable number of women left work altogether in response to the poor jobs picture (Hartmann *et al.*, 2004). Some economists predict that such fundamental shifts will continue to press women's employment downward so that future labor force participation fluctuation will occur around a declining trend. This suggests that for years to come, even in good times, the labor market will continue to be an unreliable route out of poverty for many women (Aaronson, Fallick, Figura, Pingle, & Wascher, 2006).

Falling Wages

For years many employed women's low wages fell far below those of men. However, during the 1980s (1979–89) women's real weekly wages rose by $30 compared to a $25 loss for men—fueled by the expansion of jobs in the low-wage service sector and the gains won by the women's movement. In contrast, during the next decade (1989–97), women's real weekly earnings rose by only $6 and men's continued to fall. During the economic upturn in the late 1990s (1995–2002), tight labor markets pressed the weekly earnings of full-time women workers up—including those paid the least (Hartmann & Whittaker, 1998). However the good times were short-lived. By 2002 as the jobless recovery set in, the gains simply faded. Despite continued economic productivity from 2002 to 2003 wage growth fell by 0.2% for women in the bottom half of the pay scale—the first decline in women's real earnings since 1995. Even the gains made by higher-paid women dropped to less than half the growth from the earlier period (Bernstein & Mishel, 2004). The fall in women's wage growth picked up speed in 2002, dropping by 0.6% from 2003 to 2004 (Economic Policy Institute, 2004b), by 1.0% from 2004 to 2005 (Economic Policy Institute, 2005a) and by 1.3% from 2005 to 2006 (Bernstein & Gould, 2006; Institute for Women's Policy Research, 2006).

In 2005, the median weekly income for full-time women workers equaled $573 or $29,796, a year. This was several thousand dollars below 200% of the 2005 federal poverty line for a family of three or $32,180 a year (Bureau of Cash Assistance, 2005). Women of color earned even less. The median weekly earnings amounted to $505 for Black women and $419 for Latina women, compared to $584 for White women and $613 earned by Asian women (U.S. Department of Labor, Women's Bureau, 2006a).

The Gender Wage Gap

Women's low wages contributed to the persistent gender wage gap. Initially it took nearly 20 years for the male–female pay differential to begin to close once Congress passed the Equal Pay Act. Indeed, although women earned only 59 cents for every dollar earned by men, this rate did not budge from 1963 to the 1980s. In the 1980s, women's economic plight improved and the female-to-male wage ratio jumped from 60.2% in 1980 to 71.6% in 1990, a rise of 11.4% in 10 years. Although women continued to gain ground on their male counterparts, the good days were limited. During the next 15 years (1990–2005) the gender wage gap narrowed by only 6.4%, significantly less than the prior 11.4 point reduction in just 10 years. Moreover, since 2000 the narrowing of gender wage ratio stemmed less from women's upward strides than from falling male wages. From 2003 to 2004, although employers still paid men more than women, male wages dropped by 2.3% compared to a 1.0% decline for women (Institute for Women's Policy Research, 2006). Between 2004 and 2005, the relative loss was 1.8% for men and 1.3% for women (Institute for Women's Policy Research, 2006).

The gender wage gap cuts across occupational lines. In 2000, in 300 occupations men earned more than women—even in those where women made up the majority (National Committee on Pay Equity, 2001). In 2005, the median weekly earnings of women relative to men amounted to 61% for women doctors, 63% for women in sales, 79% for women in construction and 86% for women in computers and mathematical occupations (National Women's Law Center, 2006a). The wage gap also widened with education. In 2001, the median annual earnings gap for women 25 years and older equaled 24% for those with less than a ninth-grade education, 27% for women with a high school degree, 28% for those with a master's degree, and 40% for women with professional degrees (Lips, n.d.). For women with an associate, bachelors or a master's degree the gap equaled 25% (Lips, n.d.). Likewise with age: in 2004, college-educated women aged 45–49 earned 38% less per year than their male counterparts, up from an 11% gap when the cohort was in their 20s (Economic Policy Institute, 2005b). Women of color fared worse. In 2005, compared to every dollar earned by all men, Latina women earned 68.5 cents, Black women earned 71.7 cents, and Asian American women earned 87.2 cents (National Committee on Pay Equity, n.d.).

The slow progress for women would have been slower if the gender wage gap calculation did not overstate women's gains by including only full-time, year-round workers. If the mix included part-time, part-year workers—more common among women then men—the wage gap would have been considerably wider. Even with the exclusion of part-time work from 1960 to 2000 the wage gap narrowed by less than half a penny. The persistent wage gap has been costly for women. Over the past 40 years, the real median earnings of women have fallen short by an estimated $523,000. Over a lifetime (47 years of full-time work), this gap equals a wage loss of $700,000 for female high school graduates, $1.2 million for college graduates, and $2 million for professional school graduates (National Committee on Pay Equity, n.d.). Even when they work hard and "play by the rules", women lose out. To this day, the gender wage gap in the United States is larger than in most western industrialized countries and much larger than in Australia, Denmark, and Spain, where women make roughly 90% of what men make (Leonhardt, 2003).

Sex-Segregated Jobs

The clustering of women and persons of color in certain occupations that pay less also keeps women poor. Some economists argue that this "occupational sex-segregation" arises because women freely choose low-wage jobs to avoid more dangerous work and to secure the more flexible schedules required for caregiving work in the home. Others argue the women "choose" to become teachers, child-care workers, home health aides, and secretaries and men to become truck drivers, judges, orderlies, and surgeons due to sex-role socialization, sex discrimination, and the gender division of labor. In any case, while women occupy a wider range of jobs and careers today, they remain concentrated in "women's jobs." These jobs carry low wages, few fringe benefits, limited job ladders, little or no union protection, and tasks that parallel the care work done by women in the home (Boraas, 2003).

The crowding of women into a small number of low-paid women's jobs declined very little from 1900 to 1960 (Wells, 1998). The sex segregation of jobs shifted slowly during the1960s and declined more rapidly during the 1970s (Wells, 1998), but during the 1980s and 1990s the pace of change slowed. Despite the substantial inroads women made into occupations previously filled by men, as late as 2005 occupations remained highly sex-segregated. In 10 of the 20 leading occupations, woman made up more than 85% of the total number of workers (U.S. Department of Labor, Women's Bureau, 2006a). The median weekly wage paid in eight out of 10 of these "women's jobs" fell below the average median weekly wage for all full-time women workers (U.S. Department of Labor, Women's Bureau, 2006c). As a group, all workers of color comprise a far smaller percentage of the labor force then all women workers: 23.1% versus 46.6%. However, fueled by racial discrimination, the market channels women of color into particular low-paid, low-status service occupations "reserved" for them, such as nurses' aides, licensed practical nurses, private household workers, as well as kitchen workers and hospital orderlies (Figart, n.d.).

The concentration of White women and women of color into "women's jobs" contributes to the gender wage gap. Sociologist Paula England (2005) reports that the segregation of jobs and women's responsibility for childrearing each contribute heavily to the wage gap. Hartman and Triemann (1981, as cited in King, 1992) state that occupational differences alone account for 35–40% of male–female wage disparity. A key longitudinal study of Black and White women aged 34–44 found that the segregation of Black women into low-paying occupations played a larger role in creating the racial wage gap than the worker's schooling and job experience, which together accounted for only one-fifth of the difference. The concentration of women in low-paying "women's jobs" profits employers. Other things being equal, paychecks get smaller as the percentage of female and persons of color on a job rises (Figart, n.d.). Thus, for women, the segregation of jobs by sex and race reduces the effectiveness of employment as a route out of poverty.

Sexual Harassment

Less often discussed, sexual harassment also limits women's earnings. Sexual harassment refers to unwelcome sexual conduct at the workplace that causes an employee to lose a job or a promotion, or creates a hostile, offensive, or intimidating workplace. Workplace sexual harassment is not a new problem, although legal liability for it is. No occupation is immune from sexual harassment. Half of all women surveyed say they have experienced some form of harassment at work, a proportion that did not budge until after the 1991 Anita Hill hearings (National Women's Law Center, 2000). From 1992 to 2003, sexual harassment claims increased by 5% among Whites, 42% among Blacks, an astonishing 120% among Hispanic women and 14.7% for men (National Partnership for Women and Families, *Workplace discrimination*, n.d.). Women experience more harassment in the better-paid occupations that have traditionally excluded them—both blue collar jobs and professions (National Women's Law Center, 2000).

Despite the frequency and harm of sexual harassment, most cases—as many as 95% of all incidents—go unreported (Roberts & Mann, n.d.). Even with the recent jump, only 5–15% of women formally reported harassment to their employers or fair employment agencies. Most fear the loss of their job, harm to their careers, not being believed, and/or that nothing can or will be done about the harassment. Embarrassment or shame at being harassed also stands in their way (National Women's Law Center, 2000).

Reported or not, sexual harassment impairs women's physical and emotional health. Well-known reactions include anxiety, depression, sleep disturbance, weight loss or gain, loss of appetite, headaches and post-traumatic stress disorder (National Women's Law Center, 2000). Harassment also affects women's financial status. To avoid the harassing behavior, victimized women may take sick leave, leave without pay, or transfer to new jobs—all of which can lead to a loss of wages or considerable unemployment. The ongoing practice of harassment represents still another reason why women cannot confidently rely on work to lift them out of poverty.

Lack of Work Supports

Caregiving labor is critical to families, society, and the employment of women. However, the workplace has not kept pace with changes in women's work patterns during the last 50 years. The resulting lack of work supports is still another reason why the labor market is an unreliable source of income for women.

For one, women's near-exclusive responsibility for care work, even when they work outside the home, limits chances in the job market. The presence of children needing care causes more women than men to lose time from work or status at work (Boushey, 2005a). Nationwide, 22.4 million families provide care for elderly relatives (National Partnership for Women and Families, Workplace flexibility, n.d.). According to Hochschild and Manchung (2002), the "second shift," lands middle-class married women workers on the (lower-paid) "Mommy Track." The double day also exhausts single mothers who end up in the bottomless pit of poverty (Albeda & Tilly, 1997).

Women also face enormous challenges trying to balance work and family responsibilities. Nearly 75% of mothers with children under age 18 work for pay either full- or part-time, seven million as single mothers; the same is true for 1.5 million single fathers (McCrate, 2002). Faced with stagnating wages, many have increased the *number of hours* on the job just to make end meet. From 1979 to 2000, working wives alone added close to 500 hours of work per year, or more than 12 weeks of full-time work. Middle-income wives added the most hours—up by 535—the equivalent of over three months of full-time work (Mishel, Bernstein, & Allegretto, 2006). Not surprisingly, the average mother (and father) now spends 22 fewer hours every week with their children than parents did in 1969 (Career Evolution, 2000).

Despite a "24/7" work environment and the mounting rhetoric about "family values," few companies offer the flexibility or the supports needed by working women and men to care for their families, to pursue their careers, or just to hold on to their jobs. Furthermore, since the mid-1970s, many of the work supports women won have became less available. Pregnancy discrimination is on the rise, family leave policies have been threatened, and childcare services are harder to come by. One economist (Boushey, 2005b, p. 1) concluded that the nation's failure to address the ongoing conflict between market and family needs is, "the result of the deliberate neglect of the needs of families in favor of the desire of employers to control workers' time." Boushey suggests that the unmet need for supports for care work represent a form of labor market discrimination.

Pregnancy Discrimination

The Pregnancy Discrimination Act of 1978 protects employees against discrimination that is in any way related to pregnancy, childbirth, or pregnancy-related conditions. Surprisingly, in recent years, complaints have soared. From 1992 to 2003, the number of pregnancy discrimination charges filed with the federal Equal Employment Opportunity Commission (EEOC) rose by 39% although the nation's birthrate dropped by 9% (Armour, 2005). Pregnancy discrimination is now one of the fastest-growing types of employment discrimination charges filed with the EEOC, outpacing the rise in sexual harassment and sex discrimination claims.

The increased complaints reflect changes in the female workforce, employer's views of pregnant women, and their effort to improve the bottom line. More women of childbearing age now work, more employed women work while pregnant, and more pregnant women stay at work further into the pregnancies. The number of women who quit their jobs upon pregnancy fell from more than half prior to 1978 to just 26.9% in the early 1990s (National Partnership for Women and Families, Pregnancy Discrimination Act, n.d.). Yet, employers still view pregnant women stereotypically as overly emotional and less competent. Also, they regard pregnant women as a financial liability due to the costs of maternity leave, health care, and flexible work arrangements. Meanwhile, the pregnant women pressing charges—ranging from entry-level jobs through high-paid executives—claim they have been fired unfairly, denied promotions and, in some cases, urged to terminate pregnancies in order to keep their jobs (National Partnership for Women and Families, Pregnancy Discrimination Act, n.d.). Unfortunately, the number of cases women have lost rose from 49.2% of the total in 1992 to 55.6% in 2005 (U.S. Equal Employment Opportunity Commission, 2006).

Family Leave

Since 1993, the Family and Medical Leave Act (FMLA) has enabled more than 50 million workers to take leave to care for a new baby or seriously ill family member, or to recover from their own serious illness without fear of losing their jobs (National Partnership for Women and Families, 2006). The FMLA requires employers with 50 or more permanent employees to allow employees of either sex up to six weeks of unpaid leave in a 12-month period for the birth or adoption of a child, up to two weeks of leave in a 12-month period for the care of a child, spouse or parent with a serious health condition, and up to two weeks of leave in a 12-month period for the employee's own serious health condition.

Although numerous surveys indicate that at least one-third of workers believe that women's main work-related problem is finding ways to balance work and family demands (Lovell & Rahmanou, 2000), the current policy offers very little help. For one, small firms that employ large numbers of women are not covered, so that less than half of all workers benefit from the FMLA. Second, unlike 163 other nations, only the United States and Australia do not provide paid leave. Close to 80% of U.S. employees do not take family leave because they need a paycheck (National Partnership for Women and Families, Paid family leave, n.d.). Other women take the shortest leave possible, which can be highly stressful, or take leave without pay, which has led to bankruptcy or public assistance applications. Longer-term strategies include fewer hours, part-time work, and jobs with schedules that accommodate family responsibilities. To the extent that women take time out from work, they place their current earnings, future promotions, and retirement income at risk (Lovell & Rahmanou, 2000).

To manage conflicting demands, women want flexibility at work, such as extended family leave, high-quality part-time employment, flextime programs and alternative personal and sick days policies to deal with unexpected contingencies. Such flexibility is especially important for low-paid single mothers and low-paid women of color who tend to have the most rigid work schedules and employers with near absolute control over their worktime (McCrate, 2002).

Not surprisingly, when surveyed, 80% of workers support paid parental leave, 85% favor paid leave to care for a new child or seriously ill family member, and nearly 75% think the government should do more to help. Some states use unemployment insurance (baby UI benefit) or temporary disability programs to expand paid medical and family leaves—a practice that is supported by 84% of all adults (Lovell & Rahmanou, 2000). In contrast, the Department of Labor proposed to scale back the FMLA by changing the definition of serious illness, restricting intermittent leave use, and otherwise eroding the protection (National Partnership for Women and Families, 2005). Advocates fear such changes will scale back the program, eliminate hard-won gains and generally make the labor market less friendly to women and their families.

Childcare

It is well known that access to stable, affordable and quality childcare helps women stay employed (Lee, 2004; Lempke, Witte, Queralt, & Witt, 2000). Yet childcare services elude many women. Cost is particularly important to low-income mothers. In 2004, only 7% of low-income mothers received any help with childcare cost from government, employers, or family members (Lee, 2004). Lacking support, low-income mothers must pay market prices or settle for inferior or no services (Boushey, 2005c).

The supply of services also presents a problem. In 2005, programs funded by the Childcare Development Block Grant (CCDBG) served 1.78 million children from birth to age 13 each month, and up from 1.47 million in 2000 (Administration for Children and Families, n.d.). Although 44,000 more children needed childcare than in 2004, the number served by CCDBG remained relatively flat (Administration for Children and Families, n.d.). When programs funded by TANF and Social Service Block Grants (SSBG) are counted, an estimated 2.2 million children are served—still less than the 2.5 million served each month in 2000 (CLASP, 2006).

The lack of affordable childcare makes the labor market a less reliable route out of poverty, especially for low-income women (National Women's Law Center, 2006b). In the words of one working mother, "if you're telling people that they cannot have childcare, they probably will not be able to work. For every two steps forward, you're being dragged backward" (Henry, Wershkul, & Rao, 2003).

The State

The state is the third major source of income for women. However, like marriage and the market, the welfare state has become a less reliable route out of poverty. Instead of growing to fill the gap created by the declining capacities of marriage and the market to support women, the economic backup once provided by government programs has become threadbare.

The 1935 Social Security Act (SSA; PL 74-271) spawned the U.S. welfare state by legalizing federal responsibility for social welfare. From the New Deal to the Great Society, the welfare state expanded, driven by prosperity, population growth, the emergence of new needs, and the demands made by the increasingly militant trade union, civil rights, women's liberation and other movements (Abramovitz, 1992). The growth of income support, health, education, housing, nutrition, social services, and other programs provided a minimum standard of living that, among other things, reduced economic security, supported women's care work in the home, and eased the tension between work and family life.

However, since the mid-1970s tax and spending cuts have weakened the state's capacity to protect women from poverty. In contrast to the 1930s, when the nation's leaders saw government action as the solution to the problems caused by the collapse of the economy, in the mid-1970s they concluded that government was part of the problem. Faced with the second major economic crisis of the twentieth century, they blamed their economic woes on "big government," and called for a restructuring of the postwar social, economic, and political institutions along the old laissez-faire lines (Abramovitz, 2004).

The shift was neither accidental nor simply mean-spirited. Rather it was part of a broader economic recovery strategy designed to promote economic growth by increasing investment and savings by the wealthy. Known as Reaganomics, supply-side economics or neoliberalism, the strategy to redistribute income upwards and downsize the state first surfaced in the mid-1970s under President Carter. It was launched in full by President Reagan and has been followed by every administration since.

The strategy sought to systematically undo the New Deal by: (1) limiting the role and regulatory power of the federal government; (2) shrinking the welfare state; (3) lowering labor costs, and (4) weakening the influence of popular movements best positioned to resist the resulting austerity plan. At the same time, the far right got a grip on U.S. public policy, leading to an effort to restore so-called "family values" and a color-blind social order. The now familiar retrenchment tactics include: (1) tax cuts and a less progressive tax code; (2) budget reductions; (3) devolution (shifting social welfare responsibility from the federal government to the states); (4) privatization (transferring public programs to the private sector); and (5) undoing the historic gains won by the trade union, civil rights, women's liberation and gay rights movements.

We were promised that the benefits of this pro-market/pro-family strategy would trickle down to the average person. Instead, dismantling the welfare state weakened government intervention as a route out of poverty for women, especially those who turn to the nation's key income support programs: AFDC/TANF, food stamps and UI, Earned Income Tax Credit (EITC) and the minimum wage.

Welfare Reform

The program known as the Aid to Families with Dependent Children (AFDC) was created in 1935 (as ADC) to enable single mothers to stay home with their children. In 1996 Congress replaced AFDC with a new program called Temporary Aid to Needy Families (TANF) that included time-limited benefits, required work and otherwise restricted eligibility. Once the rolls fell by half this historic public assistance program became less reliable as a source of income for women who comprise the overwhelming majority of adult recipients. Chapter 4 discusses these programs in detail.

Food Stamps

The current version of the national food stamp program began in 1974 to help low-income individuals purchase food and obtain a nutritious diet. Women comprised nearly 60% of all adult recipients in 2004 (Barrett, 2006, Table A-27). Of all households, 45% were White, 31.3% Black, 13% Hispanic and 1.3% Asian (Barrett, 2006, Table A-21).

Like TANF, food stamps serves low-income women less well than in the past. The number of eligible households using the program rose from 52.5% in 1980 to a pre-TANF peak of 69.6% in 1994, after which it fell to a low of 48% in 2001 (U.S. Department of Health and Human Services, 2006). By 2004, the participation rate rose to 54.7% of eligible households due to a loosening of some eligibility criteria (Barrett & Poikolainen, 2006). Meanwhile the real purchasing power of food stamps (in 2004 dollars) fell from a high of $236 in 1992 to $209 in 2004 (Barrett, 2006, Table A-26).

Unemployment Insurance (UI)

The UI program was created in 1935 to provide a safety net for workers who lose their jobs through no fault of their own. However, in recent years, the labor force became more female and less White and the percentage of workers receiving UI benefits declined (Wenger, 2001). The number of unemployed workers receiving UI benefits—the recipiency rate—has dropped steadily since the mid-1950s.

From an average of 49% in the 1950s, the rate plummeted steadily to 33% in the 1980s, reaching a low of 28.5% in 1984 (Wandner & Stettner, 2000). Despite some fluctuations, it has remained below 30% in most years since then (Stettner, Boushey, & Wenger, 2005).

The downward trend affected all workers, but in general jobless men were more likely to qualify for benefits than jobless women. In 2003, 41% of men and 39% of women received benefits nationwide (Economic Policy Institute, 2004a), down from 46.9% (men) and 40.0% (women) in 2001 (Smith, McHugh, Stettner, & Segal, 2003). In 2004, 41 states provided UI benefits to more men than women. The gender gap reached 17% in some states (National Employment Law Project, 2004) and was more than three times as large as the national average in others. Women in Illinois, Michigan, Ohio and, Washington were 20% less likely to receive benefits than men (Emsellem, Goldberg, McHugh, et al., 2002).

The gender gap in participation rates reflects the UI system's failure to adequately account for overall workforce changes, especially the prevalence of part-time and temporary workers and women's unique work patterns (Economic Policy Institute, 2004a). Women are less likely to qualify for UI benefits because low wages and part-time work make it harder to meet minimum earnings require-ments. In 2000, twice as many low-wage workers (where women predominate) as high-wage workers faced unemployment, but only 18% of workers earning $8.00 or less an hour received UI benefits compared to 40% of those earning more than $8.00. Likewise, four times more women than men work part-time during their prime earning years, yet 24 states categorically deny UI benefit to part-time workers. The lack of union representation also plays a role in women's lack of coverage (U.S. Department of Labor, Bureau of Labor Statistics, 2006).

The UI program does not recognize many of the family responsibilities incurred by more women than men. Most states do not provide UI benefits when workers leave a job to deal with childcare or health emergencies. Yet these urgent personal matters are the very reasons that low-wage women workers—without paid sick leave, paid family leave, or health care benefits—leave work (Stettner, Boushey, & Wenger, 2005). Women are also more likely than men to leave a job without "good cause" to follow a relocating spouse, when work schedules make childcare arrangements impossible, and when ill or aged family members need care. Finally, some women quit work to escape a violent partner, to avoid a partner who is stalk-ing them at work, or to avoid sexual harassment (Smith et al., 2003). Women who must leave their jobs for these kinds of reasons are 32% less likely to receive UI benefits than men (National Employment Law Project, 2004).

Like TANF and food stamps, the value of the UI benefit has fallen. From1990 to 2001 the percentage of lost income replaced by UI benefits fell by 5%. In 1999, UI benefits replaced only 33% of an average worker's lost earnings. Replacing only one-half or one-third of lost income means more certain poverty for a low- than a middle-income earner. In 2001, a single working parent with two children receiving UI benefits faced $1,317 less than needed to maintain a minimal, no-frills living standard. For a two-parent, two-child family with one full-time and one part-time worker, the gap was still $334 (Boushey & Wenger, 2001).

Earned Income Tax Credit (EITC)

Finally, the EITC, established in 1975 to offset the effects of federal payroll taxes on low-income families, has become the main antipoverty program for the working-age population. In fiscal year 2005, the $34 billion in federal EITC spending exceeded the $24 billion spent on TANF and other family support programs. Reaching 21.5 million taxpayers, the EITC program lifts four to five million people out of poverty each year (Greenstein, 2005; Llobrera & Zahradnik, 2004).

However, even this popular and effective program has faltered. First, government spending for EITC has slowed (Office of Management and Budget, 2006). Second, since it is tied to a worker's earnings, stagnant wages have yielded both a flat EITC and reduced buying power. Third, although Congress adjusts the EITC income limits and benefit ceilings for inflation, the adjustments do not compensate for the deterioration of the minimum wage (Office of Management & Budget, 2006). Indeed, the after-tax income of EITC-eligible families with a full-time, minimum-wage worker and children has not increased since 2004 and will not increase again until the minimum wage is raised (Office of Management & Budget, 2006).

The Minimum Wage

The federal minimum wage, first enacted in 1938 as part of the Fair Labor Standards Act, is part of a long tradition of regulations intended to protect workers from unfair and unsafe working conditions. From 1938 to 1981, Congress regularly increased the wage floor to keep pace with inflation and the benefits accrued disproportionately to low-income workers, where women predominate. However, this practice ended when President Reagan failed to increase the minimum wage from January1981 to April 1990 (Bernstein & Shapiro, 2006).

The federal minimum wage was stuck at $5.15 an hour or $10,300 a year from 1997 to 2007—its lowest level since 1955 and the second-longest period without a hike (Ettlinger, 2006). Meanwhile, inflation increased by 26% overall due to rising gasoline costs (134%), childcare (52%), medical care (43%), food (29%), housing (23%) and other necessities (Bernstein & Shapiro, 2006). The wage floor is not tied to inflation, so its real purchasing power declined steadily as a percentage of both the federal poverty line and as a percentage of the average wage. From 90% of the poverty level in 1968, the real wage floor fell steadily to 51% of the poverty line for a four-person family in 2006, the lowest level since 1955 (Bernstein & Shapiro, 2006; Levitis & Johnson, 2006). Similarly, in the 1950s and 1960s, the minimum wage ranged from 44 to 56% of the average wage, then plummeted to 31% in 2006—the lowest share since at least the end of World War II (Ettlinger, 2006). Fortunately, some states have picked up some of the slack. Through the end of 2005, 17 states and the District of Columbia raised their minimum wages to a median average of $6.55, ranging from $5.70 an hour in Wisconsin to $7.35 in Washington State (Wolfson, 2006). Most recently, in May 2007, Congress raised the minimum wage to $7.25 over three years.

Conclusion

The historical record suggests that structural changes in family arrangements, the economy and the state have reduced the capacity of each institution to protect women from poverty. Solutions, which are not out of reach, require political will, not rocket science. Conservatives hope to end women's poverty by restoring traditional "family values." They favor marriage promotion and some work training for male breadwinners. Liberals prefer to reduce women's poverty through labor market reform (e.g. enforcing laws banning unequal pay and sexual harassment and expanding programs to help women manage work and family life, such as childcare, paid family leave and ending pregnancy discrimination) and expanding the welfare states taxes and spending. More long-term or radical solutions to women's poverty challenge basic labor market structures, such as occupational segregation by sex and race, the upward redistribution of income and the declining progressivity of the U.S. tax system.

Since even in the best of times the market cannot guarantee a job to everyone ready and willing to work, women would benefit if the state reclaimed its role as provider of last resort ensuring an economic backup for those in need. In the long run, women would stand to gain from a broader agenda that defines access to jobs, income, education, and health as human rights rather than charity. The current attack on the welfare state makes it seem as if such reforms are impossible. Yet U.S. and western European records demonstrate that such programs do not exceed the limits of a market economy. Many western industrial nations have adopted some or all of this agenda. Moreover, since the 1930s, mainstream political leaders and social movements in the United States have proposed, endorsed, and pushed a human rights agenda only to be stymied by opponents whose interests were threatened by any move toward greater social justice. Our job is to once again to create conditions for social change! In the words of Martin Luther King, Jr. (1967), "History will have to record that the greatest tragedy of this period of social transition was not the strident clamor of the bad people, but the appalling silence of the good people."

References

Aaronson, S., Fallick, B., Figura, A., Pingle, J., & Wascher, W. (2006). *The recent decline in labor force participation and its implications for potential labor supply* (preliminary draft). The Brookings Institution. Available HTML: http://www.brookings.edu/es/commentary/journals/bpea_macro/200603bpea_aaronson.pdf#search=%22female%20labor%20force%20participation%202005%22\ (accessed 30 November 2006).

Abramovitz, M. (1992). The Reagan legacy: Undoing the class, race and gender accords. *Journal of Sociology and Social Welfare, 19*, 91–110.

Abramovitz, M. (2004). Saving capitalism from itself: Whither the welfare state? *New England Journal of Public Policy, Fall/Winter*, 21–32.

Administration for Children and Families. (n.d.). *Program data and statistics, childcare and development fund data tables, 1998 to 2005*. Childcare Bureau. Available HTML: http://www.acf.hhs.gov/programs/ccb/data/index.htm (accessed 3 December 2006).

Albeda, R. & Tilly, C. (1997). *Glass ceilings and bottomless pits: Women's work, women's poverty*. Boston: South End Press.

American Institute on Domestic Violence. (n.d.). *Domestic violence in the workplace statistics.* Available HTML: http://www.aidv-usa.com/Statistics.htm (accessed 7 January 2006).

AmeriStat. (2003). *Diversity, poverty characterize female-headed households, number and percent of households by household type and race/ethnicity, 1970–2002* (March). Available HTML: http://www.prb.org/Articles/2003/DiversityPovertyCharacterizeFemaleHeadedHouseholds.aspx (accessed 18 November 2006).

Armour, S. (2005, 17 February). Pregnant workers report growing discrimination. *USA Today* (online) Available HTML: http://www.usatoday.com/money/workplace/2005-02-16-pregnancy-bias-usat_x.htm (accessed 22 December 2006).

Aron-Dine A. & Shapiro, I. (2006). *In first half of 2006, wages and salaries captured smallest share of income on record.* Center on Budget and Policy Priorities. Available HTML: http://www.cbpp.org/8-31-06inc.htm (accessed 10 November 2006).

Barrett, A. (2006a). *Characteristics of food stamp households, fiscal year 2005.* U.S. Department of Agriculture, Food and Nutrition Services FSP-06, Table A-21: Distribution of Participating Households with Selected Household Characteristics by the Race of the Household Head; Table A-26: Comparison of Average Nominal and Real Values of Key Food Stamp Household Characteristics for Fiscal Years 1989 to 2005; Table A-27: Comparison of Number of Food Stamp Participants by Gender and Age for Fiscal Years 1989 to 2005. September. Available HTML: http://www.fns.usda.gov/OANE/menu/Published/FSP/FILES/Participation/2005Characteristics.pdf (accessed 14 November 2006).

Barrett, A. & Poikolainen, A. (2006). *Food stamp program participation rates: 2004.* Available HTML: http://www.fns.usda.gov/oane/MENU/Published/FSP/FILES/Participation/FSPPart2004.pdf (accessed 13 November 2006).

Bernstein, J. (2006). *Jobs recovery at five reveals uniquely weak expansion. Economic snapshot.* Economic Policy Institute. Available HTML: http://www.epi.org/content.cfm/webfeatures_snapshots_2006 1213 (accessed 15 December 2006).

Bernstein, J. & Furman, J. (2006). *A tough recovery by any measure: New data show consumer expenditures lag for low and middle income families.* Center on Budget and Policy Priorities, Economic Policy Institute. Available HTML: http://www.epi.org/issuebriefs/230/ib230.pdf (accessed 15 December 2006).

Bernstein, J. & Gould, E. (2006). *Working families fall behind.* Economic Policy Institute. Available HTML: http://www.epi.org/content.cfm/webfeatures_econindicators_income20060829 (accessed 17 December 2006).

Bernstein, J. & Mishel, L. (2004). *Weak recovery claims new victim: Workers' wages* (Issue Brief #196). Washington, DC: Economic Policy Institute.

Bernstein, J. & Price, L. (2005). *An off-kilter expansion slack job market continues to hurt wage growth* (Economic Policy Institute Briefing Paper #164). Washington, DC: Economic Policy Institute.

Bernstein, J. & Shapiro, I. (2006). *Nine years of neglect: Federal minimum wage remains unchanged for ninth straight year, falls to lowest level in more than half a century.* Center on Budget and Policy Priorities, Economic Policy Institute. Available HTML: http://www.cbpp.org/8-31-06mw.htm (accessed 4 January 2006).

Boraas, S. (2003). How does gender play a role in the earnings gap? An update. *Monthly Labor Review, 126,* 3–15.

Boushey, H. (2005a). *Are women opting out? Debunking the myth.* Executive Summary, Center for Economic and Policy Research. Available HTML: www.cepr.net/publications/opt_out_2005_11.pdf (accessed 18 November 2006).

Boushey, H. (2005b). *Who pays for today's families.* Center for Economic and Policy Research. Available HTML: http://www.cepr.net/columns/boushey/2005_03.pdf#search=%22women%20labor%20market%20%22 (accessed 18 November 2006).

Boushey, H. (2005c). *The effects on employment and wages when Medicaid and childcare subsidies are no longer available.* Center for Economic and Policy Research. Available HTML: http://www.cepr.net/publications/labor_markets_2005_01_26.pdf (accessed 19 November 2006).

Boushey, H. & Wenger, J. (2001). *Coming up short: Current unemployment insurance benefits fail to meet basic family needs.* (Economic Policy Institute Issue Brief #169). Washington, DC: Economic Policy Institute.

Bureau of Cash Assistance. (2005). *2005 emergency program income guidelines for Emergency Safety Net Assistance (ESNA) and Emergency Assistance to Needy Families with Children (EAF)*. Available HTML: http://www.otda.state.ny.us/main/gis/2005/05DC010.rtf (accessed 5 December 2006).

Career Evolution. (2000). Career evolution: The future of work. *The Economist, 354*, 89–92.

CLASP. (2006). *Childcare and development block grant participation in 2005*. Center for Law and Social Policy. Available HTML: http://www.clasp.org/publications/ccdbgparticipation_2005.pdf.

Dorian, S. & Miller, M. (2002). *Let them eat wedding rings: The role of marriage in the promotion of welfare reform*. Alternatives to Marriage Project. Available HTML: http://www.unmarried.org/rings.php (accessed 9 November 2006).

Economic Policy Institute. (2004a). *Unemployment insurance frequently asked questions. Issue guide*. Available HTML: http://www.epinet.org/content.cfm/issueguides_unemployment_faq (accessed 17 November 2006).

Economic Policy Institute. (2004b, 26 August). *Weak 2003 labor market leads to lower incomes and higher poverty. Income Picture*. Available HTML: http://www.epinet.org/content.cfm/webfeatures_econindicators_income20040826 (accessed 22 November 2006).

Economic Policy Institute. (2005a). *Economy up, people down: Declining earnings undercut income growth. Income Picture*. Available HTML: http://www.epi.org/content.cfm/webfeatures_econindicators_income20050831 (accessed 22 November 2006).

Economic Policy Institute. (2005b). *The gender wage gap is real—Snapshots*. Available HTML: http://www.epi.org/content.cfm/webfeatures_snapshots_20050914 (accessed 13 November 2006).

Economic Policy Institute. (2006). *Share of all workers earning poverty level wage 1973–2005. Data Zone*. Available HTML: http://www.epi.org/datazone/06/poverty_wages.pdf (accessed 15 November 2006).

Edin K. (2000). A few good men: Why poor mothers don't marry or remarry? *The American Prospect, 28*, 26–31.

Emsellem, M., Goldberg, J., McHugh, R., *et al.* (2002). *Failing the unemployed: A state-by-state evaluation of unemployment insurance systems* (Economic Policy Institute Briefing Paper #122). Washington, DC: Economic Policy Institute.

England, P. (2005). Gender inequality in labor markets: The role of motherhood and segregation. *Social Politics: International Studies in Gender, State & Society, 12*, 264–88.

Ettlinger, M. (2006). Securing the wage floor: Indexing would maintain the minimum wage's value and provide predictability to employers. (Economic Policy Institute Briefing Paper #177). Washington, DC: Economic Policy Institute.

Fein, D. (2004). *Married and poor: Basic characteristics of economically disadvantaged married couples in the U.S.* (Supporting Healthy Marriage Working Paper SHM-01). Available HTML: http://www.mdrc.org/publications/393/workpaper.pdf (accessed 15 November 2006).

Figart D. (n.d.). *Race and pay equity, policy brief*. National Committee on Pay Equity. Available HTML: http://www.pay-equity.org/info-racebrief.html (accessed 10 January 2006).

Fox, J. (2006, 18 December). More cream for the fat cats. *Fortune, 154* (online). Available HTML: http://money.cnn.com/magazines/fortune/fortune_archive/2006/12/25/8396760/index.htm?postversion=2006121805 (accessed 10 January 2007).

Greenstein, R. (2005, 17 August). *The earned income tax credit: Boosting employment, aiding the working poor*. Center on Budget and Policy Priorities. Available HTML: http://www.cbpp.org/7-19-05eic.htm (accessed 5 January 2006).

Greenhouse, S. & Leonhardt, D. (2006, 28 August). Real wages fail to match a rise in productivity. *New York Times*. Available HTML: http://www.nytimes.com/2006/08/28/business/28wages.html?pagewanted=1 (accessed 9 December 2006).

Halle, T. (2002). *Charting parenthood: A statistical portrait of fathers and mothers in America*. Washington, DC: Child Trends, Inc.

Hartmann, H. & Whittaker, J. (1998). *Stall in women's real wage growth slows progress in closing the wage gap* (Institute for Women's Policy Research Briefing paper). Washington, DC: Institute for Women's Policy Research.

Hartmann, H., Lovell, V., & Wershckul, M. (2004, 24 October). *Women and the economy: Recent trends in job loss, labor force participation and wages* (Institute For Women's Policy Research, Publication #B425). Available HTML: http://www.iwpr.org/pdf/B245.pdf (accessed 9 December 2006).

Henry, C., Wershkul, M., & Rao, M. (2003, October). *Childcare subsidies promote mothers' employment and children's development* (Institute for Women's Policy Research Briefing Paper #G714). Washington, DC: Institute for Women's Policy Research.

Hochshild, A. & Manchung, A. (2002) *The Second Shift* (2nd ed.). New York: Penguin Group.

InfoPlease. (2006). *Unmarried-partner households by sex of partners and race and Hispanic origin of householder, 2000*. Available HTML: http:/www.infoplease.com/ipa/A0908648.html (accessed 18 November 2006).

Institute for Women's Policy Research (2006, August). *The gender wage ratio in women and men's earnings* (#C350). Available HTML: http://www.iwpr.org/pdf/Updated2006_C350.pdf (accessed 7 December 2006).

King, M. (1967, April). *Beyond Vietnam: A time to break the silence.* Available HTML: http://www.americanrhetoric.com/speeches/mlkatimetobreaksilence.htm (accessed 5 December 2006).

King, M. (1992). Occupational segregation: Race and sex 1940–1988. *Monthly Labor Review, 115*, 30–6.

Lee, S. (2004, 4 November). *Women's work supports, job retention and job mobility* (Institute for Women's Policy Research Brief #C359). Available HTML: http://www.iwpr.org/pdf/C359.pdf (accessed 7 December 2006).

Lempke, R., Witte, A., Queralt, M., & Witt, R. (2000). *Childcare and the welfare to work transition* (National Bureau of Economic Research Working Paper #7583). Cambridge, MA: National Bureau of Economic Research.

Leonhardt, D. (2003, 17 February). Gap between pay of men and women smallest on record. *New York Times.*

Levitis, J. & Johnson, N. (2006, 20 November). *Together, state minimum wages and state earned income tax credits make work pay.* Center on Budget and Policy Priorities. Available HTML: http://www.cbpp.org/7-12-06sfp.htm? (accessed 28 November 2006).

Lips, H. (n.d). *The gender wage gap: Debunking the rationalizations.* Available HTML: http://www.womensmedia.com/new/Lips-Hilary-gender-wage-gap.shtml (accessed 26 November 2006).

Llobrera, J. & Zahradnik, B. (2004). *A hand up: How state earned income tax credits help working families escape poverty in 2004.* Center on Budget and Policy Priorities. Available HTML: http://www.cbpp.org/5-14-04sfp.htm (accessed 5 January 2006).

Lovell, V. (2000). *Paid family and medical leave: Supporting working families in Illinois* (Institute for Women's Policy Research Publication #B235). Available HTML: http://www.iwpr.org/pdf/IL%20testimony%209-00.pdf (accessed 14 December 2006).

Lovell, V. & Rahmanou, H. (2000). *Paid family and medical leave: Essential support for working women and men* (Institute for Women's Policy Research Publication #A124). Available HTML: http://www.iwpr.org/pdf/famlve2.pdf (accessed 15 January 2006).

McCrate, E. (2002). *Working mothers in a double bind: Working moms, minorities have the most rigid schedules, and are paid less for the sacrifice* (Economic Policy Institute Briefing Paper #124). Washington, DC: Economic Policy Institute.

Mishel, L., Bernstein, J., & Allegretto, S. (2005). *The state of working America 2004/2005: Higher inequality leads to uneven progress.* Washington, DC: Economic Policy Institute.

Mishel, L., Bernstein, J., & Allegretto, S. (2006). *The state of working America 2006/2007, family income: New economy drives a wedge between productivity and living standards.* Economic Policy Institute. Available HTML: http://www.stateof workingamerica.org/swa06-01-family_income.pdf (accessed 11 December 2006).

Nakosteen, R. & Zimmer, M. (1997). Man, money, and marriage: Are high earners more prone than low earners to marry? *Social Science Quarterly, 78*, 66–82.

National Committee on Pay Equity. (2001). *Profile of the gender wage gap by selected occupations for the year 2000.* Available HTML: http://www.pay-equity.org/PDFs/occupation2000.pdf (accessed 1 December 2006).

National Committee on Pay Equity. (n.d.). *The wage gap remains.* Available HTML: http://www.pay-equity.org/info-time.html (accessed 1 December 2006).

National Employment Law Project. (2004). *Why unemployment insurance matters to working women and families: An important tool in the work–family balance. A changing workforce, changing economy fact sheet.* Available HTML: http://www.nelp.org/ui/initiatives/family/uiwomenfam121704.cfm (accessed 1 December 2006).

National Partnership for Women and Families. (n.d.). *Paid family leave*. Available HTML: http://www.nationalpartnership.org/Default.aspx?tabid=116 (accessed 1 December 2006).

National Partnership for Women and Families. (n.d.). *Pregnancy Discrimination Act 25 years later: Pregnancy discrimination persists*. Available HTML: http://www.nationalpartnership.org/site/DocServer/Pregnancy25thAnnivFacts.pdf?docID=1202 (accessed 1 December 2006).

National Partnership for Women and Families. (n.d.). *Workplace discrimination: Sexual harassment*. Available HTML: http://www.nationalpartnership.org/site/PageServer? pagename=ourwork_wpd_SexualHarassment (accessed 1 December 2006).

National Partnership for Women and Families. (n.d.). *Workplace flexibility*. Available HTML: http://www.nationalpartnership.org/site/PageServer?pagename=ourwork_wpf_WorkplaceFlexibility (accessed 1 December 2006).

National Partnership for Women and Families. (2005). *Family and medical leave Act protections need to be expanded, not undermined*. Available HTML: http://www.nationalpartner ship.org/Portals/p3/NewsRoom/PressStatements/2005/FMLARegulationsFeb05.pdf (accessed 1 December 2006).

National Partnership for Women and Families. (2006, 20 November). *Labor Department's request for information on the family and medical leave act is alarming, nation's leading expert says*. Available HTML: http://www.nationalpartnership.org/Portals/p3/NewsRoom/PressStatements/2006/FMLA_Info_RequestNov30_06.pdf (accessed 1 December 2006).

National Women's Law Center. (2000). *Sexual harassment in the workplace*. Washington, DC: Author.

National Women's Law Center. (2006a). *The paycheck fairness act: Helping to close the wage gap for women*. Washington, DC: Author.

National Women's Law Center. (2006b). *Childcare remains out of reach for many low-income families*. Washington, DC: Author.

Office of Management and Budget. (2006). *Budget of the Government of the United States, fiscal year 2007, historical tables*: Table 8.5: Outlays for mandatory and related programs: 1962–2011. Available HTML: http://www.Whitehouse.gov/omb/budget/fy2007/pdf/hist.pdf (accessed 30 December 2006).

Ooms, T. (2002, 7 April). Marriage plus. *The American Prospect*. Available HTML: http://www.prospect.org/cs/articles?article=marriage_plus (accessed 10 January 2006).

Price, L. (2006). *Why people are so dissatisfied with today's economy* (Economic Policy Institute Issue Brief #219). Washington, DC: Economic Policy Institute.

Roberts, B. & Mann, R. (n.d.). *Sexual harassment in the workplace: A primer*. Available HTML: http://www3.uakron.edu/lawrev/robert1.html (accessed 1 December 2006).

Roberts, S. (2007, 16 January). 51% of women are now living without a spouse. *New York Times*. Available HTML: http://www.nytimes.com/2007/01/16/us/16census.html? ex=1169614800&en=f4c43dd44de05994&ei=5070&emc=eta1 (accessed 16 January 2007).

Smith, R., McHugh, R., Stettner, A., & Segal, N. (2003). *Between a rock and a hard place: Confronting the failure of state unemployment insurance systems to serve women and working families*. National Employment Law Project. Available HTML: http://www.nelp.org/docUploads/Between%20a%20Rock%20and%20a%20Hard%20Place%20070103%5F071503%5F092511%2Epdf (accessed 18 November 2006).

Statistical Abstract of the United States. (2006). *Marital status of the population, 1900–2004*. Available HTML: http://www.infoplease.com/ipa/A0193922.html (accessed 7 December 2006).

Stettner, A. & Allegretto, S. (2005). *The rising stakes of job loss: Stubborn long-term joblessness amid falling unemployment rates* (Economic Policy Institute Briefing Paper #162). Washington, DC: Economic Policy Institute.

Stettner, A., Boushey, H., & Wenger, J. (2005). *Clearing the path to unemployment insurance for low-income workers: An analysis of alternative base period implementation*. National Employment Law Project and the Center for Economic and Policy Research. Available HTML: http://www.nelp.org/ui/initiatives/low_wage/abpreport.cfm (accessed 8 December 2006).

U.S. Census Bureau, Historical Poverty Tables. (n.d.). Table 13: Number of families below the poverty level and poverty rate, 1959 to 2005. Available HTML: http://www.census.gov/hhes/www/poverty/histpov/hstpov13.html (accessed 27 November 2006).

U.S. Census Bureau, Historical Poverty Tables. (n.d.). Table 7: Poverty of people, by sex: 1966 to 2005. Available HTML: http://www.census.gov/hhes/www/poverty/histpov/hstpov7.html (accessed 5 December 2006).

U.S. Department of Health and Human Services, National Center for Health Statistics. (n.d.).: *Marriages and divorces, 1900–2005*. Available HTML: http://www.infoplease.com/ipa/A0005044 .html (accessed 5 January 2006).

U.S. Department of Health and Human Services. (2006). *Annual report to Congress: Indicators of welfare dependence 2006*, Table IND 4b: Number and percentage of eligible households participating in the food stamp program, selected years. Available HTML: http://aspe.hhs.gov/hsp/ indicators06/ch2.pdf (accessed 3 December 2006).

U.S. Department of Labor, Bureau of Labor Statistics. (n.d.). *Civilian labor force participation rate— 20 yrs. and over, women, 1948–2006*, Table A—1 Series Id: LNS11300026. Available HTML: http://www.bls.gov/cps/cpsatabs.htm (accessed 13 December 2006c).

U.S. Department of Labor, Bureau of Labor Statistics. (2006, 20 January) *Union members in 2005* (USDL 06-99). Available HTML: http://www.bls.gov/news/news,release.union2.nr0.htm (accessed 13 January 2006).

U.S. Department of Labor, Women's Bureau. (2006a). *Twenty leading occupations of employed women*. Available HTML: http://www.dol.gov/wb/factsheets/20lead2006.htm (accessed 25 May 2007).

U.S. Department of Labor, Women's Bureau. (2006b). *Women in the labor force: A data book* (Report #996), Table 16—Median usual weekly earnings of full-time wage and salary workers in current dollars by race, Hispanic or Latino ethnicity, and sex, 1979–2005 annual averages. Available HTML: http://www.bls.gov/cps/wlf-table16-2006.pdf (accessed 13 December 2006c).

U.S. Department of Labor, Women's Bureau. (2006b). *Women in the labor force: A data book*. (Report #996), Table 18—Median usual weekly earnings of full-time wage and salary workers by detailed occupation and sex, 2005 annual averages. Available HTML: http://www.bls.gov/cps/wlf-table18-2006.pdf (accessed 14 December 2006).

U.S. Equal Employment Opportunity Commission. (2006 Aug.). *Pregnancy discrimination charges: EEOC & FEPA combined: FY 1992–FY 2005*. Available HTML: http://www.eeoc.gov/stats/pregnanc .html (accessed 12 December 2006).

Wandner, S. & Stettner, A. (2000). Why are many jobless workers not applying for benefits? *Monthly Labor Review*, 123, 21–32.

Wells, T. (1998). *Changes in occupational sex segregation during the 1980s and 1990s*. (Center for Demography and Ecology Working Paper #98-14). Madison: University of Wisconsin.

Wenger, J. (2001). *Divided we fall: Deserving workers slip through America's patchwork unemployment insurance system*. Washington, DC: Economic Policy Institute.

Wolfson, P. (2006). *State minimum wages: A policy that works* (Economic Policy Institute Briefing Paper #176). Washington, DC: Economic Policy Institute.

Critical Thinking Questions

1   According to Abramovitz, current social structures work to trap women in poverty. How might increased emphasis on marriage result in greater stigma and discrimination against single mothers and their children?

2   Explore online resources and newspapers to find out how much it costs to rent a two-bedroom apartment in your area. Next, using your own diet as an example, calculate how much it would cost to feed a single mother and her two children. Multiply the amount you spend for your own food and the amount you calculated to feed a family of three by three (as Mollie Orshansky did when she developed the official poverty measure that is still used today). Compare your figures to the poverty threshold figures for a family of one and a family of three presented in Table 1.1. Could you survive?

3   For years, minimum-wage workers have reported that they feel invisible. Think about where you encounter minimum-wage workers in your community. Are the services they provide different from services provided by moderate or high-income workers? Many low-income workers are women. What is the connection between "women's work" and low wages? If you have every worked in a low-wage job, reflect on your experiences.

4 Life After Welfare Reform

Karen Seccombe

Chris and her three children are among the nearly three million "successful" families that have left Temporary Assistance for Needy Families (TANF), the cash assistance program created in 1997 in the wake of welfare reform (U.S. Department of Health & Human Services, 2005). Chris left welfare for work, and has been steadily employed for nearly three years – a model TANF leaver in every way. Yet on closer scrutiny, her story does not ring of success.

Chris is a slight woman, 38 years old, who has been raising her three children alone since her husband left more than five years ago. He pays no child support and rarely sees the children, who are now aged seven, nine, and 12. Chris and her children live in a cramped two-bedroom apartment in a rundown section of town, but it is all they can afford on Chris's pay of $9.00 an hour. Her workday begins early—her job begins at 7:30 a.m., but the commute by bus adds another hour each way. She pays her neighbor to help get her children to school, which takes a chunk out of her already small paycheck.

Her feelings about leaving welfare for work are mixed. On the one hand, she is pleased with herself for finding and maintaining work: "good-paying" work that is significantly above minimum wage, and she believes she is a good role model for her children. Yet, on the other hand, Chris is extremely worried about her inability to pay basic bills despite her full-time employment. In particular, she and her children have no health insurance, and her children are all in need of medical or dental care. Her employer does not offer insurance and her single year of transitional Medicaid benefits given to her when she left TANF has now expired. She earns too much to qualify for continued Medicaid benefits, but not enough to purchase insurance privately. Consequently, Chris and her children join the other 47 million Americans who are completely uninsured (DeNavas-Walt, Proctor & Lee, 2006). Chris and her family, like millions of others, are at grave risk for suffering needlessly because they cannot afford to pay their medical bills.

On the day we met, Chris was particularly worried about her 12-year-old daughter who has a serious dental condition, is in chronic pain and needs immediate attention. Her daughter needs a permanent crown, but with no way to pay for it, she instead had to choose the less expensive, temporary treatment:

> What she needed was a crown to be put on there permanently. I couldn't afford a crown, so that's why the temporary was placed in there. It shouldn't

be in there as long as it has, or it's going to affect her gum and rot it out, and the teeth are going to be rotten. I couldn't afford the crown so the doc has to hold off until I figure out something. It's been terrible. We had appointments. I've got letters saying you have to finish your appointments, yet I don't have the coverage. I'm asking for help.

When asked what she will do, she began to cry, feeling the pain of watching her young child suffer. Through her tears she explained that this stress is new to her, because in the past her Medicaid was automatically included with her welfare check. Now, since leaving welfare for work, she has to find her own health insurance, yet knows that few potential employers would offer it to her. Instead of a secure job with benefits, she can only find temporary work, which offers no protection for her family,

> I could have gone the rest of my life without feeling the stress I'm going through, worrying about what I'm going to do. . . . I don't know, how can you prepare for it? My main priority was getting as much work as I can to keep a roof over our heads. Now they hire more temps. . . . I know I've proven myself. I feel like I'm being used right now through my work. I was willing to give up part of my pay to be able to be permanent and have medical coverage. I don't care about vacation or sick leave. What have I got to fall back on? What have my kids got to fall back on?

We may not hear a lot about poverty these days; however, we do hear about welfare and welfare reform. Americans tend to view welfare with suspicion, fearing that it discourages work incentives and motivation. Many believe that welfare recipients are lazy, content to live off the "public dole." One survey found that about one half of persons who live relatively comfortably on an income of at least twice the poverty level believe that, "the primary cause of poverty is that poor people lack motivation." They also believe that, "poor people have it easy because they can get so many government benefits without doing anything in return" (NPR Online, 2001). These attitudes are important because they shape public discourse about welfare and welfare reform. They become "public facts"—grand statements about social events that we do not or cannot experience personally—regardless of their accuracy (Gusfield, 1981).

Welfare programs have been around for many years and reflect societal attitudes toward poverty and toward the worthy and unworthy poor. "Welfare," as we have come to call it, was created in 1935 as Title IV of the Social Security Act, a critical piece of legislation produced during the New Deal, when millions of families were suffering financial hardship. Unprecedented numbers of families were homeless and hungry, and children joined their parents begging in the streets. Private charities and churches stepped up their efforts to help the needy, but the problem had become so rampant that their efforts could not keep pace with the need. Under President Franklin D. Roosevelt, responsibility for social welfare was transferred from individual states or charity work to the federal government.

Welfare programs were primarily targeted toward women and children because they were seen as more vulnerable than men to conditions of poverty, and therefore more deserving of assistance. The first national welfare programs were designed to help single mothers stay home and take care of their children. Reformers were concerned about children's lack of supervision when their mothers worked, fearing that children roamed the streets, took jobs themselves, or got into trouble in their mothers' absence. They argued that the future of our nation depended on the proper upbringing of children by their mothers at home (Abramovitz, 1996a, b; Gordon, 1994; Mink, 1995).

A lot has changed over the past 75 years. Today, our society expects single mothers to work for pay rather than stay home to care for their children (Seccombe, 2007b). Single mothers are no longer deemed to be uniformly worthy of assistance and excused from work. The trend of mothers' employment has grown steadily; however, beginning in the 1970s, their numbers spiraled quickly upwards. Today, working mothers are the norm rather than the exception. About three-quarters of single mothers and two-thirds of married mothers are employed outside the home for pay (U.S. Census Bureau, 2006). Although mothers of school-age children have the highest rates of labor force participation of all mothers, over half (53%) of mothers with infants under one year are also employed (U.S. Department of Labor, 2006).

With so many mothers working, politicians began to feel uncomfortable continuing to pay women to stay home to care for their children. They framed welfare as problematic, arguing that benefits had become too attractive and that many mothers were opting to receive welfare rather than to work for pay. Various welfare reforms were implemented over the years, with only minimal success at reducing the size and scope of welfare programs. However, in 1996 the U.S. Congress passed important legislation that drastically changed welfare as an entitlement program.

"Ending Welfare as We Know It"

By 1996, under President William J. Clinton's administration, approximately 13 million persons or nearly five million families with children received Aid to Families With Dependent Children (AFDC), the principal cash welfare program of the time (U.S. Department of Health & Human Services, 2007). Congress, mirroring public sentiment concerning welfare, wrestled with ways to reduce the size of welfare caseloads.

President Clinton advocated reforming the welfare system, believing that the federal government should institute a comprehensive series of reforms to prevent what has been described as "long-term dependence" on the system. He stressed that the focus of welfare should be in getting people back to work, as employment "gives hope and structure and meaning to our lives" (Clinton, 1997). Rather than creating programs that focused on increasing welfare recipients' education level or training so that they could improve their human capital, he argued instead for an assortment of services, including health insurance and childcare to support lower-wage workers. He acknowledged in a 1994 speech, that, without these services, welfare recipients are unable to leave welfare for work:

> There are things that keep people on welfare. One is the tax burden of low wage work; another is the cost of childcare; another is the cost of medical care . . . today you have this bizarre situation where people on welfare, if they take a job in a place which doesn't offer health insurance, are asked to give up their children's healthcare, and go to work. . . . That doesn't make any sense.
>
> (Clinton, 1997a)

The Republican-led Congress went to President Clinton twice with welfare reforms that he considered too punitive and inadequate to support families. However, at the time of their third attempt Clinton was up for reelection and his Republican opponent could make the most of the fact that Clinton had twice vetoed Republican-initiated welfare reform. Consequently, on 22 August 1996 President Clinton signed the bill before him to eliminate AFDC and to revamp welfare "as we know it." Although noting that the legislation was not his ideal, he claimed that the legislation met his general criteria for moving people from welfare to work, offered benefits such as childcare and health care (although, only temporarily), and would further enforce child support payments on the part of absent parents. It supported his belief that welfare recipients must find jobs, and it offered some degree of help in doing so.

Through the Personal Responsibility and Work Opportunity Reconciliation Act (PRWORA; PL 104–193), the former AFDC program was abolished. Instead, Temporary Assistance for Needy Families (TANF) was created and went into effect as federal law on 1 July 1997 (Coven, 2005). In a nutshell, PRWORA was designed to move families from welfare to work. Proponents hailed the legislation as a powerful way to decrease welfare dependency. Critics, including Clinton himself, felt many of the changes were highly punitive.

How TANF Works

Under the 1996 TANF rules, cash assistance is no longer an entitlement program available to parents who otherwise meet the financial criteria—today TANF programs provide cash assistance to fewer than half of the families who meet eligibility requirements (Coven, 2005; Parrott & Sherman, 2006). Instead, under federal guidelines, states are expected to move people from welfare to work quickly, and divert new welfare cases whenever possible.

The federal government provides $16.6 million in block grants to states per year to meet the four purposes set out in federal law, which are to: (1) provide assistance to needy families so that children may be cared for in their own homes or in the homes of relatives; (2) end the dependence of needy parents on government benefits by promoting job preparation, work, and marriage; (3) prevent and reduce the incidence of out-of-wedlock pregnancies and establish annual numerical goals for preventing and reducing these pregnancies; and (4) encourage the formation and maintenance of two-parent families (Coven, 2005). States can spend TANF funds in a number of ways, including cash assistance and wage supplements, childcare subsidies, education and job training, transportation assistance, and other services. To receive TANF funds, states must also spend some of their own dollars on programs for needy families, known as the "maintenance of effort," or the MOE requirement.

Important change ushered in by PRWORA include a lifetime welfare cap of five years and work requirements that demand that able-bodied recipients work within two years, with only a few exceptions granted. Other changes under this reform include some childcare assistance, one year of transitional Medicaid benefits, required identification of the children's biological fathers so that child support could more easily be pursued, and the requirement that unmarried minors live at home and stay in school to receive benefits.

Furthermore, more power was granted to individual states, and under these general federal parameters states could amend the policies to best meet their individual needs. Some hail this as a boon to local control; others fear that poor states have little to offer their poorest residents and consequently either eliminate some families who were previously deemed eligible, or else siphon off money from other state-funded programs such as education or job training programs.

State Policies and State Variation

Under the old AFDC program, all families that met federal income eligibility criteria were entitled to receive cash assistance. Under TANF, eligibility is primarily determined by state rules, and families are no longer automatically entitled to assistance even if they meet financial criteria. States now decide who can receive assistance, under what circumstances, and for how long. Yet these decisions are complex because of federal mandates, fiscal constraints at the state level, conflicting TANF goals and the myriad exemptions to work requirements or time limits that may be granted because of extenuating circumstances.

Since the passage of PRWORA, some states have enacted time limits that are more stringent than the five years imposed by the federal government. There are two types of limits states can impose. The first is a *lifetime* limit, which states when benefits can be permanently eliminated. While the federal government established a five-year limit, nine states opted for shorter limits. For example, the limit in Arkansas is 24 months, the limit in Florida is 48 months and the Utah limit is 36 months. Exemptions may be granted in hardship cases, defined differently across states. For example, 17 states will provide an exemption to verifiable victims of domestic violence and seven states will provide an exemption if caring for an infant under a few months old (Rowe & Russell, 2004).

Thirteen states impose an additional type of time limit that limits benefits *temporarily* for a specific period of time. For example, in Nevada, families who receive TANF for 24 months are then ineligible to receive benefits for the next 12 months, even though ultimately they could receive five years of lifetime benefits.

The federal government enacted work requirements that require recipients to work as soon as the state determines they are able, or after 24 months of benefit receipt, whichever is earlier. Most states require recipients to begin work or finish their high school education immediately and to work a minimum of 30 hours per week. Generally, post-secondary education is no longer allowed, despite the fact that a college degree would significantly improve job prospects, pay, and job benefits like health insurance coverage. Again, some exemptions are allowed and these vary by state. Thirty-seven states provide an exemption to care for an ill or incapacitated person and 45 states allow exemptions to care for a young infant, usually defined as less than 12 months old, but 11 states require work after the child is three months old. A few states offer no exemptions at all for young children (Rowe & Russell, 2004). Noncompliance with work requirements may reduce the adult portion of the benefits or terminate benefits for the entire family for six months or longer.

The pressure exerted on TANF recipients to "just get a job" is keenly felt. Recipients feel they must take any job that becomes available to them, regardless of pay or benefits. This mentality can deflect attention from gathering needed information for planning to find a "good job"—one with a livable wage and benefits such as health insurance. In the interviews conducted with families leaving TANF for work in Oregon, respondents reported having experienced pressure from their caseworkers to take "any job" to get off TANF, even jobs without health insurance, while receiving little information from the caseworkers regarding the qualifications for Medicaid eligibility after the transitional year of coverage expires (Hartley, Seccombe, & Hoffman, 2005; Seccombe, & Hoffman, 2007; Seccombe & Lockwood, 2003).

Twenty-one states imposed family cap policies that limit or deny additional benefits to families who have a child while on TANF, even though this policy was not part of the federal mandate. These states have special treatment for families that have an additional child while receiving benefits. For example, in California, if a child is born within 10 months after a family begins TANF, there will be no increase in the cash benefit for that child (Rowe & Russell, 2004). These policies are popular because many people worry that families will deliberately have additional children to increase the size of their welfare check. Although TANF benefits vary across states, a typical monthly benefit would increase by only about $50 to compensate for an additional child; therefore it is questionable whether very many women would deliberately have a child for the extra money.

Other TANF Policies and Regulations

There are many other TANF rules and regulations. For example, PRWORA retains a federal requirement that those receiving assistance must assign their child support rights over to the state; furthermore, enforcement has become more stringent, with fewer exemptions available. As in the past, to receive assistance recipients must cooperate with the state in establishing paternity (if this is in question), obtaining a support order and enforcing that order. A mother must appear at all relevant court or administrative agency hearings, and turn over to the state any child support payments received directly from the father. However, in the past there was room for "good cause" exemptions (i.e. the child was conceived as the result of a forcible rape or incest, pursuing support could result in physical or emotional harm, or adoption was under consideration or was pending). PRWORA has now established stricter child support enforcement policies (U.S. Department of Health & Human Services, 2004). Recipients must assign child support rights and cooperate with paternity establishment efforts. States have the option to either deny cash assistance or reduce assistance by at least 25% to those individuals who fail to cooperate. These policies have the potential to either help or to harm women and their children, depending on the situation surrounding paternity.

Policies toward assets also vary among states. Families are allowed to have a vehicle while receiving TANF funds, although most states allow only one per family (including two-parent families). Twenty-three states limit the value of the vehicle, often to under $5,000. For example, in New York, the fair market value of an allowable vehicle is capped at $4,650. These policies severely restrict the mobility and transportation needs of families. Other allowable assets are even more meager. In 33 states a family can have no more than $2,000 in assets, above and beyond their vehicle (Rowe & Russell, 2004).

Reauthorization in 2006

Although the TANF block grants were only authorized until the end of fiscal year 2002, Congress temporarily extended TANF funding several times while working on legislation to reauthorize the block grants and make some modifications to the rules and funding levels. President George W. Bush and his appointees are strong believers in the merits of PRWORA. Dr. Wade F. Horn, HHS assistant secretary for children and families, reports, "The Bush Administration is dedicated to welfare reform because it replaces dependency with self-sufficiency" (U.S. Department of Health and Human Services, 2005, p. 1). As part of the Deficit Reduction Act of 2005 (passed in July 2006), Congress reauthorized the TANF block grant program through 2010. Work requirements have been intensified. States now face a higher hurdle to maintain federal TANF funding by meeting a 50% participation rate for all families and a 90% participation rate for two-parent families. This means that fewer persons are now exempt from work requirements, or they are exempt for a more limited duration, for reasons related to domestic violence, the presence of very young children, mental or physical health, or other issues. States must document that they are meeting the 50%/90% rule, or face penalties.

Moreover, activities defined as work or work-related have narrowed as well. For example, all higher education, as well as the time a student spends doing homework for her vocational education training program, can no longer count as "work" unless it is done in a supervised study session. The reauthorization continues its focus on marriage and includes $150 million to support programs designed to encourage couples to form and sustain marriage (U.S. Department of Health and Human Services, 2006a; Work, Welfare and Families, 2006).

What are possible results of changes in TANF regulation? Several possibilities loom (Work, Welfare and Families, 2006). First, states may cut services to meet the 50%/90% participation rate. A decrease in the number of families receiving TANF may be interpreted as a decrease in need, resulting in even further restrictions. Second, states may be forced to increase state budgets to ensure federal TANF funding. Third, states penalized for not meeting the 50%/90% participation rate will face federal funding reductions and may need to make up welfare budget deficits.

Measuring "Success"

The press often reports how "successful" the monumental 1996 changes in the welfare system have been. From January 1998 to September 2000, the top 50 U.S. newspapers published 250 stories about welfare reform. Of the articles, 52% portrayed welfare reform and the decline in caseloads as positive, or positive with caveats, and only 24% portrayed welfare reform as negative, or negative with caveats. The remaining 24% of stories were neutral and gave equal weight to the pros and cons of welfare reform (Schram & Soss, 2001).

How has success been defined? News stories eschew investigative journalism in favor of presentations using government statistics. In the case of welfare reform, the specific goals or markers of success have rested squarely on *declining caseloads* rather than other markers, such as poverty reduction, or a decrease in the number of persons suffering from food insecurity. The focus on declining caseloads arose because of the increasing attention to so-called welfare dependency, intergenerational poverty and long-term use from the 1960s through the 1990s. The resulting 1996 reform sought to address these issues, but did so in a way that ignored the sources of poverty, such as increasing income inequality, the erosion of the purchasing power of minimum wages, racial and sex discrimination in the workplace, and other forms of social injustice. Declining caseload data as the sole indicator of welfare success has now become a "public fact," rarely questioned or debated (Gusfield, 1981).

If the purpose of reform was simply to move families off assistance, then welfare reform policies have been a resounding success. Welfare caseloads were immediately reduced, prompting President Clinton to hail welfare reform a triumph and to announce that the debate about it was over. By June 2005, welfare caseloads had decreased by 60% since 1997, declining from about five million to under two million families (U.S. Department of Health and Human Services, 2006b).

However, these statistics only indicate that the number of people on welfare was reduced. It tells nothing about whether welfare reform "works," in the sense of whether poverty has declined. "You can't tell whether welfare reform is working simply from caseload numbers," argues Wendell Primus, a welfare expert who quit the Clinton administration in protest over his signing of the welfare legislation. "Those figures do not tell how many former recipients moved from welfare to work, or simply from dependency to despondency. You have to look at where these people went," he suggested (Broder, 1997).

What has happened to families who left welfare? Initially, many Americans applauded the changes, resolute in their opinions that welfare erodes the work ethic and that families become dependent upon public aid. They worried about whether their tax dollars were being spent subsidizing people who were unwilling to work for a living.

Others feared that welfare reform would erode the social safety net for vulnerable individuals and families. They wondered what would happen to the many poor people who may not be able to find work when they reach the government's time limit. They questioned whether good jobs were available for all the people now on assistance and lamented that most would likely be paid wages that fail to bring their incomes above the poverty line. They were concerned about the lack of investment in human capital and wanted to know why welfare recipients were no longer allowed to go to college to further their education. They asked who would care for the children, worried about both availability of care and quality of care, given the inadequacy of childcare reimbursements. Finally, they wondered how the health care needs of the new class of low-income workers and their children would be met after their transitional Medicaid expired.

Two-parent welfare families were targeted as the first to be cut off from welfare assistance. By 1 October 1997, a little over one year after welfare reform became law, the federal government mandated that 75% of two-parent welfare families either have jobs or be in job training programs. Yet, in this first real test of welfare reform, approximately half the states fell short of these employment goals (DeParle, 1997). Work requirements in two-parent families seems easy, requiring a total of 35 hours per week between two adults, and while one is working, the other should presumably be able to provide childcare. Yet there are extenuating circumstances in these families that had made TANF a necessity: for example, mental or physical health problems, substance abuse, or some other compelling problem. If the difficulties of employing two-parent households have been so seriously underestimated, why, then, do we now expect 90% of them to be employed? Moreover, what does this suggest about the other, more challenging, cases involving single parents?

How Is TANF Really Working?

Today, 10 years after TANF was created, there is a burgeoning amount of research that shows us what has happened to families in the aftermath of welfare reform. I will summarize some of the key findings here.

• *States spend an increasing portion of their budgets on services rather than cash assistance.* In 1997, when states implemented TANF, the focus was largely on restructuring welfare programs for compliance with the new federal law. Initially, state officials spent the majority of funds on cash assistance. However, since that time, funding has shifted substantially, with a declining emphasis on cash assistance. Cash assistance spending has declined by nearly $4 billion, while funding on childcare, work-related activities, or social services has more than doubled. Declines in cash assistance expenditures vary across states; for example, declining by 39% in Ohio and 23% in Pennsylvania from 1998 to 2004, but only 7% in Wisconsin (Waller & Fremstad, 2006). The emphasis on childcare, work-related activities, and social services means that many families, who are diverted from TANF and must find work, may also receive some noncash help to do so. Yet they are not reflected in caseload data, which include only people who receive cash assistance through TANF. Therefore, official statistics are misleading. Even the US Government Accountability Office (GAO) acknowledges that caseload figures grossly underestimate the numbers of families who receive benefits and services funded fully or in part through TANF, possibly by nearly 50% (US GAO, 2002; Waller & Fremstad, 2006). Thus the often-touted "success" of welfare reform, using caseload data, has been greatly exaggerated.

• *Poverty rates among families that leave TANF are very high.* Former recipients had a median income of $7.75 an hour in 2002, not enough to lift a small family out of poverty (Loprest & Zedlewski, 2006). Many studies report that 50–75% of families remain poor even two to three years after leaving welfare (Blank, 2002; Loprest & Zedlewski, 2006). Using national data, Loprest and Zedlewski report that, in 2002, one in three welfare leavers had incomes below 50% of the poverty level.

• Moreover, even those families with incomes above the poverty threshold have very low incomes. About 90% of TANF leavers in one state study lived below 185% of poverty—they are therefore not counted in official statistics, but continue to live on the margins of society (Acs & Loprest, 2004). Although poverty rates decline over time, it is at a very modest rate. For example, a California study sponsored by the Department of Health and Human Services that looked at leavers at two points in time—first 5–10 months after leaving welfare and again 11–16 months after leaving welfare—found that income gains averaged only $60 to $70 per month (Macurdy, Marruto, & O'Brien-Strain, 2003). Another HHS-sponsored study of welfare reform in Wisconsin reported that the net income of welfare leavers in the year after they left welfare was actually lower than their income prior to leaving welfare. Although their earned income was significantly higher, their benefits declined by more than their earned income (Cancian, Haveman, Meyer, & Wolfe, 2003).

• *A large share of very poor and needy families does not receive TANF and their numbers are increasing.* Data indicate that about 52% of families who would have been eligible for cash assistance under the old rules do not receive assistance, up from only about 20% in the first half of the 1990s (Parrott & Sherman, 2006). Why has program participation dropped so sharply? Many families are actively discouraged from applying for aid and are diverted from TANF. A report based on data from Boston, Chicago, and San Antonio found that 77% of welfare applicants experience some type of diversion, including formal gatekeeping policies or informal practices (Moffitt & Winder, 2003). The few studies on those persons who are diverted show some interesting trends: for example, TANF applicants who were diverted from the program were more likely to have significantly lower or higher educational levels than TANF recipients (London, 2003; Moffitt & Winder, 2003). While it may be argued that more highly educated applicants may have more alternatives available to them, it is perplexing why those with very low education levels also are diverted, as they may be most vulnerable and in need of aid. Likewise, other studies have found that persons diverted from TANF were more likely to be Black, were more likely to speak Spanish as their primary language, and were more likely to be disabled or have other health problems (Fremstad, 2004).

• *Employment rates among single mothers are falling and the number of "disconnected families" is on the rise.* The focus of welfare reform on work and employment rates among single mothers rose during the late 1990s from 62% just prior to welfare reform to 73% in 2000. Nonetheless, since 2000, employment rates have fallen, reaching 69% in 2005 (Parrott & Sherman, 2006). Since 2000, the labor market for low-skilled workers has weakened. There are fewer new jobs and supports for low-income workers have stagnated. Not surprisingly, employment rates have fallen. Between fiscal years 1996 and 2004, the number of single mothers receiving TANF fell by two million, yet employment among single mothers increased by only about one million. "Disconnected welfare leavers"—families that leave TANF but are not working—rose to 21% of TANF leavers in 2002, up from 17% in 1997 (Loprest & Zedlewski, 2006). These disconnected families generally face multiple barriers to work and have significant economic hardship. Their average income (including boyfriends' income, if any) was just $6,178 in 2002, averaging only about one-third of the income of other families who left TANF. Over a third have at least three significant barriers to employment, such as a health condition that limits work, poor mental health, a child under 12 months, no high school diploma, a disabled child, little or no work experience, or limited English skills. This represents a three-fold increase in the number of persons with multiple barriers since 1997 (Loprest & Zedlewski, 2006). These families report that they are "barely making it from day to day" and many suffer from hunger and food insecurity (Seccombe & Hoffman, 2007; Wood & Rangarajan, 2003; Zedlewski, 2003).

• *Families leaving TANF face many significant challenges to their well-being.* In their national study comparing the well-being of recent TANF leavers, those who are still on welfare and those who have never received welfare, Loprest and Zedlewski (2006) report that the lives of TANF leavers are not appreciably better than are those who are still on the system. For example, nearly 44% of families who recently left TANF reported being unable to pay rent or utilities in the past year, compared to 40% of those still on TANF. Over a quarter of both groups have used a food bank or have had two or more bouts of food insecurity. Almost one-quarter report that their children have many behavioral or emotional problems, compared to 16% of current recipients. Furthermore 80% report that their child (or children) is not engaged in school and 20% report problems with skipping school. These kinds of problems can bring tremendous stress to families as they attempt to negotiate new work and family balances.

• *Families leaving welfare are more likely to have significant health problems compared to other families and have less access to health care. These problems interfere with their ability to obtain and maintain steady employment.* In a statewide study in Oregon, I found that 24% of adults who had recently left TANF for work rated their health as only fair or poor (Seccombe & Hoffman, 2007), compared to 22% of poor adults nationally and 9% of adults overall (Schiller, Adams, & Coriaty Nelson, 2005). Likewise, I found that 15% of parents who had recently left welfare reported having at least one child in fair or poor health. This compares to 5% of poor children, and 2% of children nationally, who are in fair or poor health (Dey & Bloom, 2005; Seccombe & Hoffman, 2007). Families who leave TANF for work have poorer health that can impede their ability to find or keep a job and they are also significantly less likely to have health insurance. I found that, 18 months after leaving welfare for work, 40% of sampled adults and 20% of their children were completely uninsured (Seccombe & Hoffman, 2007). These adults and children use the health care system less often and are more likely to delay or forgo needed health care because they have no way to pay for it (Seccombe & Hoffman, 2007). This exacerbates their health problems, further compromising their ability to work.

There is a strong relationship between health (of adult or child) and employment (Powers, 2003; Zedlewski, 2003). A Michigan study found that physical and mental health problems, as well as child health problems, are each related to lower employment durations over a five-year period, even after controlling for important factors that affect employability, such as job skills, work experience, or transportation availability (Corcoran, Danziger, & Tolman, 2003).

• *Childcare assistance is crucial to helping families move from welfare to work.* Concern over the lack of safe and affordable childcare emerged as a common reason why women turned to, or remained on, welfare. Childcare is often patched together in a fashion that leaves mothers anxious (Seccombe, 2007a). While extended families are often the preferred childcare provider, relatives cannot always be counted upon. Living in high-density and high-crime areas, poor families worried about the safety of their children in daycare centers or with other babysitters that they did not know well. As one woman argued, "I'm not going to leave him with someone I don't know until he's old enough to tell me what happened." They also worried about the psychological effects of inadequate care—crowded, dirty, or impersonal conditions—upon their children. These concerns have largely been overlooked in quantitative studies that focus on the daycare availability—are there enough daycare slots for the children who need them? My in-depth interviews reveal that the availability of childcare slots is not the primary consideration; rather, it is the quality of care that is most imperative.

Mothers also worried about childcare costs. Costs vary dramatically across the country, but they are beyond the reach of most poor and low-income families. One quarter of families with young children earn less than $25,000 per year, while childcare can cost $10,000 per child (Children's Defense Fund, 2005). Providing subsidized, high-quality childcare increases the likelihood that current and former welfare recipients leave welfare and work full-time (Danziger, Ananat, & Browning, 2004; Fuller, Kagan, Caspary, & Gauthier, 2002; Scott, London, & Hurst, 2005). Childcare subsidies are associated with higher employment rates, an increase in full-time employment, and decreased likelihood of returning to welfare. However, subsidies are generally low, often less than $2.00 an hour, and therefore limit what type of childcare a family can realistically use. Yet research indicates that higher subsidies are further associated with increased employment (Fremstad, 2004).

Consequently, funds to increase the number (and in some states the dollar amount) of childcare subsidies were an important component of TANF and the initial funding seemed promising. However, since 2002, funding has been stagnant though need is increasing. President Bush's 2008 budget proposes to freeze childcare funding for the sixth year in a row. Only one in seven children eligible for childcare assistance actually receives it (Children's Defense Fund, 2007). Moreover, with caseloads inching up again and with the inflationary erosion of TANF block grants to states, at least 23 states have reduced childcare funding for low-income families since 2003. For example, Nebraska cut 1,600 children off subsidies when it reduced the income cutoff from 185% to 120% of poverty (Friedlin, 2004). The number of children receiving help declined by about 200,000 in 2004 and is expected to decline by 500,000 in 2010. At least one-third of states place eligible families who apply for assistance on waiting lists or turn them away without even taking their names because there are not enough funds to provide services (Schulman & Blank, 2004).

Conclusion

Where do these findings leave us—can the radical alterations in the welfare system that changed it from an income-based entitlement program to one that directly promotes work and discourages cash assistance be deemed a success? It depends on how "success" is framed. If the purpose of reform is simply to move families off public aid, then welfare reform policies should be applauded. By June 2006, welfare caseloads had decreased to just over 4.1 million recipients or 1.7 million families, a reduction of about 65% since PRWORA was signed into law in 1996, and at the lowest level since 1964 (U.S. Department of Health and Human Services, 2006b). The media report that welfare reform has been an unqualified success because caseload reductions have been so dramatic.

However, if the goal of welfare reform is to reduce poverty and genuinely improve lives, one could argue that welfare reform has been a relative failure. By most measures, including revised caseload data that correctly take into account the number of people still using TANF services if not its cash income, welfare reform has not considerably improved the lives of former recipients. Their incomes are still low and most families continue to teeter on the brinks of impoverishment. They suffer in silence, unable to buy adequate food for their children, unable to afford to heat their homes or procure health insurance for their families.

Chris and her children, introduced in the opening of this chapter, are one of these families. While government statistics count them as an unqualified welfare reform success story, a qualitative evaluation would offer a deeper assessment. For Chris, and millions of others, welfare reform is not a resounding success.

References

Abramovitz, M. (1996a). *Regulating the lives of women: Social welfare policy from colonial times to the present* (rev. ed.). Boston: South End Press.

Abramovitz, M. (1996b). *Under attack, fighting back: Women and welfare in the United States*. New York: Monthly Review Press.

Acs, G. & Loprest, P. (2004). *Leaving welfare: Employment and well-being of families that left welfare in the post-entitlement era*. Kalamazoo, MI: W. E. Upjohn Institute for Employment Research.

Blank, R. (2002, Dec.). Evaluating welfare reform in the United States. *Journal of Economic Literature, 40*, 1105–66.

Broder, J. (1997, 17 Aug.). Big social changes revive the false god of numbers. *New York Times*, Week in Review Section.

Cancian, M., Haveman, R., Meyer, D., & Wolfe, B. (2003, Jan.). *The employment, earnings, and income of single mothers in Wisconsin who left cash assistance: Comparisons among three cohorts*. Madison, WI: Institute for Research on Poverty.

Children's Defense Fund. (2005). *Childcare and head start organizers tool kit*. Available HTML: http://www.childrensdefense.org/site/DocServer/cc_hs_toolkit.pdf?doc ID=201 (accessed 3 June 2007).

Children's Defense Fund. (2007). *Children and low-income families continue to be left behind: A look at the President's 2008 budget and children*. Available HTML: http://www.childrensdefense.org/site/PageServer?pagename=policy_budget#education (accessed 5 June 2007).

Clinton, B. (1997). Welfare should be reformed. In C. Cozic (Ed.), *Welfare: Opposing viewpoints* (pp. 26–7). San Diego: Greenhaven Press.

Corcoran, M., Danziger, S., & Tolman, R. (2003). *Long-term employment of African-American and White welfare recipients and the role of persistent health and mental health problems* (Working Paper Series #03–5). Washington, DC: National Poverty Center.

Coven, M. (2005). *An introduction to TANF*. Center on Budget and Policy Priorities. Available HTML: http://www.centeronbudget.org/1-22-02tanf2.htm (accessed 3 January 2006).

Danziger, S., Ananat, E., & Browning, K. (2004). Childcare subsidies and the transition from welfare to work. *Family Relations, 52*, 219–28.

DeNavas-Walt, C., Proctor, B., & Lee, C. (2006, August). *Income, poverty, and health insurance coverage in the United States: 2005* (Current Population Reports No. P60-231). Washington, DC: U.S. Census Bureau.

DeParle, J. (1997, 6 February). A sharp decrease in welfare cases is decreasing speed. *New York Times*.

Dey, A. & Bloom, B. (2005). Summary health statistics for U.S. Children: National health interview survey, 2003. *Vital Health Statistics, 10* (223). Available HTML: http://www.cdc.gov/nchs/data/series/sr_10/sr10_223.pdf.

Fremstad, S. (2004). *Recent welfare reform research findings*. Center on Budget and Policy Priorities. Available HTML: http://www.centeronbudget.org/1-3004wel.htm (accessed 3 January 2007).

Friedlin, J. (2004, August). Welfare series: Childcare promises fall through. *Women's eNews*. Available HTML: http://www.womensenews.org/article.cfm/dyn/aid/1947 (accessed 8 January).

Fuller, B., Kagan, S., Caspary, G., & Gauthier, C. (2002). Welfare reform and childcare options for low-income families. *The Future of Children, 12*, 97–119.

Gordon, L. (1994). *Pitied but not entitled*. New York: Free Press.

Gusfield, J. (1981). *The culture of public problems*. Chicago: University of Chicago Press.

Hartley, H., Seccombe, K., & Hoffman, K. (2005). Planning for and securing health insurance in the context of welfare reform. *Journal of Health Care for the Poor and Underserved, 16*, 536–54.

London, R. (2003). *Which TANF applicants are diverted and what are their outcomes?* Cited in S. Fremstad, *Recent welfare reform research findings*. Center for Budget and Policy Priorities, 2004. Available HTML: www.cbpp.org/1-30-04wel.htm.

Loprest, P. & Zedlewski, S. (2006). *The changing role of welfare in the lives of low-income families with children* (Occasional Paper # 73). Washington, DC: The Urban Institute.

Macurdy, T., Marruto, G., & O'Brien-Strain, M. (2003). *What happens to families when they leave welfare?* San Francisco: Public Policy Institute of California.

Mink, G. (1995). *The wages of motherhood: Inequality in the welfare state 1917–1942.* Ithaca, NY: Cornell University Press.

Moffitt, R. & Winder, K. (2003). *The correlates and consequences of welfare exit and entry: Evidence from the three-city study* (Welfare, Children and Families: A Three-City Study Working Paper #03-01). Baltimore, MD: Johns Hopkins University Press.

NPR Online. (2001, May). Poverty in America. In *NPR/Kaiser/Kennedy School poll.* Available HTML: http://www.npr.org/programs/specials/poll/poverty (accessed 1 December 2005).

Parrott, S. & Sherman, A. (2006). *TANF AT 10: Program results are more mixed than often understood.* Washington, DC: Center on Budget and Policy Priorities.

Powers, E. (2003). Children's health and maternal work activity: Static and dynamic estimates under alternative disability definitions. *Journal of Human Resources, 38,* 522–66.

Rowe, G. & Russell, V. (2004). *The welfare rules databook: State policies as of July 2002.* Washington, DC: The Urban Institute.

Schiller, J., Adams, P., & Coriaty Nelson, Z. (2005). Summary health statistics for the U.S. population: National health interview survey, 2003. *Vital Health Statistics 10* (224).

Schram, S. F. & Soss, J. (2001). Success stories: Welfare reform, policy discourse, and the politics of research. *Annals of the American Academy of Political and Social Science, 577,* 49–65.

Schulman, K. & Blank, H. (2004). *Childcare assistance policies 2001–2004: Families struggling to move forward, states going backward.* Washington, DC: National Women's Law Center.

Scott, E., London, A., & Hurst, A. (2005). Instability in patchworks of childcare when moving from welfare to work. *Journal of Marriage and Family, 67,* 370–86.

Seccombe, K. (2007a). *Families in poverty.* Boston: Allyn & Bacon.

Seccombe, K. (2007b). *So you think I drive a Cadillac? Welfare recipients' perspectives on the system and its reform* (2nd ed.). Needham Heights, NJ: Allyn & Bacon.

Seccombe, K. & Hoffman, K. (2007). *Just don't get sick: Access to health care in the aftermath of welfare reform.* Piscataway, NJ: Rutgers University Press.

Seccombe, K. & Lockwood, R. (2003). Life after welfare in rural communities and small towns: Planning for health insurance. In J. Kronenfeld (Ed.), *Research in the sociology of health care,* Vol. 20. Greenwich, CT: JAI Press.

U.S. Census Bureau. (2006). *The 2006 statistical abstract: The national data book.* Washington, DC: Author.

U.S. Department of Health and Human Services. (2004). *Temporary Assistance for Needy Families (TANF). Sixth Annual Report to Congress.* Office of Family Assistance. Available HTML: http://www.acf.hhs.gov/programs/ofa/annualreport6.htm.

U.S. Department of Health and Human Services. (2005). *Welfare rolls continue to fall* (Press Release [Online]). Available HTML: http://www.acf.hhs.gov/news/press/2005/TANFdeclineJune04.htm.

U.S. Department of Health and Human Services. (2006a). *Temporary Assistance for Needy Families (TANF). Seventh Annual Report to Congress.* Office of Family Assistance. Available HTML: http://www.acf.hhs.gov/programs/ofa/annualreport7.htm.

U.S. Department of Health and Human Services. (2006b). *TANF: Total number of families (fiscal year 2005).* Available HTML: http://www.acf.hhs.gov/programs/ofa/caseload/2005/family05tanf.htm (accessed 4 April 2006).

U.S. Department of Health and Human Services, Administration for Children and Families. (2007). *Temporary Assistance for Needy Families: Separate state program-maintenance of effort aid to families with dependent children caseload data.* Office of Family Assistance. Available HTML: http://www.acf.hhs.gov/programs/ofa/caseload/caseloadindex.htm (accessed 26 April 2007).

U.S. Department of Labor, Women's Bureau (2006). *Women in the labor force in 2005.* Available HTML: http://www.dol.gov/wb/factsheets/Qf-laborforce-05.htm (accessed 6 June 2006).

U.S. General Accounting Office. (2002). *Welfare reform: States provide TANF-funded work support services to many low-income families who do not receive cash assistance* (GAO-02-615T). Washington, DC: Author.

Waller, M. & Fremstad, S. (2006). *New goals and outcomes for temporary assistance: State choices in the decade after enactment.* Washington, DC: Brookings Institution.

Wood, R. & Rangarajan, A. (2003). *What's happening to TANF leavers who are not employed?* Washington, DC: Mathematica Policy Research, Inc.

Work, Welfare and Families. (2006). *Welfare (TANF) reauthorization.* Available HTML: http://www. workwelfareandfamilies.org/home/TANF.html (accessed 4 June 2006).

Zedlewski, S. (2003). *Work and barriers to work among welfare recipients in 2002.* Washington, DC: Urban Institute Press.

Critical Thinking Questions

1   Based on everything you have read, do you believe that TANF has been effective in reducing poverty? How do you think welfare recipients might answer this question? Are some parts of TANF policies better than others? Which parts do you support? How would you improve on TANF?

2   Chapters 3 and 4 argue that market forces make it difficult for women to achieve economic independence. Do you agree with this argument? Why, or why not? If not market forces, then what is it? Do you know women who are struggling to be independent? How would you explain their situations?

3   What are the biggest challenges in getting out of poverty for single mothers? Explain your answer.

5 The Dynamics of Rural Family Poverty

Karen Slovak and Karen Carlson

Poverty is unevenly distributed throughout the United States with the highest concentrations in the most rural and most urban areas of the country. For decades, urban poverty has received far more research and policy attention than rural poverty, diverting interest away from the 7.5 million poor Americans who live in rural areas. More than 14% of rural residents live in poverty compared to 12.1% of urban residents (U.S. Department of Agriculture, Economic Research Service (USDA/ERS), 2004). According to the USDA/ERS, 2004 family poverty rates were higher for rural families of all compositions, with female-headed households faring worst (see Fig. 5.1). Consequently, poor families in rural areas face special challenges that are often left unaddressed. Since more families in rural areas are poor and more often in single-parent households, rural children tend to fare less well than urban children (USDA/ERS, 2004). Rogers (2005) reported that in 2003, rural child poverty was 21% compared to 18% in metropolitan areas. That year rural children represented 36% of the rural poor.

Rural poverty is also differentiated from urban poverty by its persistence over time. According to the USDA/ERS (2004, Persistence of Poverty, para 1):

> An area that has a high level of poverty this year, but not next year, is likely better off than an area that has a high level of poverty in both years. In order to shed light on this aspect of poverty, ERS has defined counties as being persistently poor if 20 percent or more of their populations were living in poverty over the last 30 years.

Out of 386 persistently poor U.S. counties in 2004 (USDA/ERS, 2004), 340 or 88% were nonmetropolitan counties. Karger and Stoesz (2006) blame chronic, persistent rural poverty for high illiteracy, low educational levels, lack of highly trained workers, low-skill and low-paying employment, and a deficient physical infrastructure.

Not surprisingly, minorities in rural areas, like their urban counterparts, are at greater risk for poverty (USDA/ERS, 2004). In 2003, Blacks experienced a poverty rate of 30.5% and among Hispanics, the fastest growing nonmetropolitan minority, the rate was 25.4%, more than twice the rate for Whites (11.1%).

Though there is a common notion that rural life is peaceful and idyllic, rural communities face pervasive poverty along with associated mental and behavioral

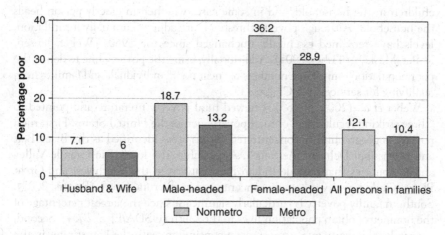

Figure 5.1 Poverty Rates by Family Type and Residence, 2003.

Note: Percentage of people in families, either primary or related subfamilies, who are poor.

Source: Prepared by the Economic Research Service using data from the U.S. Census Bureau's 2004 Current Population Survey, March Supplement.

health issues. Furthermore, poor rural families face serious service barriers and include diverse cultural characteristics that present persistent challenges to service provision. With rural families faring less well than their urban counterparts, the lack of attention to families in rural communities is disheartening. Most policies and programs are modeled on urban areas and often do not translate well to rural areas. This chapter highlights differences between rural and urban poverty in terms of numbers and characteristics, impact, rural TANF programs, and barriers to addressing poverty. Throughout the chapter, we illustrate the unique nature of rural poverty and point to strengths that operate to reduce the impact of poverty in rural communities.

Defining Rural Poverty

Researchers have long faced problems defining the term rural (Rios, 1988), though most definitions tend to consider geographic and population density. Consequently, size estimates for the U.S. rural population have varied. Both the U.S. Census Bureau and the Office of Management and Budget estimate the U.S. rural population at about 21% (North Dakota State University, 2001). Other sources, including the U.S. Government Accountability Office (USGAO, 2004), estimate that 17% or 49 million people live in rural areas, defining a third of the population in 18 states as rural. By any estimate, the rural population is a sizeable portion of the U.S. population.

Who are the rural poor? In general, rural families with an annual before-tax income that falls below the poverty threshold are considered poor. As noted in Chapter 1, the poverty threshold varies according to family size, the number of children in the household, and in some cases whether an elderly person heads the household. Although poverty thresholds are adjusted annually for inflation, levels have remained essentially unchanged since the 1960s (Weber, Jensen, Miller, Mosley & Fisher, 2005). Additionally, using the poverty line to define the poor population omits large numbers of "near poor" individuals and families from qualifying for services (see Chapter 1).

Weber *et al.* (2005, p. 383) reviewed rural poverty literature and pointed to "three striking regularities" of rural poverty across the United States. First, rural poverty is geographically concentrated within areas identified as the Black Belt and Mississippi Delta in the South, Appalachia, the lower Rio Grande Valley and in counties that include Indian Reservations in the Southwest and Great Plains. Child poverty is heavily concentrated in the rural South (Rogers, 2005). Southern family poverty is particularly significant since the largest percentage of the nonmetropolitan population lives in the south (USDA/ERS, 2004). Second, county-level poverty rates vary across a continuum, with the lowest rates in the suburbs and the highest rates in remote rural areas.

Third, the studies Weber *et al.* (2005, p. 383) reviewed confirmed USDA/ERS findings that rural areas have disproportionate rates of high poverty and persistent poverty. Additionally, in 2003, the Annie E. Casey Foundation (National Conference of State Legislators, 2003) reported that 195 of the 200 persistently poor U.S. counties (with continuous poverty rates of 30% or higher) were rural. Duncan (1996) links poverty persistence in Appalachia to oppression by the coal industry, a growing elderly population, and a dwindling younger population with little political influence. Other researchers link its persistence in rural areas to negative attitudes toward welfare (Osgood, 1977) and dependence on nontraditional agricultural employment, part-time work, seasonal and service industry employment, and other nonbenefit jobs (Albrecht, Albrecht, & Albrecht, 2000; Cochran *et al.*, 2002). Clearly, there are a number of unique characteristics in rural areas that contribute to high poverty and persistent poverty.

Based on their review, Weber *et al.* (2005) identified three major factors in addition to demographics and local economies that differentiate rural from urban poverty. First, poor rural families are relatively isolated from social institutions such as schools, county offices, and the labor market. Second, rural residents with power and privilege use their influence to manipulate the local social structure to maintain their privileged positions and subjugate the poor. Third, individuals who live in "good job households," those described as stable and well-paying, with more benefits and greater flexibility, are more able to pursue other economic opportunities to supplement their incomes, doubly advantaging them over those in "bad job" structures. Typically, families supplement their incomes through moonlighting or entrepreneurship or with a secondary earner.

It is well known that poverty and near poverty are both intimately linked to employment, unemployment, and underemployment. According to Prause and Dooley (1997, p. 243), using the unemployment rate as the primary indicator of hardship in the labor market obscures both rates and glosses over problems associated with underemployment. Prause and Dooley (p. 244) define underemployment as "involuntary part time employment, intermittent unemployment, and inadequate income (including both full-year and non-full-year poverty wage earners)." They argue that while unemployment is likely to be transient, underemployment tends to be persistent, affecting career development and several measures of well-being. Underemployment rates, perhaps another way to talk about "bad job structures," are higher in nonmetropolitan areas compared to all metropolitan areas. In 2000, for example, underemployment rates were 16.2% in rural areas, higher than suburban rates (11.3%) and higher than all metropolitan areas, including city centers, where the underemployment rate was 15.5% (Jensen & Slack, 2003). It is important to note that underemployed people in rural areas are less likely than those in urban areas to become "adequately employed" (Jensen, Findeis, Hsu & Schachter, 1999, p. 417).

In their research, Fisher and Weber (2004) compared urban to rural poverty and discovered an important contextual difference. Urban residents are more likely to be poor in terms of net worth, while rural residents are more likely to be poor in terms of liquid assets. Thus, rural residents may be vulnerable to particular hardship because they are unable to convert assets, like homes and farms, to cash during economic downturns.

TANF as a Response to Poverty in Rural Areas

The concept of welfare changed upon PRWORA implementation in 1996, because it resulted in TANF, a program geared toward self-sufficiency, with time limits and work requirement stipulations (See Chapter 4). Rural areas with higher poverty concentrations and poor local economies face serious barriers to meeting TANF work requirements. As a result, TANF rates tend to be lower than should be expected in rural areas. According to GAO (2004) statistics, only about 14% of all TANF families across the United States were rural in 2004, while the rural portion of individual states' TANF cases ranged from a low of 0.2% to a high of 77%.

Experts have examined TANF rates as a measure of success for moving poor families to self-sufficiency. While urban and rural TANF caseloads have declined at a similar rate since 1997 (GAO, 2004), rural areas with high unemployment have continued to face significant challenges implementing TANF. Therefore, using TANF rates as a success measure in rural areas is problematic. Indeed, as the U.S. Department of Health and Human Services (2005, p. 1) reported, "rural TANF recipients face additional barriers in moving from welfare to work, such as a lack of public transportation systems, few child care services, and limited employment and training opportunities." Further, rural TANF families are not evenly distributed and tend to be concentrated in communities that face high unemployment and low educational attainment (GAO, 2004). The rural economy continues to be a primary challenge for rural families since it remains fragile and uneven, and is dominated by low-wage industries (Fluharty, 2000; Harley, Savage & Kaplan, 2005). Even finding a job may be difficult and most jobs will not pay wages that enable workers to remain above the poverty level for long. Mother-only families in rural areas are even more likely to be affected by underemployment because rural women may be more likely to work in part-time and/or low-paying jobs than their urban counterparts (McKernan *et al.*, 2001).

Despite the challenges, rural TANF programs have been cited as strengthening community connection and collaboration. For example, TANF clients often receive personal attention that may help them overcome problems and find jobs (GAO, 2004). This is echoed by Murty (2004), who reported that many rural communities have tightly knit, dense social networks that enhance the sense of taking care of each other informally. Also, faith-based organizations, strong family values, and resourcefulness add to a sense of connection and collaboration in rural communities (Templeman & Mitchell, 2004).

While it is apparent that TANF can work in rural areas as an impetus towards self-sufficiency, we cannot forget that poverty rates have fallen little since its implementation. Many people have been unable to escape poverty and are still dependent on food stamps, Medicaid and other public assistance programs (Danziger, 2002). Therefore, evidence of declining TANF caseloads in rural areas does not represent a universal decline in rural family poverty. Long-term escape from poverty for rural families is still an elusive goal and extreme hardship remains.

The Impact of Poverty on Rural Family Well-Being

Mental and Physical Health

Harley *et al.* (2005) reviewed the rural community literature and found that rural residents experience more mental and physical health problems than their urban counterparts. In the rural poverty context, poorer mental and physical health may be associated with work-related disabilities, mental illness, economic disadvantage, and limited community resources. A number of studies have considered the relationships among poverty, unemployment, and underemployment and various mental and physical health factors. Prause and Dooley (1997), using data from the National Longitudinal Survey of Youth, found that several employment status factors were significantly related to lower self-esteem. School-leavers with the lowest self-esteem levels were:

- unemployed/discouraged (no longer looking for work)
- underemployed, including:

    o   involuntarily employed part-time
    o   earning wages at poverty level
    o   experiencing intermittent unemployment.

In addition to lower self-esteem, some studies have found strong relationships between employment status and depression. Dooley, Prause & Ham-Rowbottom (2000) found adverse employment changes—from adequate to inadequate employment and inadequate employment to unemployment—resulted in significant increases in depression incidence. And in their research on employment status and mental health among poor rural women, similarly, Kim, Seiling, Stafford and Richards (2005) found a significant relationship between employment status and depression incidence, which led them to conclude that the severe imbalance between employment demand and employment availability jeopardizes mental health and contributes to increased depression.

While research shows that poverty is linked to poor mental health outcomes in urban communities, rural residents are at a special disadvantage because they are more likely to experience difficulty in accessing care. In rural areas, more often than not, the primary care physician is the contact point for care (Fox, Blank, Rovnyak, & Barnett, 2001). One reason the rural poor turn to their primary care physicians for mental health issues is that individuals often seek treatment for physical complaints (National Rural Mental Health Association, 1999). Moreover, the stigma associated with mental illness in rural communities may lead rural residents to turn to their primary care physicians rather than to seek out mental health providers. Unfortunately, most primary care physicians are not trained to assess or provide mental health services.

While most of the research addresses the relationship between mental health and poverty, the physical health of poor families is also compromised. Unfortunately, however, most research in this area has been conducted in urban areas (see Malloy & Eschbach, 2007; Melchior, Moffitt, Milne, Poulton, & Caspi, 2007). Regarding the association between rural poverty and employment status, Dooley and Prause (2005) found maternal employment changes among pregnant women, especially shifts from adequate employment to underemployment, were related to giving birth to significantly lower birthweight babies.

Violence and Trauma

In recent years, studies in urban areas have pointed to poverty as a possible contributor to violence exposure (Bolland, 2003; Gelles, 1992; Greene, 1993; Korbin, 2003). In both the 1975 and 1985 versions of the Family Violence Survey, Gelles (1992) found that while violence occurs in all social classes and across the full range of family income, severe violence toward children occurs more frequently in households with below poverty incomes. Korbin (2003, p. 433) lists general violence exposure among the "harms that befall children as a result of poverty, inequality, lack of opportunity, and local, national and global hostilities." Greene (1993) suggests that violence is a frequent occurrence in poor sections of urban centers. Youth in these settings witness violence frequently, seeing people beaten up, stabbed, shot, or killed. Often victims are known to the witness and may include family, friends, classmates, or neighbors. Adolescents may imitate what they see and become involved in violence themselves. Bolland (2003), in a study of 2468 inner city adolescents living in high-poverty neighborhoods, found significant relationships between hopelessness and a long list of behaviors, including violent and aggressive behaviors, substance abuse, sexual behaviors, and accidental injury. Along these lines, Garbarino, Hammond, Mercy and Yung (2004, p. 303) suggest that risk factors related to poverty and family disruption have a great deal of power to, "permanently distort children's beliefs about ... safety." If children do not believe adults can keep them safe, they are more likely to engage in activities like gang membership and gun culture participation.

Other research demonstrates that students who participated in a means-tested school lunch program for four years were more likely to externalize problems, experience peer relationship problems and to have lowered self-esteem (Ackerman, Brown, & Izard, 2004, pp. 368–9). In their six-year longitudinal study that assessed children at four time-points (preschool, first, third, and fifth grade), they found that family income had a significant impact on externalizing and internalizing behaviors and on academic competence. An interesting dimension in their research is the finding that "maximum persistence" (income adversity over all three of the measured intervals) showed no stronger effects than minimum persistence (income adversity over two consecutive intervals).

Unfortunately, there has been little such research completed in rural settings. Most of these studies and others that address violence and poverty have focused on urban locations or have combined data for all locations. Only recently have some studies suggested that rural violence is a significant issue. Despite a 44% overall drop in the violent crime rate from 1993 to 2000, both adolescent violence and general violence in rural areas have risen (Spano & Nagy, 2005). Arcus (2002, p. 175) discussed major correlates of endorsing and using corporal punishment in school settings, noting that poverty, religious views, and geographic region are "interwoven with each other and with aggression and violence." Moreover, she argued that the chronic stresses associated with poverty may intensify the inclination to use aggression.

More recently, Carlson (2006) examined poverty, violence exposure, and aggression in rural schools and found that the poverty rate (as indicated by the proportion of students who received free or reduced-price lunches) was a significant predictor of direct exposure to school violence. The poverty rates at the schools in her sample ranged from 32 to 59%. Students sensed that violence was an everyday occurrence and considered violence to be "no big deal." Also, poverty was significantly positively associated with aggressive behaviors and ideas, including damaging property and "comfort with guns." These relationships were especially strong for male students.

While domestic violence occurs in all community types, it is an understudied phenomenon in rural America and can be influenced by poverty as reported by the Federal Office of Rural Health Policy (Johnson, 2000):

> Very few data-based studies of rural battered women exist, but the already significant problems of battered women are likely exacerbated by rural factors. Poverty, lack of public transportation systems, shortages of health care providers, under-insurance or lack of health insurance, and decreased access to many resources (such as advanced education, job opportunities and adequate child care) all make it more difficult for rural women to escape abusive relationships.
>
> (Background And Significance, Para 3)

In 1997, Mulder and Chang reviewed literature that addressed domestic violence, service barriers, and interventions in rural areas. In their study, increased economic dependence was associated with increased abuse frequency and severity. In addition, Mulder and Chang reported that rural economies were often unfavorable toward women for several reasons, including lack of jobs, low-paying jobs, undereducation and sex-role stereotyping, all of which limit their economic independence.

Indeed, despite the myth that rural areas are peaceful and idyllic, living in a rural area does not protect poor youth or their families from violence exposure and this stereotype has acted as a barrier to our knowledge of violence and to the implementation of child and family services in rural communities. Whether as victims or witnesses, violence exposure profoundly impacts youth through associated physical and psychological repercussions, and repeated violence exposure over time reaps cumulative psychological consequences (Slovak & Joseph, 2001; Slovak & Singer, 2002).

Substance Abuse

Substance abuse is often intertwined with poverty and plagues both rural and urban families, though some differences do exist. According to a report on rural substance abuse by Karen Van Gundy (2006), poverty may play a unique role in rural substance abuse and subsequent treatment. Gundy reported that unemployed rural residents were seven times more likely than unemployed urban residents to meet the criteria for stimulant abuse. Further, alcohol abuse among rural youth was greater than their urban counterparts and was exacerbated by parent absence from the household. Sadly, Gundy also reported that rural adults living with children were more prone to abuse stimulants than similar urban adults.

Barriers to Service in Rural Communities

Lack of Services, Community Culture, and Knowledge

While there are many barriers to service in rural communities, the primary problem is lack of services (Amundson, 2001; Letvak, 2002; McCabe & Macnee, 2002; New Freedom Commission on Mental Health, 2003). Poverty compounds insufficient services by creating substantial barriers to accessing resources that do exist, as well as information and relationships that could increase personal power (Manning & Van Pelt, 2005). For example, while a rural community strength is a greater sense of community and cooperation (Harley *et al.*, 2005), the greater tendency to know people in the community may serve as a reason to avoid services. The gossip, stereotyping and stigma associated with mental health and social services may prevent poor people from seeking help (Manning & Van Pelt, 2005).

Two additional stigma-related barriers in rural communities may be the lack of mental health knowledge and distorted perceptions of the helping process. In an attempt to understand what motivates and prevents impoverished rural residents from using services, Fox *et al.* (2001) reported that 99% of their overall sample stated they would seek help if they thought it would help them. However, when a subsample of participants screened positive for mental health disorders and received an educational intervention, the main reason given for not seeking help was they felt there was no need to contact a service provider. Fox *et al.* (p. 435) argue that there is a "need for massive and targeted educational programs designed to inform and convince impoverished rural individuals that they can effectively be treated for depression and anxiety and that treatment will be relevant."

Regarding alcohol treatment, Van Gundy (2006) reported that rural states tended to have the greatest unmet need, which she attributed to a number of barriers, including inadequate resources for treatment overhead, law enforcement and prevention programs, and the large geographic regions over which such programs must be stretched. This is in addition to long waiting lists, understaffed regional hospitals, and the great distances rural residents might have to travel for treatment.

Another alcohol/drug-related treatment barrier in rural areas appears to be lack of health insurance coverage to treat the primary issue of substance abuse and related disorders. In a 2001 statement, the Congressional Rural Caucus (as cited in Harley *et al.*, 2005) noted that rural residents were more likely to lack health insurance coverage and that rural communities were more likely to be designated as Health Professional Shortage Areas.

Fox *et al.* (2001) studied perceived barriers to mental health care among rural impoverished residents and found that rural residents' perceptions confirmed Caucus findings. The most frequently endorsed barriers keeping the respondents from getting health care were cost of care (40%) and lack of health insurance (30.4%).

Informal Assistance

There is a strong value in rural communities of "taking care of our own" through informal means (Fetke *et al.*, 1998; McCoy, McCoy, Lai, Weatherly, & Messiah, 1999). This value often incorporates suspicion toward outsiders who offer help, resistance to change, and distrust of institutions (Harley *et al.*, 2005; Jones, 1991). Fox *et al.* (2001) demonstrated the importance of this value in their study when participants reported that a friend or family member and their minister were among the top five types of helpers that rural impoverished residents would consider consulting for any mental health concern. Watkins (2004) also cited the central role of the church in the helping nature of rural communities.

Geography and Transportation

Travel presents a significant barrier to accessing services and resources for rural families (Anderson & van Hoy, 2006; Davis, 2004; Moulding, 2005). Davis points to several problem levels. First, families often must travel long distances to receive services. This requires access to reliable transportation, since public transportation in rural communities is limited or nonexistent. Not surprisingly, poor rural families may not be able to afford the expense of buying and maintaining a vehicle. Second, service providers' ability to offer services may be affected, since they too must travel greater distances to provide services.

Recruitment and Retention of Service Providers

A crucial barrier to accessing services is recruitment and retention of qualified service providers (Merwin, Hinton, Dembling, & Stern, 2003). Most rural areas have few practitioners and many rural practitioners are inadequately prepared for their rural clientele. Gumpert, Saltman, and Sauer-Jones (2000) suggest that a generalist training approach (rather than training narrowly focused specialists) along with a focus on community assessment systems is needed. Practitioners must: (1) understand community assessment systems in terms of cultural norms and values; (2) understand practice implications; and (3) be sensitive to local culture.

Finally, ethical considerations are relevant in preparing practitioners to work with poor rural families. Rural practitioners face challenges that are different from those faced by urban or suburban practitioners. According to Burkemper (2005), professional ethical codes are generally geared toward urban professional practice. Common ethical challenges for rural practitioners include:

> conflicts of interest and dual relationships, otherwise referred to as boundary dilemmas; informed consent and confidentiality; fees, including bartering; sharing information between agencies and with other professionals; protection of confidentiality related to office location and procedures; and cultural and practice competence including access to supervision and consultation.
>
> (p. 186)

Despite recruitment, retention, and practice issues, it is important to note that there are also positive dimensions to working in rural communities. For example, rural practitioners experience more autonomy and independence, more rapid promotion and prestige, and a greater opportunity to see the results of their efforts (Ginsberg, 2005).

Conclusion

While urban families have been the focus of most poverty research and discussions, rural families constitute a significant group that must face poverty and associated outcomes. Indeed, the characteristics of rural communities often result in pervasive poverty that is hard to overcome and often leaves the communities in greater need than urban areas. Research, policy, and practice tend to be developed with urban communities in mind, then altered slightly and applied in rural communities. While programs and practices for addressing urban poverty can be used in rural communities, they must be adapted to rural culture and community characteristics. Unless we modify research, policy, and practice to address rural issues, rural families living in poverty will continue to fare less well than poor families in urban communities.

At the same time, we cannot forget that rural families possess multiple strengths and resiliency characteristics that offer advantages for addressing poverty and concomitant issues. According to Scales and Streeter (2004, p. 1), by viewing rural communities as asset-rich, we can, "begin to see the depth of the human spirit and the richness of the creative potential that exists in rural communities."

References

Ackerman, B., Brown, E., & Izard, C. (2004). The relations between persistent poverty and contextual risk and children's behavior in elementary school. *Developmental Psychology, 40*, 367–77.

Albrecht, D., Albrecht, C., & Albrecht, S. (2000). Poverty in nonmetropolitan America: Impacts of industrial, employment, and family structure variables. *Rural Sociology, 65*, 87–103.

Amundson, B. (2001). America's rural communities as crucibles for clinical reform: Establishing collaborative care teams in rural communities. *Families, Systems and Health, 19*, 13–23.

Anderson, E. & van Hoy, J. (2006). Striving for self-sufficient families: Urban and rural experiences for women in welfare-to-work programs. *Journal of Poverty, 10*, 69–91.

Arcus, D. (2002). School shooting fatalities and school corporal punishment: A look at the states. *Aggressive Behavior, 28*, 173–83.

Bolland, J. (2003). Hopelessness risk behaviour among adolescents living in high-poverty inner-city neighbourhoods. *Journal of Adolescence, 26*, 145–58.

Burkemper, E. (2005). Ethical mental health social work practice in the small community. In L. Ginsberg (Ed.), *Social work in rural communities* (4th ed.) (pp. 175–88). Alexandria, VA: Council on Social Work Education.

Carlson, K. (2006). Poverty and youth violence exposure: Experiences in rural communities. *Children and Schools, 28*, 87–96.

Cochran, C., Skillman, G., Rathge, R., Moore, K., Johnston, J., & Lochner, A. (2002). A rural road: Exploring opportunities, networks, services and supports that affect rural families. *Child Welfare, 81*, 838–48.

Danziger, D. (2002). Approaching the limit: Early national lessons from welfare reform. In B. Weber, G. Duncan & L. Whitener, (Eds.), *Rural dimensions of welfare reform*. Kalamazoo, MI: W. E. Upjohn Institute for Employment Research.

Davis, T. (2004). Using wraparound services to build rural communities of care for children with serious emotional disturbance and their families. In T. Scales & C. Streeter (Eds.), *Rural social work: Building and sustaining community assets* (pp. 132–46). Belmont, CA: Brooks/Cole/Thompson Learning.

Dooley, D. & Prause, J. (2005). Birth weight and mothers' adverse employment change. *Journal of Health and Social Behavior, 46*, 141–55.

Dooley, D., Prause, J., & Ham-Rowbottom, K. (2000). Underemployment and depression: Longitudinal relationships. *Journal of Health and Social Behavior, 41*, 421–36.

Duncan, C. (1996). Understanding persistent poverty: Social class context in rural communities. *Rural Sociology, 61*,103–24.

Fetke, D., Bond, G., McDonel, E., Salyers, M., Chen, A., & Miller, L. (1998). Rural assertive community treatment: A field experiment. *Psychiatric Rehabilitation Journal, 21*, 371–9.

Fisher, M. & Weber, B. (2004). Does economic vulnerability depend on place of residence? Asset poverty across metropolitan and nonmetropolitan areas. *Review of Regional Studies, 34*, 137–55.

Fluharty, C. (2000, 8 March). *Oversight hearing regarding the National Rural Development Partnership*. Testimony of Chuck Fluharty before the Subcommittee on Forestry, Conservation, and Rural Revitalization Senate Committee on Agriculture. Available HTML: http://agriculture.senate .gov/Hearings/ Hearings_2000/March_8__2000/00308flu.htm (accessed 28 November 2007).

Fox, J., Blank, M., Rovnyak, V., & Barnett, R. (2001). Barriers to help seeking for mental disorders in a rural impoverished population. *Community Mental Health Journal, 37,* 421–36.

Garbarino, J., Hammond, W., Mercy, J., & Yung, B. (2004). Community violence and children: Preventing exposure and reducing harm. In K. Maton & C. Schellenbach (Eds.), *Investing in children, youth, families, and communities: Strengths-based research and policy* (pp. 303–20). Washington, DC: American Psychological Association.

Gelles, R. (1992). Poverty and violence toward children. *American Behavioral Scientist, 35,* 258–74.

Ginsberg, L. (2005). *Social work in rural communities* (5th ed.). Alexandria, VA: Council of Social Work Education.

Greene, M. (1993). Chronic exposure to violence and poverty: Interventions that work for youth. *Crime and Delinquency, 39,* 106–24.

Gumpert, J., Saltman, J., & Sauer-Jones, D. (2000). Toward identifying the unique characteristics of social work practice in rural areas: From the voice of practitioners. *Journal of Baccalaureate Social Work, 6,* 16–35.

Harley, D., Savage, T., & Kaplan, L. (2005). Racial and ethnic minorities in rural areas: Use of indigenous influence in the practice of social work. In L. Ginsberg (Ed.), *Social work in rural communities* (4th ed.) (pp. 367–85). Alexandria, VA: Council on Social Work Education.

Jensen, L. & Slack, T. (2003). Underemployment in American: Measurement and evidence. *American Journal of Community Psychology, 32,* 21–31.

Jensen, L., Findeis, J., Hsu, W., & Schachter, J. (1999). Slipping into and out of underemployment: Another disadvantage for nonmetropolitan workers? *Rural Sociology, 64,* 417–38.

Johnson, R. (2000). *Rural health response to domestic violence: policy and practice issues* (Federal Office of Rural Health Policy, Order # 99–0545(P)). U.S. Department of Health and Human Services, Health Resources and Services Administration. Available HTML: http://ruralhealth.hrsa.gov/pub/domviol.htm (accessed 11 December 2007).

Jones, L. (1991). Appalachian values. In B. Ergood & B. Kuhre (Eds.), *Appalachia: Social context* (3rd ed.) (pp. 169–73). Dubuque, IA: Kendall/Hunt.

Karger, H. & Stoesz, D. (2006). *American social welfare policy: A pluralist approach* (5th ed.). Boston, MA: Allyn and Bacon.

Kim, E., Seiling, S., Stafford, K., & Richards, L. (2005). Rural low-income women's employment and mental health. *Journal of Rural Community Psychology, E8*(2). Available HTML: http://www.marshall.edu/jrcp/8_2_Eun.htm (accessed 11 December 2007).

Korbin, J. (2003). Children, childhoods, and violence. *Annual Review Anthropology, 32,* 431–46.

Letvak, S. (2002). The importance of social support for rural mental health. *Issues in Mental Health Nursing, 23,* 249–61.

Malloy, M. & Eschbach, K. (2007). Association of poverty with sudden infant death syndrome in metropolitan counties of the United States in the years 1990 and 2000. *Southern Medical Journal, 100,* 1107–13.

Manning, S. & Van Pelt, E. (2005). The challenges of dual relationships and the continuum of care in rural mental health. In L. Ginsberg (Ed.), *Social work in rural communities* (4th ed.) (pp. 259–82). Alexandria, VA: Council on Social Work Education.

McCabe, S. & Macnee, C. (2002). Weaving a new safety net of mental health care in rural America: A model of integrated practice. *Issues in Mental Health Nursing, 23,* 263–78.

McCoy, V., McCoy, C., Lai, S., Weatherly, N., & Messiah, S. (1999). Behavior change among crack-using rural and urban women. *Substance Use and Misuse, 34,* 667–84.

McKernan, S., Lerman, R., Pindus, N., & Valente, J. (2001). *The relationship between metropolitan and non-metropolitan locations, changing welfare policies, and the employment of single mothers* (Poverty Research Working Paper #192). Washington, DC: The Urban Institute.

Melchior, M., Moffitt, T., Milne, B., Poulton, R., & Caspi, A. (2007). Why do children from socio-economically disadvantaged families suffer from poor health when they reach adulthood? *American Journal of Epidemiology, 166,* 966–74.

Merwin, E., Hinton, I., Dembling, B., & Stern, S. (2003). Shortages of rural mental health professionals. *Rural Mental Health, 17,* 42–51.

Moulding, P. (2005). Fare or unfair? The importance of mass transit for America's poor. *Georgetown Journal on Poverty Law and Policy, 12,* 155–80.

Mulder, P. & Chang, A. (1997). Domestic violence in rural communities: A literature review and discussion. *Journal of Rural Community Psychology, E1*(1). Available HTML: http://www.marshall .edu/jrcp/vole1/vol_e1_1/vole1no1.html (accessed 11 December 2007).

Murty, S. (2004). Mapping community assets: The key to effective rural social work. In T. Scales & C. Streeter (Eds.), *Rural social work: Building and sustaining community assets* (pp. 278–89). Belmont, CA: Brooks/Cole/Thompson Learning.

National Conference of State Legislators. (2003). A different landscape: Rural poverty in America. *State Legislatures, 29,* 7.

National Rural Mental Health Association. (1999). *Mental health in rural America, 1999.* Available HTML: http://www.nrharural.org/advocacy/sub/issuepapers/ ipaper14.html (accessed 28 November 2007).

New Freedom Commission on Mental Health. (2003). *Achieving the promise: Transforming mental health care in America: Final report* (DHHS Pub. No. SMA-03-3832). Rockville, MD: Department of Health and Human Services.

North Dakota State University, North Dakota State Data Center. (2001). *Rural/urban/metro/nonmetro and frontier discussion: Definitions and North Dakota maps.* Available HTML: http://www.ndsu.edu/ sdc/data/ruralurbanmetrononmetro.htm#census (accessed 16 August 2006).

Osgood, M. (1977). Rural and urban attitudes toward welfare. *Social Work, 22,* 41–7.

Prause, J. & Dooley, D. (1997). Effects of underemployment on school-leavers' self esteem. *Journal of Adolescence, 20,* 243–50.

Rios, B. (1988). *Rural: A concept beyond definition* (Eric Clearinghouse on rural education and small schools #ED296820). Las Cruces, NM: Eric Digest.

Rogers, C. (2005, March). *Rural children at a glance* (Information Bulletin No. EIB1). Washington, DC: U.S. Department of Agriculture, Economic Research Service.

Scales, T. & Streeter, C. (2004). Introduction: Asset building to sustain rural communities. In T. Scales & C. Streeter (Eds.), *Rural social work: building and sustaining community assets* (pp. 1– 6). Belmont, CA: Brooks/Cole/Thompson Learning.

Slovak, K. & Joseph, A. (2001). Violence and mental health issues among Student Assistance Program participants in a rural county. *School Social Work Journal, 25,* 9–25.

Slovak, K. & Singer, M. (2002). Children and violence: Findings and implications from a rural community. *Child and Adolescent Social Work Journal, 19,* 36–56.

Spano, R. & Nagy, S. (2005). Social guardianship and social isolation: An application and extension of lifestyle/routine activities theory to rural adolescents. *Rural Sociology, 70,* 414–37.

Templeman, S. & Mitchell, L. (2004). Utilizing an asset-building framework to improve policies for rural communities: One size does not fit all for families. In T. Scales & C. Streeter (Eds.), *Rural social work: Building and sustaining community assets* (pp. 196–205). Belmont, CA: Brooks/Cole/ Thompson Learning.

U.S. Department of Agriculture, Economic Research Service. (2004). *Rural income, poverty, and welfare: Rural poverty.* Available HTML: http://www.ers.usda.gov/Briefing/IncomePovertyWelfare/ ruralpoverty/ (accessed 29 August 2006).

U.S. Department of Health and Human Services (2005). *The 2005 Report to the Secretary: Rural health and human services issue.* Washington, DC: The National Advisory Committee on Rural Health and Human Services.

U.S. Government Accountability Office. (2004). *Welfare reform: Rural TANF programs have developed many strategies to address rural challenges* (GAO-04-921). Washington, DC: Author.

Van Gundy, K. (2006). Substance abuse in rural and small town America. *Reports on Rural America 1*(2). Durham, NH: University of New Hampshire Carsey Institute.

Watkins, T. (2004). Natural helping networks: Assets for rural communities. In T. Scales & C. Streeter (Eds.), *Rural social work: Building and sustaining community assets* (pp. 65–75). Belmont, CA: Brooks/Cole/Thompson Learning.

Weber, B., Jensen, L., Miller, K., Mosley, J., & Fisher, M. (2005). A critical review of rural poverty literature: Is there truly a rural effect? *International Regional Science Review, 28,* 381–414.

Critical Thinking Questions

1   How "fluid" (temporary versus long-term) is the incidence of poverty in rural communities? Is it the same in urban areas? What about in the nation as a whole?

2   Some critics believe that more emphasis on marriage will expose many low-income women and their children to emotional and physical abuse, especially if they are encouraged to marry or to stay in bad marriages. Do you believe this is a problem? Why, or why not?

3   Make a list of things poor rural families need to thrive. How do their needs compare to the needs of poor urban families? Are there more similarities than differences?

6 Hispanic Families in Poverty

The Hidden Contribution of Immigration

Robert Aponte and Carrie E. Foote

Hispanics or Latinos, as they are variously called, are persons of Latin-American origin. Despite varying national origins, they are widely seen as a single group and have been much in the news lately.[1] Due largely to record-breaking immigration, Hispanics have recently surpassed Blacks in sheer numbers, even though they trailed them by over 20 million persons just three decades ago. Indeed, in 2005, Hispanics came to comprise a full 14.5% of the total population, whereas Blacks[2] only accounted for 11.9% of the population that year (U.S. Census Bureau, 2006a).

Despite the record growth, Hispanics and their families have long been known to experience substantial economic hardship in the United States. At the same time, their deprivation is often seen as comparatively moderate among minority groups. For instance, it is often implied, if things are so bad here for Hispanics, why do they come in such high numbers? In addition, Hispanics and their families have almost always registered less poverty and higher incomes than Blacks and their families, despite the latter group's far greater seniority in this nation. With record-breaking Hispanic growth over the last several years, and with standard statistics on Hispanics continuing to indicate less deprivation than corresponding statistics for Blacks, the perspective that things for this group cannot be too bad is easy to sustain. Unfortunately, this perspective could not be more mistaken.

In this chapter, we undermine the view that Hispanic families are faring comparatively well in the United States, despite economic data that support the assertion. Moreover, we show the importance of disaggregating socioeconomic data for Hispanics, including their poverty rates and national origin criteria, in order to assess their situation accurately. When the economic data on Hispanics and their families are viewed by their individualized national origin categories, the indicators reveal more complexity in their well-being and begin to show the more extensive deprivation that key Hispanic groups sustain. Put bluntly, a fair amount of "hidden" deprivation surfaces.

A related critical point concerns nativity. In many instances, disaggregating data by nativity is very important. This is especially so for Mexican immigrants. As we show, not only are they inordinately deprived, many of their sufferings are even more "hidden" than those of Mexicans born in the United States. We present detailed disaggregated data when available.

Despite the complexities, the two largest groups, Mexicans and Puerto Ricans, sustain most Hispanic poverty in the United States. Together, they accounted

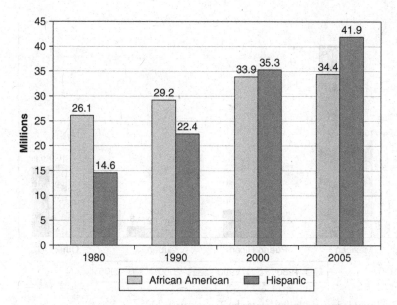

Figure 6.1 African American* and Hispanic Populations, 1980–2005.
*Non-Hispanic.
Source: Census Scope (2000) U.S. Census Bureau (2006a).

for roughly 73% of all Hispanics in the U.S. in 2005 and for 78.2% of all Hispanic poor that year (U.S. Census Bureau, 2006a). Because they are the poorest groups, this chapter will focus primarily on Mexicans (especially immigrants) as the data permit, and secondarily on Puerto Ricans. Data for Blacks and Whites are included for comparison.

Hispanic Growth, Income, and Poverty

The contours of recent Hispanic growth are illustrated in Fig. 6.1, which compares the relative population sizes for Blacks and Hispanics from 1980 through 2005 (Census Scope, 2000; U.S. Census Bureau, 2006a). The reversal in relative rankings, by size, is remarkable. As shown in Fig. 6.1, Hispanics trailed Blacks by over 11 million persons as recently as 1980, whereas by 2005, they led the latter group by fully 7.5 million. Indeed, Hispanics virtually doubled in number between the 1990 count (22.4 million) and the 2005 estimate (41.9 million). A doubling of this population in no more than one half of a generation[3] strongly signifies that their growth could not have resulted from natural increase (excess of births over deaths) alone. Rapid immigration is clearly implicated. Moreover, the figures do not tell the whole story, as they omit the sizable undercounts for both groups. The Hispanic undercount is almost certainly greater than the Black undercount for the obvious reason that millions of Hispanics are undocumented.

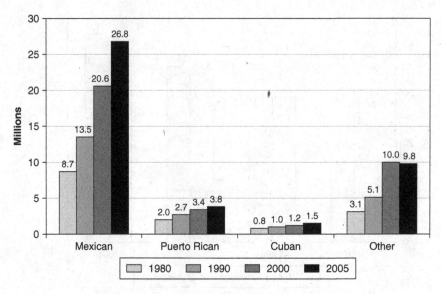

Figure 6.2 Hispanic in the United States by Types, 1980–2005.
Source: U.S. Census Bureau (2002, 2006a).

Indeed, the latest Immigration and Naturalization Services' (INS, 2003) estimates for the nation's total undocumented population, as of 2000, peg the Mexican contingent at 4.8 million persons (69% of the nation's total), with five additional Latin American nations: El Salvador, Guatemala, Colombia, Honduras, and Ecuador (along with China), contributing between 100,000 and 200,000 undocumented persons apiece. The vast majority are almost certainly working-class or labor migrants who bear more than a passing resemblance to Mexican immigrants. A more recent estimate by a top researcher at the PEW Hispanic Institute pegged the Mexican contingent at six million persons in 2004 and noted that some 80–85% of all migration from Mexico in recent years has been undocumented (Passel, 2005). Hence the belief that Hispanic growth is largely fueled by immigration is strongly supported by these data, as is the belief that Hispanics likely sustain a larger undercount than any other group in the United States.

Fig. 6.2 shows Hispanic growth patterns over the past two decades (1980–2005) by nationality group (Mexican, Puerto Rican, Cuban, and others). The pattern is clear: Mexicans are the largest group and dominate the growth by a substantial margin (U.S. Census Bureau, 2000, 2002, 2006a). Thus the idea that immigrants, especially Mexicans, are disproportionately contributing to phenomenal Hispanic growth is further supported.

That Hispanic growth draws heavily on undocumented Mexican immigration is very important for this chapter. First, it facilitates focusing primarily on Mexicans, by far the largest subgroup within the Hispanic camp. Second, and just as important, a significant proportion of this population is very vulnerable. Aside from fearing deportation and the accompanying loss of livelihood, this

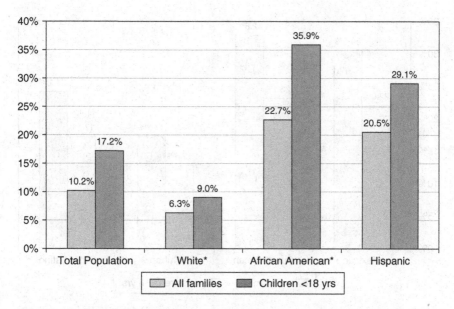

Figure 6.3 Poverty Rates for Families and Children by Race and Hispanic Origin, 2005.
*Non-Hispanic.
Source: U.S. Census Bureau (2006a).

subgroup is highly susceptible to employer exploitation and, as is well known, generally possesses extremely modest educational credentials (Aponte, 1996; Crowley, Lichter, & Qian, 2006; Suro & Passel, 2003). This vulnerability has great implications for family well-being, even if the consequences are not always apparent in conventional economic measures.

Among the most heavily used measures of family economic well-being are median family income, median household income, and the percentage of the population below the official U.S. poverty line. These measures are especially meaningful for our arguments because they are sometimes significantly misleading. For Hispanics, this is certainly true. Fig. 6.3 provides 2005 poverty rates for families and children separately, and by four categories (U.S. population, Whites, Blacks and Hispanics). The story the data tell is, on the one hand, shocking, but on the other, consistent with conventional wisdom.

The foremost message in Fig. 6.3 is that racial and ethnic inequality and lack of child well-being continue at high levels (U.S. Census Bureau, 2006a). While fewer than one in 10 White families and children separately are below the poverty line, over two in 10 of the corresponding minority groups are so impoverished. As contrasted with the 6.3% poverty rate for White families shown in Fig. 6.3, the Hispanic rate is slightly greater than 20% and for Blacks it approaches 23%. The data are devastating for minority children. The poverty rate for White children (9%) is dwarfed by over three times greater rates for Hispanic and Black children. While nearly three of 10 (29.1%) Hispanic children are poor, over one third of Black children (35.9%) live in poverty.

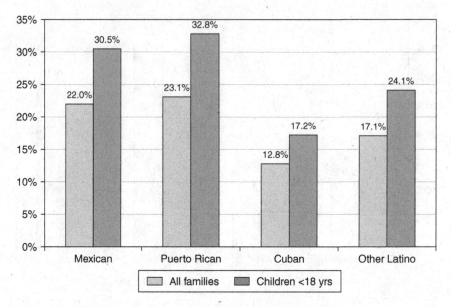

Figure 6.4 Poverty Rates for Families and Children by Hispanic Type.
Source: U.S. Census Bureau (2006a).

Each of these indicators for minority children's poverty constitutes an incredible and unconscionable statistic. Notably, also, the child poverty rate exceeds the poverty rate for families in each group, which indicates that poor families tend to be larger than nonpoor families. Finally, Fig. 6.3 shows, in keeping with conventional wisdom and in spite of the factors going against them, Hispanics *appear* to fare better than Blacks.

Disaggregating Hispanic indicators by group changes the Hispanic poverty portrait considerably. Fig. 6.4 shows the 2005 poverty rates of Hispanics divided out by the top three nationalities in population size and residual grouping (U.S. Census Bureau, 2006a). As expected, in the pattern that emerges, the two largest groups, Mexicans and Puerto Ricans, show substantially greater poverty than the aggregated Hispanic poverty rate indicates (Fig. 6.3). Conversely, the remaining categories of Hispanics show significantly less impoverishment, particularly Cubans.

Fig. 6.4 shows that poverty rates for Mexican families (22.0%) and Black families (22.7%, see Fig. 6.3) are nearly identical. Puerto Rican families show a slightly higher poverty rate (23.1%) than Black families. The 35.9% poverty rate for Black children, however, remains unchallenged by the top two Hispanic groups, although rates for both groups are higher than 30%. Nonetheless, it is clear that the disaggregated statistics provide a substantially different story than the indicators for all Hispanics.

An even more popular set of indicators of family well-being are median household income and median family income. Figs. 6.5 and 6.6 provide these indicators for Whites, Blacks, and Hispanics in 2005 (U.S. Census Bureau, 2006a). These figures tell a story similar to the one offered by poverty statistics. Whereas

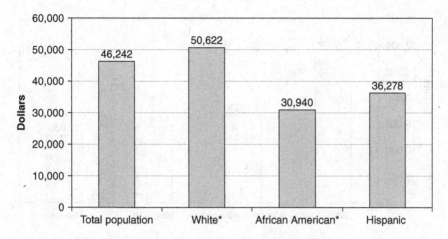

Figure 6.5 Median Household Income by Race and Hispanic Origin, 2005.
*Non-Hispanic.
Source: U.S. Census Bureau (2006a).

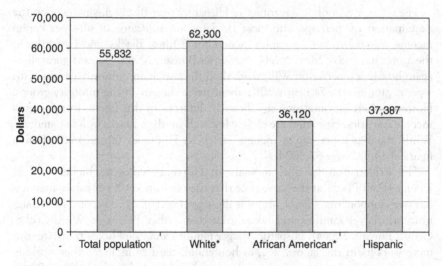

Figure 6.6 Median Family Income by Race and Hispanic Origin, 2005.
*Non-Hispanic.
Source: U.S. Census Bureau (2006a).

White median household and family incomes are 50.6K and 62.3K, respectively, the corresponding figures for Blacks are 30.9K and 36.1K, and for Hispanics 36.3K and 37.4K, considerably lower. In this instance, however, the Hispanic advantage over Blacks is larger. According to median household income, Hispanics enjoy about a 5.4K advantage over Blacks (36.3K over 30.9K), while in the corresponding comparison of median family income, the advantage (37.4K over 36.1K) is smaller, but still formidable (1.3K).

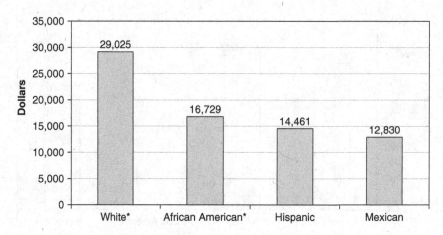

Figure 6.7 Per Capita Income by Race and Hispanic Origin, 2005.
*Non-Hispanic.
Source: U.S. Census Bureau (2006a).

The relative economic advantage of Hispanics over Blacks dissipates upon the examination of, perhaps, the most fundamental indicator of all—per capita income. Fig. 6.7 shows per capita income for Whites, Blacks, and Hispanics in the aggregate, and of Mexicans (U.S. Census Bureau, 2006a). These figures show again how much better-off Whites are than the two major minority groups, with a per capita income of nearly 30K, about twice the size of the minority groups. However, there is something significantly different in this figure. In per capita income statistics, Hispanics are clearly less well-off than Blacks by a fair amount. While the Black per capita income is 16.7K, Hispanics (aggregated) show a figure of 14.5K, over $2,000 less.

The explanation for the anomaly of Hispanics enjoying higher median incomes than Blacks at the same time that they sustain lower per capita incomes has two components, one of which is illustrated by Fig. 6.8. Hispanics have significantly larger families and households than either Blacks or Whites (U.S. Census Bureau, 2006a). Hispanics' larger families and households translate into more workers in the labor force, as households tend to include other working adults, in addition to the main householder(s). Additional workers bring in more dollars per household, on average, than the workers in Black families. Hence, Hispanic households show higher median family incomes, but because the earnings must support a larger number of individuals, Hispanic families end up with lower earnings per capita than Black families.

Still more revealing is the per capita figure for Mexicans (Fig. 6.7). The largest of the Hispanic group, Mexicans register an even lower figure than Hispanics as a whole (12.8K). The Puerto Ricans figure (not shown) is 16.5K—virtually identical to Blacks' per capita income (U.S. Census Bureau, 2006a). Hence, Mexicans are easily the major driving force behind the exceptionally low showing by Hispanics as a whole. In addition, there is good reason to believe that,

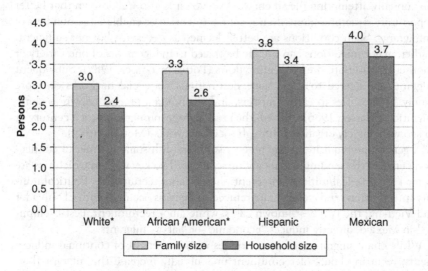

Figure 6.8 Average Family and Household Size by Race and Hispanic Origin, 2005.
*Non-Hispanic.
Source: U.S. Census Bureau (2006a).

within the Mexican population, it is the immigrant contingent that drives down the statistics for the whole group.

Also, it is notable that the larger families and households of Hispanics as a group are largely a function of Mexicans, who show an average family size of four persons. Even more pointed are the 2002 census figures for Hispanic family size (Ramirez & de la Cruz, 2003). These data estimate how many family households have five or more members. Mexican families show by far the largest number at 30.8%. In contrast, only 10.8% of White families had more than four members and other Hispanic groups' family sizes fell between Whites and Mexicans.

Recently, Aponte (2003) compared family size data from the 1990 and 2000 censuses. His findings showed that the average household size of Mexicans actually inched upward across the 1990s, in sharp contrast to White and Black family sizes. Clearly, this is attributable to the record-breaking influx of Mexican families during the 1990s. Immigrant families have been consistently larger than U.S.-born Mexican families. In fact, Crowley *et al.* (2006) reviewed 2000 census microdata and found that Mexican immigrant families were larger than U.S.-born Mexican families in every U.S. region.

Immigrants and Hidden Hispanic Family Hardships

Immigrants from Mexico come to the United States for many reasons, but most come to obtain more lucrative employment and improve family well-being either in the United States or back in Mexico. Such migrants typically earn far more in the United States than they can earn in Mexico, despite their relative concentration in the lowest-paying sectors of the U.S. labor market. Indeed, hundreds die annually attempting illegal entry. However, it is also well known that better opportunity structures alone do not suffice to entice or enable large numbers of immigrants. Such conditions are better deemed as necessary, but not sufficient. Rather, major migrations can usually be traced to inducements of one variety or another that initiate the pioneering flows (Portes & Borocz, 1989). Subsequent migrants are steered to these same destinations via social networks or, more simply, by their ties to earlier movers, and so on, via a process known as chain migration (Massey, 1986). Indeed, the great European migrations of a century or so ago were largely organized through social networks (Moretti, 1999).

A general prerequisite to the process is to establish some manner of connection between the sending and receiving societies. Two key ways in which ties are formed are political/military intervention and labor recruitment. Political/military intervention tends to generate refugee streams, as occurred with El Salvador and Vietnam, the two best-known cases, while labor recruitment, best exemplified in Mexico, directly induces "economic" or "labor" migrants.

While chain migration often continues without benefit of continual inducements, recurring bouts of recruitment undoubtedly increase the migrant flow. Moreover, it is clear that while foreign worker recruitment to the United States has been highly restricted for decades, illegal recruitment is almost certainly carried out with some frequency (Aponte 2003; Johnson-Webb, 2003). In the very recent past, for example, the corporate giant Tyson Foods, and some of its executives, were indicted by a federal grand jury on charges relating to illegal recruitment of Mexican workers during the 1990s (Grimsley, 2001). As recently detailed by Aponte (2003), the areas where the plants that were specified in the Tyson indictment were located witnessed Hispanic growth (overwhelmingly Mexican) that was nothing short of astounding.

Even the most cursory glance at a few of the examples provided by Aponte (2003) yields sufficient cause for accepting the recruitment hypothesis. In Monroe City, North Carolina (NC), the (overwhelmingly Mexican) Hispanic population grew from 215 to 5,611 persons from 1990 to 2000. In Union County, NC, where Monroe is located, the corresponding numbers were 675 persons (1990) and 7,637 (2000). In Springdale City, Arkansas (AK), the corresponding increase was from 446 to 9,005 persons (a growth of 8,559), and in nearby Benton County, AK, the increase was from 1,359 to 13,469 (a growth of 12,110). Similarly astounding examples of growth ensued in many of the other areas in question.

This leads to the following points. First, we assume that recruitment efforts, whether direct or indirect, are an important element in recent Mexican migration. Without recruitment, many fewer migrants would come, though migration would not end. Second, we assume further that the vulnerability of the undocumented migrants is what makes them so highly desirable and sought-after. If these assumptions are valid, we might expect to find that immigrant workers are indeed poorly paid at undesirable jobs, that they endure dangerous worksites, and that they turn up in areas where recruitment was undertaken. Some of this has already been illustrated and the rest follows. What is clear is that immigration has fueled Hispanics' phenomenal population growth and is a major force in the enduring poverty of Hispanic families. But, as we will see, the deprivations sustained by the group go beyond readily observable, standard, economic deprivations.

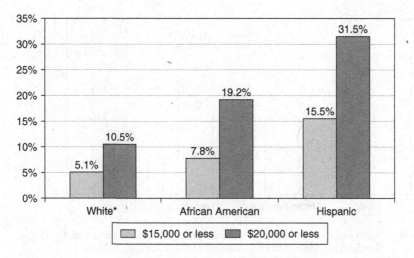

Figure 6.9 Low Income Earners as Percentage of All Full-Time, Year-Round Workers 15 Years and Over by Race and Hispanic Origin, 2003.

*Non-Hispanic.

Source: U.S. Census Bureau (2006a).

Earlier we showed that Mexicans and their families clearly sustain the lowest per capita income of all groups examined. Fig. 6.9 illustrates this point from a different angle. It shows the percentage of full-year, full-time workers who toil at rock bottom wages at two levels, by three groups: Whites, Blacks and Hispanics (U.S. Census Bureau, 2006b). The first of the indicators gives the percentage of such workers that earn 15K or less for a full year's labor. Whereas only 5.1% of White workers and 7.8% of Black workers earn such meager wages, some 15.5% of Hispanic workers do so. The second indicator shows what proportion earn 20K or less for a year's labor. The same rankings are maintained. While the figures for Whites and Blacks are 10.5% and 19.2%, respectively, the Hispanic figure is a whopping 31.5%. Almost certainly, wage discrimination is at play here.

There are other workplace-related forms of hardship that affect Hispanic families more than other families, and immigrants almost surely are disproportionately represented among the deprived in these instances. No doubt the most serious example concerns health coverage. In the United States the vast majority of individuals obtain health insurance through employment. However, not all jobs provide health coverage and some require voluntary employee contributions that employees cannot afford. Hence, aside from the unemployed, most adults (and their dependents) who lack coverage do so because they work for organizations that do not offer health insurance coverage or because the coverage available is beyond their ability to pay.

The population lacking coverage has grown to record numbers in recent years and the issue has been the subject of many headlines. What such headlines do not often divulge is that the Hispanic group is by far the most undercovered of the three major minority groups. As Fig. 6.10 shows, in 2004 some 12% of

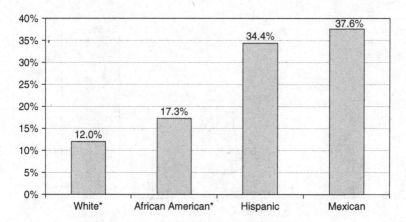

Figure 6.10 Percentage of Population Lacking Health Insurance Coverage for People Under 65 by Race and Hispanic and Mexican Origin, 2004.

*Non-Hispanic.

Source: NCHS (2006).

Whites and 17.3% of Blacks lacked health insurance coverage, but the figure for Hispanics was 34.4% (National Center for Health Statistics, 2006). Moreover, in this instance, separate data for Mexicans indicate that fully 37.6% lacked insurance coverage in 2004. Immigrants are likely to be most affected by this problem. A recent analysis of survey data from California, the state with the most Mexicans, revealed that Hispanic immigrants were more likely than U.S.-born Hispanics to do without insurance (Greenwald, O'Keefe, & DiCamillo, 2005).

No form of oppression sustained by Hispanic families, however, surpasses the dangers employed family members often endure at their jobsites. As suggested earlier, they are often recruited to perform work considered quite dangerous, even by veterans in the particular occupations. In addition, they often receive insufficient training for such jobs and are additionally ill-prepared because of language barriers. The results are as predictable as they are tragic: Hispanics lose their lives at work far more frequently than other workers, and the fatality rate gaps are increasing (see Figs. 6.11 and 6.12).

Fig. 6.11 compares 2001 workplace fatality rates for non-Hispanic Whites, Blacks, and Hispanics (Bureau of Labor Statistics, 2002). Whereas Blacks suffered 3.8 workplace deaths per 100,000 workers and Whites show a corresponding rate of 4.2 deaths, Hispanics experienced a remarkable 6.0 such deaths. The 1999 figures (not shown) revealed similar, though closer, rankings among the three groups. From 1999 to 2001 rates held constant for Whites, fell for Blacks, and actually rose for Hispanics.

Fig. 6.12 shows the recorded number of fatalities at work sustained by Hispanic workers from 1992 to 2005 (U.S. Department of Labor, 2007). Over that period, their deaths increased from 533 to 917. Ironically, this was a period when the

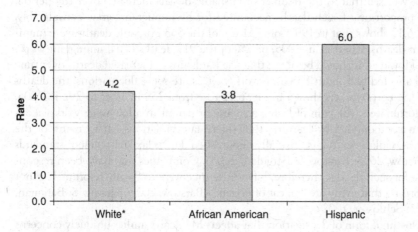

Figure 6.11 Workplace Fatality Rates in the United States by Race and Ethnic Origin, 2001 (Per 100,000 Workers).

*Non-Hispanic.

Source: Bureau of Labour Statistics (2002).

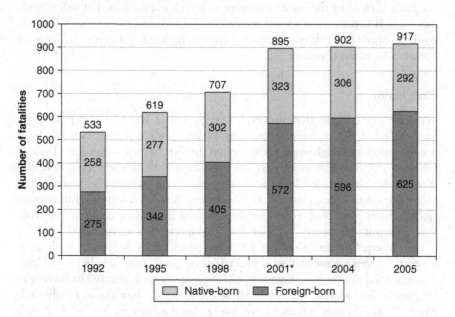

Figure 6.12 Number of Fatal Work Injuries Involving Hispanic Workers, 1992–2005.

*Excludes fatalities resulting from the September 11 terrorist attacks.

Sources: U.S. Department of Labour (2007).

overall number of deaths at work was actually decreasing (Bureau of Labor Statistics, 2002). Fig. 6.12 provides a crucial piece of evidence for the ideas presented here. It shows the number of Hispanic deaths by nativity for each year. It is easy to see that as the number of Hispanic deaths increased over the period, the proportion of such deaths accounted for by immigrants grew considerably. Fig. 6.12 shows that in 1992 some 51.6% of the 533 Hispanic deaths were immigrant deaths, whereas, in 2005, 68.2% of the 917 deaths befell immigrant workers. However, it should be noted that the hardships of increased deaths over time also affected U.S.-born Hispanic workers. Despite some fluctuations, the deaths of U.S.-born workers shown in Fig. 6.12 rose from 258 in 1992 to 292 in 2005. Unfortunately, the pain of losing a spouse or parent in a low-wage workplace is often compounded by learning that safety law violations led to many of the deaths, violations that go virtually unpunished due to lax enforcement standards (Barstow, 2003; Barstow & Bergman, 2003). Companies that have been responsible for such deaths, therefore, have little incentive to "really reform." It is not surprising that many are "repeat offenders" (Barstow, 2003; Barstow & Bergman, 2003; Schlosser, 2002).

One final form of deprivation that affects Mexican families uniquely concerns border crossings. Aponte (2003) found that from about 1996 to 2001, over 300 deaths per year were recorded as having occurred to Mexicans attempting to cross into the United States. The culmination of hazards confronted by at least some migrating families seems to defy reality. Indeed, to put it bluntly, such are the hazards faced by the workers desperate enough to take jobs that will provide just enough income to stave off starvation, but will sometimes also kill them. And, we should add, these are only some of the hidden deprivations of poor Mexican immigrant families.

Conclusion

We have argued here that the explosive growth of the Hispanic population in the United States, fueled mainly by Mexican-origin immigrants, has been accompanied by heightened, albeit often hidden, deprivations for Hispanic families. The data presented here are consistent with this interpretation. We have shown that while Mexican immigrants appear to bear the brunt of the increasing misfortunes, Hispanic family poverty is more than just an immigrant phenomenon. This chapter has barely scratched the surface of the many problems confronting Hispanic families; many complex issues remain unaddressed.

Our interpretations, although far from providing a definitive analysis of Hispanic poverty, nevertheless support various generalizations about problems and potential solutions. Immediate policy responses are warranted in three specific areas. Two address life and death issues, while also bearing on family well-being. First, Hispanic families have inadequate health care access. Although expanding access to health care is a well-recognized national issue, we show that Hispanic families have the least access to and the most to gain from true reforms. Inadequate health care can have an enormous impact on family well-being when families face crises, such as disability or prolonged illness.

Immigration policy represents a second area in need of reform. Whatever their shortcomings, at least politicians are debating various alternatives. What is often lost in the shuffle, however, is that men, women and, tragically, sometimes children, are dying daily in border-crossing attempts. Moreover, lives are devastated and livelihoods decimated whenever hard-working people are seized and returned to Mexico by INS raids. Many are lured to the United States by corporate interests (directly or indirectly), and their lives are turned upside down when they lose a family member to a border crossing tragedy or a deportation.

Finally, workplace reforms are needed badly. Aside from the almost certain violations of rules concerning wages, Hispanic workers are subject to dangerous working conditions. As noted previously, many organizations have maintained conditions that have led to multiple worker deaths. Organizations that maintain exploitive working conditions are not the only guilty parties. Certain components of the federal government co-conspire in this tragic drama. While some agencies of government (and individuals within them), such as investigators from the Department of Labor and the Occupational Safety and Health Administration (OSHA), do attempt to enforce wage and safety standards, sometimes heroically, their efforts are often thwarted by other government entities.

Political appointees, bureaucrats, and others in power steadfastly endeavor to undermine efforts to tighten regulations, stiffen sanctions and carry out prosecutions. In this way, authorities facilitate, encourage, and otherwise abet fundamentally criminal conduct. The source of the problem is almost certainly political. The solution is almost certainly political as well. Countless lives and family livelihoods are hanging in the balance.

Notes

1 The notion that "Hispanics" or "Latinos" constitute a meaningful collectivity is not without controversy. A full discussion of the issues is beyond the scope of this Chapter. Suffice to say that we accept the designation as sufficiently meaningful for the purpose at hand. Moreover, the individual nationality groups in question at any given point in the Chapter are sufficiently identified to avoid any misrepresentations or misinterpretations of any key issues.
2 All references to Black and White refer to non-Hispanics except where noted.
3 The length of time separating birth cohorts that is generally considered a "generation" is 30 years (Costello, 1992).

References

Aponte, R. (1996). Urban employment and the mismatch dilemma: Accounting for the immigrant exception. *Social Problems, 43,* 268–83.

Aponte, R. (2003). Latinos in the U.S.: The new largest minority and its discontents. *Journal of Latino-Latin American Studies, 1,* 21–33.

Barstow, D. (2003, 22 December). U.S. rarely seeks charges for deaths in the workplace. *New York Times,* p. A1.

Barstow, D. & Bergman, L. (2003, 10 January). Deaths on the job, slaps on the wrist. *New York Times,* p. A1.

Bureau of Labor Statistics. (2002). *Census of fatal occupational injuries summary.* Available HTML: www.http://bls.gov.

Census Scope. (2000). U.S. population by race and ethnicity selections, 1980–2000. *Census Scope-Population by Race.* Available HTML: http://www.censusscope.org/us/print_chart_race.html.

Costello, R. (1992). *Random House Webster's college dictionary*. New York: Random House.

Crowley, M., Lichter, D., & Qian, Z. (2006). Beyond gateway cities: Economic restructuring and poverty among Mexican immigrant families and children. *Family Relations, 55*, 345–60.

Greenwald, H., O'Keefe, S., & DiCamillo, M. (2005). Why employed Latinos lack health insurance: A study in California. *Hispanic Journal of Behavioral Sciences, 27*, 517–32.

Grimsley, K. (2001, 20 December). Tyson Foods indicted in INS probe: U.S. firm sought illegal immigrants. *Washington Post*, p. A1.

INS (2003). *Estimates of the unauthorized immigrant population residing in the United States: 1990–2000*. Available HTML: http://uscis.gov.

Johnson-Webb, K. (2003). *Recruiting Hispanic labor: Immigrants in non-traditional areas*. New York: LFB Scholarly Publishing.

Massey, D. (1986). The settlement process among Mexican immigrants to the United States. *American Sociological Review, 51*, 670–84.

Moretti, E. (1999). Social networks and migrations: Italy 1876–1913. *International Migration Review, 33*, 640–57.

National Center for Health Statistics. (2006). *Health United States, 2006*. Available HTML: http://www.cdc.gov/nchs/data/hus/hus06.pdf.

Passel, J. (2005). *Estimates of the size and characteristics of the undocumented population*. Washington, DC: Pew Hispanic Center.

Portes, A. & Borocz, J. (1989). Contemporary immigration: Theoretical perspectives on its determinants and modes of incorporation. *International Migration Review, 23*, 606–30.

Ramirez, R. & de la Cruz, G. (2003). The Hispanic population in the United States: March 2002 (P20–545). Washington, DC: U.S. Government Printing Office.

Schlosser, E. (2002). *Fast food nation: The dark side of the all American meal*. New York: HarperCollins.

Suro, R. & Passel, J. (2003). *The rise of the second generation: Changing patterns in Hispanic population growth*. Washington, DC: Pew Hispanic Center.

U.S. Census Bureau. (2000). Table DP-1 Profile of general demographic characteristics. *Demographic profiles*. Available HTML: http://censtats.census.gov/data/US/01000.pdf.

U.S. Census Bureau. (2002). *Historical census statistics on population totals by race, 1790 to 1990, and by Hispanic origin, 1970 to 1990: For the United States, regions, divisions and states*. Available HTML: http://www.census.gov/population/www/documentation/twps0056.html.

U.S. Census Bureau. (2006a). Fact finder: Selected population profile in the United States. *2005 American Community Survey*. Washington, DC: U.S. Government Printing Office.

U.S. Census Bureau. (2006b). 2005 Poverty tables. *CPS 2006 annual social and economic supplement, annual demographic survey*. Available HTML: http://pubdb3.census.gov/macro/032006/pov/toc.htm.

U.S. Department of Labor. (2007). Census of fatal occupational injuries charts, 1992–2005. *Census of fatal occupational injuries (CFOI)—Current and revised data*. Available HTTP: http://stats.bls.gov/iif/oshcfoi1.htm#2005.

Critical Thinking Questions

1   What do Aponte and Foote mean by hidden deprivation? Can you think of other examples of hidden deprivation that might constrain Hispanic families? Is hidden deprivation a problem for Black families? How about rural families and single mothers?

2   Think about the seemingly insoluble contradiction between the need for cheap exploitable labor and the "need" for a country to "control" its borders. Is there a solution that would appeal to immigrant advocates, employers, and those who are concerned with immigration laws?

3   The U.S. labor movement has been in a period of decay for the last several decades. How might the influx of hundreds of thousands of new low-wage workers revitalize the labor movement in this country?

Part II

Poverty Across the Life Span

Change, Crisis, and Resilience

7 Family Poverty, Welfare Reform, and Child Development

Elizabeth A. Segal and Michael D. Niles

Poverty status has been closely linked to poor child development (Bendersky & Lewis, 1994; Masten & Garmezy, 1985; Rutter, 1987). Poor children are more likely to have problems completing school and to score lower on measures of health, cognitive development, school achievement, and emotional well-being than children in higher-income families (Duncan & Brooks-Gunn, 1997). Years of research have demonstrated this relationship. In a review of numerous studies, Eamon (2001) identified the multiple effects of poverty, including the erosion of parental coping, marital discord, family distress, and detrimental effects on children's socioemotional development. Although U.S. child poverty has decreased from the high rates of the 1980s, in 2005 almost 18% of all children were poor; for children of color the figure was even higher at almost 35% for Black children and over 28% for Latino children (DeNavas-Walt, Proctor, & Lee, 2006).

Recent research finds that more than two-thirds of children in the United States, "34 million youth between the ages of 6 and 17, are not receiving sufficient developmental resources that put them on a path to success in adulthood" (America's Promise Alliance, 2006, p. 2) and the situation is worst for poor children. These factors include safe places to live, healthy starts to life, and effective education. When we examine research findings on improving child life outcomes, two key factors emerge that significantly impact the life course for children—family income and education. In both categories, poor children are adversely affected with significantly reduced opportunities for positive life outcomes. Thus, this chapter explores all three issues: family income, welfare, and developmental outcomes for poor children.

Family Income

Over the years, there has been sufficient research and understanding of one thing regarding poverty and child development—income matters when it comes to life outcomes. Numerous studies have concluded that increasing the incomes of poor families "enhances the cognitive development of children and may improve their chances of success in the labor market during adulthood" (Duncan & Brooks-Gunn, 1997, p. 608). In spite of economic wealth in this

Table 7.1 Poverty Rates of Children by Country

Country	Child Poverty Rate (%)
United States	20.3
Italy	19.5
United Kingdom	16.3
Canada	13.9
Australia	13.5
Spain	11.9
Germany	9.5
France	7.2
Netherlands	7.0
Switzerland	6.4
Belgium	5.1
Denmark	4.0
Norway	3.7
Finland	3.2
Sweden	2.4

Source: Rainwater & Smeeding (2003, p. 21).

country, the United States ranks highest among major nations in the proportion of children living in poverty (see Table 7.1).

In fact, while poverty is clearly linked to lack of employment, three-fourths of America's poor children live in households with one or more adult earners (Rainwater & Smeeding, 2003). National data highlight the deprivation that many American children experience. In 2003, over one-third, or 37% of U.S. households with children experienced housing problems. Those problems were defined as physically inadequate, crowded or too costly housing (Federal Interagency Forum on Child and Family Statistics, 2005). Housing costs have impacted poor families most significantly over the years, doubling the proportion of low-income families paying more than half their income for housing.

More than eight million children live in households that lack health insurance coverage (DeNavas-Walt et al., 2006). Although most children receive health insurance through their parents' employment, the coverage rate dropped from 2000 to 2005. Low-income children were hardest hit, with only 18% covered through employer-provided health insurance (Gould, 2006). Even for those children typically covered by government programs, the numbers of children covered by Medicaid or SCHIP dropped, while the need increased.

Although starvation is not a problem, American children suffer significant food insecurity. Almost one in five children (18%) experience periods of food deprivation: that is, living in homes with insufficient food due to poverty (Federal Interagency Forum on Child and Family Statistics, 2005). Inadequate nutrition, one of the outcomes of food insecurity, leads to poor health and development.

These data reveal a significant degree of economic deprivation for children. Perhaps most disheartening is that these numbers indicate that although the nation has experienced a period of economic expansion, the typical household, and particularly low-income families, did not benefit from recent economic growth (Bernstein & Shapiro, 2006). With depressed family incomes, inadequate housing, lack of health insurance, and food insecurity, poor children are at great risk of diminished development and life outcomes.

Employment and Poor Families

We may ask, if three-fourths of poor children live in households where adults are employed, why is there still family poverty? The answer rests with the types of jobs and wages in which these adults are employed. Over the past 10 years inflation has resulted in increases in the cost of food (23%), housing (29%), medical care (43%), childcare (52%) and gasoline (134%) (Bernstein & Shapiro, 2006). However, in that same 10-year span, the hourly minimum wage remained unchanged at $5.15. Poor adults are clustered in jobs at or near the federal minimum wage. This means they may be working, but their families remain poor. Families in the lowest quintile averaged a household annual income of $10,655 in 2005, which divides out to about the hourly minimum wage (DeNavas-Walt *et al.*, 2006). The low wages of families in the bottom 20% has been, in part, the result of recessions followed by jobless recoveries, which means that poor working adults have been hardest hit by labor market economic trends (Mishel, Bernstein, & Allegretto, 2005).

TANF and Welfare Reform

Public cash assistance, or welfare as we commonly refer to it, is the major federal and state support for poor families. Originally developed as part of the Social Security Administration (SSA) in 1935 as Aid to Dependent Children (ADC; amended to AFDC in 1961), the program was the target of the major welfare reform efforts in 1996. Those reform efforts created TANF and shifted the program emphasis from income support to "welfare to work." The ostensible goal of the program was to emphasize economic self-sufficiency and decrease the number of people receiving assistance by emphasizing employment. That means that the family incomes of poor households needed to be increased.

As discussed in Chapter 4, TANF is a time-limited, no-guarantee program that provides temporary cash assistance and requires work efforts for all participants. TANF recipients must participate in 30 hours a week of unsubsidized or subsidized employment, on-the-job training, community service, vocational training or childcare for other parents involved in community service (Segal, 2007). Since its inception in 1996, TANF has been successful in decreasing the number of recipients from more than 12 million, of whom 8.5 were children, to fewer than 5 million, of whom 3.6 million were children, by 2004 (SSA, 2006). While the goal of reducing the number of public cash assistance recipients was achieved by welfare reform, how successful has TANF and the welfare reforms of 1996 been in alleviating poverty and improving life outcomes for poor children?

The Success of Welfare Reform

Research findings on who left TANF and their success in securing employment are mixed. Although more women left TANF for employment, they do not seem to be better off financially. They have full-time jobs that pay seven to eight dollars an hour, and even though they may have transitional support, they eventually lose health care coverage from Medicaid (Acs & Loprest, 2004). Data reveal that while the numbers on TANF have declined, there are more families today that qualify but do not receive support. In 1995, 84% of families that met AFDC eligibility requirements participated, and by 2002 only 48% of eligible families were enrolled in TANF. The drop for poor children was even more severe. The share of children living in poverty who received AFDC/TANF dropped from a high of 62% to 31% from 1995 to 2003 (Parrott & Sherman, 2006). This means that eligible families are not receiving support, and the program covers fewer poor children. Thus the "success" in decreasing the caseloads of public cash assistance programs seems to be a result of factors that do not include reducing poverty or the need for the program. The decrease in coverage of eligible families leaves an estimated two million children living in poor households with a jobless adult and no income assistance from TANF. Even before recent data revealed the decline in TANF coverage, welfare advocates were alarmed by the impact of the 1996 welfare reform:

> As currently implemented, the welfare-to-work solution is a match made in hell. It joins together poor mothers with few resources whose family responsibilities require employment flexibility with jobs in the low-wage labor market that often are the most inflexible, have the least family-necessary benefits (vacation time, health care, sick days), and provide levels of pay that often are insufficient to support a single person, let alone a family.
>
> (Albelda, 2001, p. 68)

Poverty among U.S. children is still prevalent, especially considering the wealth and recent economic growth in the nation overall. Concurrent with this trend is the decline in public cash assistance, the primary antipoverty program for poor households. With declines in low-income families' earnings accompanied by declines in public programs, the persistence of poverty among children worsens. With deeper poverty come diminished opportunities for positive development and life outcomes.

Poverty, Child Development, and Early Childhood Intervention

Any discussion on child development and how it is affected by poverty would be incomplete without considering the role of early childhood intervention programs. In the United States, early childhood intervention is a general descriptor for a wide variety of programs (Niles, 2004; Niles, Reynolds & Nagasawa, 2006; Reynolds, 2002). Most often, it is broadly defined as formal attempts to maintain or improve the quality of life of young at-risk children (typically from 0 to 5 years). These targeted early intervention efforts primarily include programs intended to promote early child development, such as home visitation programs, parenting classes, Early Head Start, Head Start or Healthy Start, preschool and kindergarten, and Part H infant and toddler programs under the Individuals with Disabilities Education Act (Karoly *et al.*, 1998; Zigler & Muenchow, 1992). The intent of early intervention is to build the best possible foundation for future health, and for future academic and social functioning (Karoly *et al.*; Reynolds, 2000). These interventions are compensatory: that is, they are designed to prevent or mitigate poor child development in at-risk families (Reynolds, 2000; 2002). Poverty status or low-family income is noted as the primary criterion for families being considered high-risk. Young children and families who reside in poverty, or have a limited family income, are targeted because early and sustained deprivation results in impaired behavioral and brain development (Ramey & Ramey, 1998; Ramey & Sackett, 2000; Reynolds, 2000; 2002). From the start, most early interventions emphasized comprehensive services-center-based early education, multifaceted family participation (i.e. training and education oversight), and physical health and nutrition services (Niles, 2004; Niles *et al.*, 2006; Reynolds, 2000, 2002). This "whole-child" philosophy continues in the present day (Reynolds, 2000; Zigler, 1994). Children are anticipated to be "ready to learn," and as a result close the performance disparity with their more economically advantaged peers (Ramey & Ramey, 1992; Reynolds, 2000).

Importance of Early Childhood Programs on Child Development

Numerous studies have provided compelling evidence that programs of relatively good quality have short- and longer-term positive effects on key indicators of child development. This is particularly true for poor children. Research documenting shorter-term effects (i.e. increased cognitive ability, school achievement, and social adjustment in the primary grades) has been extensively reported (see Barnett, 1998; Currie, 2001; Karoly *et al.*, 1998; Niles, 2004; Niles *et al.*, 2006; Reynolds, 2000, 2002; van IJzendoorn, 1998). The positive effects of early childhood intervention on improved developmental outcomes in adolescence and beyond also are documented (Ou & Reynolds, 2006; Reynolds, 2000; Reynolds, Temple, Robertson, & Mann, 2001). Barnett (1998) and others (Currie, 2001; Karoly *et al.*, 1998; Reynolds *et al.*, 2001) have found comprehensive and culturally relevant early childhood intervention programs to be associated with higher IQ scores, higher educational attainment, lower rates of grade retention and special education placement, and lower rates of criminal activities in adolescence and into adulthood. Poverty status affects these outcomes and is considered a primary predictor of later cognitive, social, and emotional problems. Moreover, with the latest technological innovations in brain imaging, neuroscientists are studying how a combination of good nurturing and stimulation during the first five years of life may in fact help to increase neural pathways in young children (Ashford, LeCroy, & Lortie, 2006). There is general consensus that the window of opportunity for stimulating a child's potential is relatively short (i.e. 0–5 years) (Ashford, LeCroy, & Lortie, 2006; Diamond & Hopkins 1998). For families living in poverty, this window of opportunity is often smaller than for nonpoor families because of unstable social and financial supports.

Historical Overview of Early Childhood Intervention, Child Development, and the Response to Poverty

Since the early 1900s, there has been evidence that families living in poverty did not perform as well on aptitude tests when compared to nonpoor families (Condry, 1983). By the 1950s, there was also evidence that children in low-income families were more likely to perform poorly on many types of academic achievement tests (Anastasi, 1958). In the 1960s, the U.S. Office of Education agreed to conduct a nationwide study of the educational achievement of diverse ethnic groups (Coleman, Campbell, Hobson, et al., 1966). This became known as the Coleman Report. Coleman et al. found that sixth-grade Black children were more than two grades behind the average White child in a variety of subjects. This gap expanded to five years or more by early adolescence (Coleman et al., 1966). Klaus and Gray (1968) termed this "progressive retardation." Deutsch (1967) called it "cumulative deficit." Although later questioned, these findings were of particular interest to policymakers because other research at that time suggested that level of academic success was a function of the child's environment rather than genetic deficits (Brazziel, 1969).

In the1960s, social class comparison research was extended to the investigation of social class differences that could be applicable to child development (Condry, 1983). Dilemmas fundamental to this research were also revealed. There was an almost predictable confounding of socioeconomic status (SES) and race, although attempts have been made to separate the two (see Condry, 1983; Palmer, 1983). Despite mounting evidence for the impacts of neighborhood composition over and above family-level influences taken as a whole, most research of the era "suggested that neighborhood composition is confounded with family characteristics, and when family characteristics are controlled, neighborhood effects are fairly weak" (Coulton, 1996, p. 91). Even so, there was significant disagreement about how and why poverty affects child development.

In his seminal book, *Stability and change in human characteristics* (1964), Benjamin Bloom suggested that the effect of the environment is greatest during the period of most rapid normal human development and its effect is least in the periods of least rapid normal development. Although acknowledging the relative scarcity of evidence on the effects that changing the environment can have on intelligence, he argued, at a practical level, "that to ameliorate the effects of poverty, steps should be taken as early in the individual's development as possible" (p. 89). This confirms what important social theories would later corroborate: that early social environments, including home, school, peers, and neighborhoods, influence children's social and emotional development (e.g., Bronfenbrenner, 1985; Wilson, 1987).

Still, there was little agreement. In the book, *The Other America* (1962), Harrington maintained that poor families grow up with a language of poverty, a psychology of poverty, and a poverty worldview that is different from the dominant society. This was later called a "culture of poverty." This notion of a "culture of the poor" resonated with theories and research on environmental disadvantage taking place at this time (Coleman et al., 1966). The terms cultural deprivation and cultural deficit were broadly accepted by social scientists in the 1960s as a concise expression of the critical interaction between poverty and child development. Once it became generally accepted that child development could be strongly influenced by environmental factors, the term cultural deficit was gradually eliminated from research, although not completely. Since then, a variety of studies have indicated that the developmental course of children in poverty was due to environmental factors rather than being determined by heredity, as some had suggested earlier.

There were also theories, from several areas of research, which claimed that early child development was qualitatively different from later development. The presumption was made that the effects of poverty on child development would be greatest during the early years of development. During the 1960s, comparisons of the environments of economically disadvantaged and advantaged children confirmed this belief. SES differences found in children's language, motivation, IQ, and other areas of child development were clear and convincing. Despite myriad criticisms, there did appear to be evidence of developmental differences in the environments of economically advantaged and disadvantaged children. The evidence lent support to the view that the cognitive, social, and emotional differences between children from lower- and higher-income homes could be attributable to (and compensated by) at least in part, the environmental and early childhood programmatic influences.

Threats to Child Development of Children Living in Poverty

In addition to academic underachievement, low motivation, or school failure, children who are poor are at increased risk of low birthweight, child mortality, and compromised brain development (Halfon & Newacheck, 1993). Poverty is also related to increased incidence of illnesses such as asthma (Gottlieb, Beiser, & O'Connor, 1995; Malveaux & Fletcher-Vincent, 1995), upper respiratory infection (Margolis, Nichol, Wuorenma, & Von Sternberg, 1992), tuberculosis (Drucker, Alcabes, Bosworth, & Sckell, 1994; Reinhard, Paul, & McAuley, 1997) and pediatric AIDS (Klerman, 1991; Klerman & Parker, 1990). Furthermore, the differential in prevalence of asthma between poor and nonpoor families was greatest for children under age 6 (Gottlieb, Beiser, & O'Connor, 1995; Malveaux & Fletcher-Vincent, 1995). These authors also found more debilitating effects of asthma on poor children, such as more days in bed and higher rates of hospitalization (Gottlieb et al., 1995; Halfon & Newacheck, 1993;

Malveaux & Fletcher-Vincent, 1995). Other researchers have linked the high asthma rates of poor inner-city children to higher sensitivity and exposure to cockroach allergen (Rosenstreich *et al.*, 1997).

As suggested in the research outlined above, there is abundant evidence that poverty disproportionately increases the threat of negative developmental outcomes for poor children. This research also attempts to answer the fundamental question: how and why do the threats of poverty manifest themselves? Several explanations seem paramount. First, financial and environmental stressors associated with poverty negatively affect parenting behaviors and the early identification of health problems, thus having an impact on child development (Lyons-Ruth, Alpern, & Repacholi, 1993; Lyons-Ruth, Easterbrooks, & Cibelli, 1997; McLeod & Shanahan, 1993; Shaw & Vondra, 1995).

Second, the effect of poverty on parental ability to provide a supportive and stimulating early home learning environment leads to problems with subsequent school readiness in children (Brooks-Gunn, Klebanov, & Liaw, 1995; Duncan, Brooks-Gunn, & Klebanov, 1994). Third, parents who are poor have been observed to have interactions with their children that are characterized by lower overall ratings of parental sensitivity and by more hostile, intrusive and erratic responses (Pianta & Egeland, 1990; Shaw & Vondra, 1995). Such parenting styles in turn place children at risk for developing insecure or disorganized/disoriented attachment strategies (Lyons-Ruth, Connell, Grunebaum, & Botein, 1990; Lyons-Ruth, Easterbrooks, & Cibelli, 1997; Zeanah, Boris, & Larrieu, 1997) as well as at heightened risk for maltreatment (Cicchetti & Toth, 1995; Crittenden & Ainsworth, 1989). This high incidence of negative parent–child interactions, which compromise the positive child development of poor children, may be linked to a variety of parental difficulties associated with poverty status.

Fourth, the poverty stressors may severely tax and limit parents' emotional and coping resources when interacting with their children (Halpern, 1993; McLeod & Shanahan, 1993; Watson, Kirby, Kelleher, and Bradley, 1996). Furthermore, a number of studies have demonstrated a positive relationship between social support and the ability to parent effectively (Bendersky & Lewis, 1994; Hashima & Amato, 1994).

Fifth, parents living in poverty have also been found to have higher rates of mental health difficulties, including depression and alcohol and substance abuse (McLeod & Shanahan, 1993), which can severely interfere with parenting quality and child development. Moreover, parental depression has been found to co-occur with poverty status at elevated rates and may be the "most significant mediator" of child development in poor families (McLeod & Shanahan, 1993).

Yet parental stress and depression are not the only relevant factors. Children born in poverty have been documented to be at greater risk for temperaments associated with affect regulation difficulties, are more easily distracted, and display less task persistence (Brooks-Gunn *et al.*, 1995). And, as explained earlier, poverty also increases the risk of low birthweight and early infancy illnesses, which, when combined with poverty status, places them in "double jeopardy" for developing cognitive and behavioral problems (Escalona, 1982; Parker, Greer, & Zuckerman, 1988). This combination of risks poses further challenges to parental psychological distress and parent–child interactions (McLeod & Shanahan, 1993).

Sixth, the early home learning environment matters. This has been found to partially mediate the effects of poverty on young children's cognitive attainment (Reynolds, 2000).

Seventh, poverty also affects young children via its impact on their immediate environment, both directly through physical characteristics, such as increased risk of lead exposure and illnesses associated with crowded household conditions, and indirectly through social characteristics, such as the chronic strain imposed on families by community disorganization and violence. Thus, such immediate environmental characteristics operate both directly (via physical characteristics) and indirectly as moderators (via social characteristics) of the risk impact (poverty and its correlates) on developmental outcomes for poor children (Reynolds, 2000).

Summary

America's historical landscape is littered with social policies and programs for poor children and families (Zigler, 1994). Typically intervention programs, even successful ones, are seen to come and go at the whim of funders and politicians. While some policymakers continue to advocate against the involvement—any involvement—of government in the workings of family life, early childhood intervention programs with a strong focus on parental involvement have proven valuable to poor children and families and show the most far-reaching and durable benefits for all family members (Seitz, 1990).

In the relative absence of economic resources and social support, systematic early childhood interventions that provide educational, social, and family support to poor families were a major justification for the development of most social programs beginning in the 1960s and continuing today through No Child Left Behind-Title I funding. Early childhood education is assumed to promote children's later educational success through cognitive and social ability enhancement, which, in turn, improves occupational attainment (Ramey & Ramey, 1998; Zigler, 1994). Although the early belief that program participation for a relatively short period of time could produce very large improvements in cognitive and social functioning was overly optimistic, programs that extend into the later school years have been shown to promote greater continuity during a key transition in children's lives—childhood to early adolescence. Additional educational, social, and family support during this time would be expected to enhance children's scholastic and social functioning (Reynolds, 2000). In fact, the Head Start designers envisioned programs that would extend into the later schools years, although they were not implemented as part of the Head Start program.

Although there has been a complex and vital discussion among research, policy, and practice in early development and early intervention for over 40 years in the United States, serious gaps of knowledge remain. First, despite decades of research on poverty and its association with child development, no single causal process by which poverty affects child development has been identified. Indeed, this may be the reason both for the power of its effect and the relative difficulty of protecting children from its negative effects. Second, each of the mediating processes is a potential target for secondary prevention/early intervention (and each has been targeted by an array of early intervention efforts; see Shonkoff & Meisels, 2000). For some of the targets, we already have effective program models (e.g. provision of high-quality early learning experiences); but for other targets, we are still searching for adequately effective program models (e.g. how we can reduce parental stress or improve parental sensitivity of care). And while the field has assumed that comprehensive approaches aimed at multiple targets are more effective intervention strategies than more focused intervention approaches, evaluations of programs like Comprehensive Child Development Program (CCDP) (St. Pierre, Layzer, & Barnes, 1995) and New Chance (Quint, Polit, Bos, & Cave, 1994) do not support this assumption. When one compares the results of programs that combined family support with early education back in the 1970s and 1980s (Yoshikawa, 1995) to the results of more recent efforts like CCDP and New Chance, we are left wondering whether in our efforts to be more comprehensive, we have watered down the quality or intensity of individual program components. If so, then the next decade should be devoted to devising and testing more strategically targeted interventions that try to do a few key things targeted on important processes very well. These are some of the program implications we draw from the new research that has emerged over the last decade. While robust economic growth over the 1990s and an expansion of the EITC have combined to reduce child poverty in recent years, we can and must do more as a nation. Without public and private sector commitment to reducing child poverty, the enormous impact of poverty on child development cannot be reversed.

References

Acs, G. & Loprest, P. (2004). *Leaving welfare: Employment and well-being of families that left welfare in the post-entitlement era.* Kalamazoo, MI: Upjohn Institute for Employment Research.

Albelda, R. (2001). Fallacies of welfare-to-work policies. *Annals of the American Academy of Political and Social Science, 577,* 66–78.

America's Promise Alliance. (2006). *Every child, every promise: Turning failure into action.* Alexandria, VA: Author.

Anastasi, A. (1958). *Differential psychology* (3rd ed.). New York: Macmillan.

Ashford, J., LeCroy, C., & Lortie, K. (2006). *Human behavior in the social environment* (3rd ed.). Belmont, CA: Thomson/Brooks-Cole.

Barnett, W. (1998). Long-term effects on cognitive development and school success. In W. Barnett & S. Boocock (Eds.), *Early care and education for children in poverty: Promises, programs, and long-term results* (pp. 11–44). Albany, NY: State University of New York Press.

Bendersky, M. & Lewis, M. (1994). Environmental risk, biological risk, and developmental outcome. *Developmental Psychology, 30,* 484–94.

Bernstein, J. & Shapiro, I. (2006). *Nine years of neglect.* Washington, DC: Center on Budget and Policy Priorities and Economic Policy Institute.

Bloom, B. (1964). *Stability and change in human characteristics.* New York: Wiley.

Brazziel, W. (1969). A letter from the South. *Harvard Educational Review, 39,* 355.

Bronfenbrenner, U. (1985). Summary. In M. Spencer, G. Brookins & W. Allen (Eds.), *Beginnings: The social and affective development of Black children* (pp. 67–73). Hillsdale, NJ: Lawrence Erlbaum Associates.

Brooks-Gunn, J., Klebanov, P., & Liaw, F. (1995). The learning, physical, and emotional environment of the home in the context of poverty: The Infant Health and Development Program. *Children and Youth Services Review, 17*, 251–76.

Cicchetti, D. & Toth, S. (1995). Developmental psychopathology and disorders of affect. In D. Cicchetti & D. Cohen (Eds.), *Developmental psychopathology*, Vol. 2: *Risk, disorder and adaptation* (pp. 369–420). New York: John Wiley.

Coleman, J., Campbell, E., Hobson C., et al. (1966). *Equality of educational opportunity.* Washington, DC: Department of Health, Education and Welfare.

Condry, S. (1983). History and background of preschool intervention programs and the consortium for longitudinal studies. In Consortium for Longitudinal Studies Staff (Eds.), *As the twig is bent: Lasting effects of preschool programs* (pp. 1–31). Mahwah, NJ: Lawrence Erlbaum Associates.

Coulton, C. (1996). Effects of neighborhoods in large cities on families and children: Implications for services. In A. Kahn & S. Kamerman (Eds.), *Children and their families in big cities: Strategies for service reform* (pp. 87–120). New York: Columbia University Press.

Crittenden, P. & Ainsworth, M. (1989). Attachment and child abuse. In D. Cicchetti & V. Carlson (Eds.), *Child maltreatment: Theory and research on the causes and consequences of child abuse and neglect* (pp. 432–63). New York: Cambridge University Press.

Currie, J. (2001). Early childhood education programs. *Journal of Economic Perspective, 15*, 213–38.

DeNavas-Walt, C., Proctor, B., & Lee, C. (2006). Income, poverty, and health insurance coverage in the United States: 2005. *Current Population Reports*, P60–231. Washington, DC: U.S. Census Bureau.

Deutsch, M. (1967). *The disadvantaged child: Selected papers of Martin Deutsch and associates.* New York: Basic Books.

Diamond, M. & Hopkins, J. (1998) *Magic trees of the mind: How to nurture your child's intelligence, creativity and healthy emotions from birth through adolescence.* New York: Dutton/Penguin.

Drucker, E., Alcabes, P., Bosworth, W., & Sckell, B. (1994). Childhood tuberculosis in the Bronx, New York. *Lancet, 343*, 1482–5.

Duncan, G. & Brooks-Gunn, J. (1997). Income effects across the life span: Integration and interpretation. In G. Duncan & J. Brooks-Gunn (Eds.), *Consequences of growing up poor* (pp. 596–610). New York: Russell Sage Foundation Press.

Duncan, G., Brooks-Gunn, J., & Klebanov, P. (1994). Economic deprivation and early childhood development. *Child Development, 65*, 296–318.

Eamon, M. (2001). The effects of poverty on children's socioemotional development: An ecological systems analysis. *Social Work, 46*, 256–66.

Escalona, S. (1982). Babies at double hazard: Early development of infants at biologic and social risk. *Pediatrics, 70*, 670–6.

Federal Interagency Forum on Child and Family Statistics. (2005). *America's children: Key national indicators of well-being, 2005.* Washington, DC: U.S. Government Printing Office.

Gottlieb, D., Beiser, A., & O'Connor, G. (1995). Poverty, race and medication use are correlates of asthma hospitalization rates: A small area analysis of Boston. *Chest, 108*, 28–35.

Gould, E. (2006). *Health insurance eroding for working families.* Washington, DC: Economic Policy Institute.

Halfon, N. & Newacheck, P. (1993). Childhood asthma and poverty: Differential impacts and utilization of health services. *Pediatrics, 91*, 56–61.

Halpern, R. (1993) Poverty and infant development. In C. Zeanah (Ed.), *Handbook of infant mental health*, (pp. 73–86). New York: Guilford Press.

Harrington, M. (1962). *The other America: Poverty in the United States.* New York: Macmillan.

Hashima, P. & Amato, P. (1994). Poverty, social support, and parental behavior. *Child Development, 65*, 394–403.

Karoly, L., Greenwood, P., Everingham, S., et al. (1998). *Investing in our children: What we know and don't know about the costs and benefits of early childhood interventions.* Santa Monica, CA: RAND.

Klaus, R. & Gray, S. (1968). The Early Training Project for disadvantaged children. *Monographs of the Society for Research in Child Development, 33* (Serial No. 120).

Klerman, L. (1991). The health of poor children: Problems and programs. In A. Huston (Ed.), *Children and poverty: Child development and public policy* (pp. 136–57). New York: Cambridge University Press.

Klerman, L. with Parker, M. (1990). *Alive and well? A review of health policies and programs for poor young children*. New York: National Center for Children in Poverty, Columbia University of Public Health.

Lyons-Ruth K., Alpern L., & Repacholi B. (1993) Disorganized infant attachment classification and maternal psychosocial problems as predictors of hostile-aggressive behavior in the preschool classroom. *Child Development, 64*, 572–85.

Lyons-Ruth, K., Connell, D., Grunebaum, H., & Botein, S. (1990). Infants at social risk: Maternal depression and family support services as mediators of infant development and security of attachment. *Child Development, 61*, 85–98.

Lyons-Ruth, K., Easterbrooks, M., & Cibelli, C. (1997). Disorganized attachment strategies and mental lag in infancy: Prediction of externalizing problems at age seven. *Developmental Psychology, 33*, 681–92.

Malveaux, F. & Fletcher-Vincent, S. (1995). Environmental risk factors of childhood asthma in urban centers. *Environmental Health Perspectives, 103*, 59–62.

Margolis, K., Nichol, K., Wuorenma, J., & Von Sternberg, T. (1992). Exporting a successful influenza vaccination program from an academic medical center to a community health maintenance organization. *Journal of American Geriatric Sociology, 40*, 1021–3.

Masten, A. & Garmezy, N. (1985). Risk, vulnerability and protective factors in developmental psychology. In B. Lahey & A. Kazdin (Eds.), *Advances in child clinical psychology* (pp. 1–52). New York: Plenum Press.

McLeod, J. & Shanahan, M. (1993). Poverty, parenting, and children's mental health. *American Sociological Review, 58*, 351–66.

Mishel, L., Bernstein, J., & Allegretto, S. (2005). *The state of working America 2004/2005*. Washington, DC: Economic Policy Institute.

Niles, M. (2004). *Participation in early childhood intervention: Does it influence children's social and emotional development?* Unpublished dissertation, University of Wisconsin-Madison.

Niles, M., Reynolds, A., & Nagasawa, M. (2006). Does early childhood intervention affect the social and emotional development of participants? *Early Childhood Research and Practice, 8*, 34–52.

Ou, S. & Reynolds, A. (2006). Early childhood intervention and educational attainment: Age 22 findings from the Chicago Longitudinal Study. *Journal of Education for Students Placed at Risk, 11*, 175–98.

Palmer, F. (1983). The Harlem Study: Effects by type of training, age of training and social class. In The Consortium for Longitudinal Studies (Ed.), *As the twig is bent*. Hillsdale, NJ: Lawrence Erlbaum Associates.

Parker, S., Greer, S., & Zuckerman, B. (1988). Double jeopardy: The impact of poverty on early childhood development. *Pediatric Clinician, North America, 35*, 1227–40.

Parrott, S. & Sherman, A. (2006). *TANF at 10: Program results are more mixed than often understood*. Washington, DC: Center on Budget and Policy Priorities.

Pianta, R. & Egeland, B. (1990). Life stress and parenting outcomes in a disadvantaged sample: Results of the Mother–Child Interaction Project. *Journal of Clinical Child Psychology, 19*, 329–36.

Quint, J., Polit, D., Bos, H., & Cave, G. (1994). *New chance: Interim findings on a comprehensive program for disadvantaged young mothers and their children*. New York: Manpower Demonstration Research Corporation.

Rainwater, L. & Smeeding, T. (2003). *Poor kids in a rich country: America's children in comparative perspective*. New York: Russell Sage Foundation.

Ramey, C. & Ramey, S. (1992). Effective early intervention. *Mental Retardation, 30*, 337–45.

Ramey, C. & Ramey, S. (1998). Prevention of intellectual disabilities: Early interventions to improve cognitive development. *Preventive Medicine, 27*, 224–32.

Ramey, S. & Sackett, G. (2000). The early caregiving environment: Expanding views on non-parental care and cumulative life experiences. In A. Sameroff, M. Lewis, & S. Miller (Eds.), *Handbook of developmental psychopathology* (2nd ed.) (pp. 365–80). New York: Plenum Publishing.

Reinhard, C., Paul, W., & McCauley, J. (1997). Epidemiology of pediatric tuberculosis in Chicago, 1974–1994: A continuing public health problem. *American Journal of Medical Science, 313*, 336–40.

Reynolds, A. (2000). *Success in early intervention: The Chicago Child-Parent Centers.* Lincoln: University of Nebraska Press.

Reynolds, A. (2002). Early childhood interventions: Knowledge, practice, and policy. *Focus, 22,* 112–17.

Reynolds, A., Temple, J., Robertson, D., & Mann, E. (2001). Long-term effects of an early childhood intervention on educational achievement and juvenile arrest: A 15-year follow-up of low-income children in public schools. *Journal of American Medical Association, 285,* 2339–46.

Rosenstreich, D., Eggleston, P., Kattan, M., Baker, D., Slavin, R., & Gergen, P. (1997). The role of cockroach allergy and exposure to cockroach allergen in causing morbidity among inner-city children with asthma. *New England Journal of Medicine, 336,* 1356–63.

Rutter, M. (1987). Psychosocial resilience and protective mechanisms. *American Journal of Orthopsychiatry, 57,* 316–31.

Segal, E. (2007). *Social welfare policy and social programs: A values perspective.* Belmont, CA: Thomson/Brooks-Cole.

Seitz, V. (1990). Intervention programs for impoverished children: A comparison of educational and family support models. In R. Vasta (Ed.), *Annals of child development,* Vol. 7: *A research annual* (pp. 73–103). London: Jessica Kingsley.

Shaw, D. & Vondra, J. (1995). Attachment security and maternal predictors of early behavior problems: A longitudinal study of low-income families. *Journal of Abnormal Child Psychology, 23,* 335–56.

Shonkoff, J. & Meisels, S. (Eds.) (2000). *Handbook of early childhood intervention* (2nd ed). New York: Cambridge University Press.

Social Security Administration. (2006). *Annual Statistical Supplement, 2005.* Washington, DC: Author.

St. Pierre, R., Layzer, J., & Barnes H. (1995). Two-generation programs: Design, cost and short-term effectiveness. *The Future of Children, 5,* 76–93.

van IJzendoorn, M. (1998). Meta-analysis in early childhood education: Progress and problems. In B. Spodek, O. Saracho, & A. Pellegrini. *Issues in early education research,* Vol. 8: *Yearbook in early childhood education* (pp. 156–76). New York: Teacher's College Press.

Watson, J., Kirby, R., Kelleher, K., & Bradley R. (1996). Effects of poverty on home environment: An analysis of three-year outcome data for low birth weight premature infants. *Journal of Pediatric Psychology, 21,* 419–31.

Wilson, W. (1987). *The truly disadvantaged: The inner city, the underclass, and public policy.* Chicago: University of Chicago Press.

Yoshikawa, H. (1995). Long-term effects of early childhood programs on social outcomes and delinquency. *The Future of Children, 5,* 51–75.

Zeanah, C., Boris, N., & Larrieu, J. (1997). Infant development and developmental risk: A review of the past 10 years. *Journal of the American Academy of Child and Adolescent Psychiatry, 36,* 165–78.

Zigler, E. (1994). Reshaping early childhood intervention to be a more effective weapon against poverty. *American Journal of Community Psychology, 22,* 37–47.

Zigler, E. & Muenchow, S. (1992). *Head Start: The inside story of America's most successful educational experiment.* New York: Basic Books.

Critical Thinking Questions

1   To what extent should government support services be available for poor children? What should they be and who should be responsible for providing them?

2   Should support services and interventions for children be offered in the home or in out-of-home settings like Head Start? Which would be more beneficial to the children and why? Which type of interventions do you think families would prefer for their children?

3   Why are health care and cash grants available for all elders regardless of income, but not for all children? In your opinion, what attitudes and values do these policies reflect? Should something be done about this?

8 Childhood Disability, Poverty, and Family Life

A Complex Relationship

Patrick Shannon

Approximately 16% of American children, nearly 12 million, are living in poverty and 7% live in extreme poverty (Annie E. Casey Foundation, 2002). Among this population, children with developmental disabilities are overrepresented. They are significantly more likely to live in poverty than children without disabilities. In 2002, nearly 22% of families living in poverty included a child experiencing a chronic illness and/or developmental disability (Wise, Wampler, Chavkin, & Romero, 2002). Newachek and Halfon (1998) reported that while approximately 12% of all children have some type of chronic disabling condition, this number increases to nearly 23% of children living in poverty in the United States. Fujiura and Yamaki (2000) reported that 28% of children with disabilities were living in poverty compared to only 16% of children in general. Meyers, Lukemeyer, and Smeeding (1998) demonstrated that children from families receiving TANF experience disability and chronic illness at twice the rate of children from families not receiving TANF. Hebbeler *et al.* (2001) reported that 42% of children entering the early intervention system for children from birth to 36 months with developmental delays and/or disabilities were receiving some form of public assistance. Finally, one-fifth of low-income families reported that they are caring for a child with a disability or chronic illness (Hanley, 2002).

Children with developmental disabilities and their families face challenges that can be defined as oppressive. They often experience oppression and discrimination when trying to access basic services that most parents take for granted (e.g. childcare) (Levy, 1995). The presence of a child with a developmental disability can have a large impact on a family's financial stability, quality of life, available time and resources, relationships with extended family and friends, and family roles (Dewees, 2004). Disability can be stigmatizing for the children and their entire families. This stigma is made considerably worse when the family is poor, racially or ethnically diverse, or headed by a single parent (Rounds, Weil, & Bishop, 1994).

The relationship between developmental disability and family poverty is complex. Children living in poverty are exposed to multiple risk factors associated with developmental disabilities. However, the costs associated with raising a child with a developmental disability greatly increase the risk of living in poverty (Birenbaum, 2002; Peterson *et al.*, 2004). Finally, poverty has negative consequences on the health and well-being of children with developmental disabilities, their families and overall family functioning (Emerson, 2004). An important question, therefore, is: Does developmental disability cause poverty or does poverty cause developmental disability? The answer to both questions is, more than likely, yes. This chapter explores these complex relationships and attempts to provide some strategies for addressing the underlying issues that affect the quality of life for families that include children with developmental disabilities. First, I will give a brief overview of developmental disabilities.

Developmental Disability

The American Academy of Pediatrics (2001b, 2006) estimated that 12–16% of U.S. children have some type of developmental or behavioral disability. This amounts to between 6.5 and 9 million children. In 2001, nearly 250,000 children under 36 months qualified for Part C early intervention services although the U.S. Department of Education (2001) has estimated that three times this number may be eligible for services. Childhood disability, generally speaking, has been defined as "an ongoing chronic physical, developmental, behavioral, or emotional condition that requires health and related services beyond that required by peers" (Newacheck & Halfon, 1998, p. 610). This chapter, however, focuses on developmental disability because of the inclusiveness of the definition. Developmental disability used to be based solely on a diagnosis such as cerebral palsy, epilepsy, or mental retardation. In recent years, the definition has been broadened considerably to focus on functional impairment. The Administration on Developmental Disabilities (ADD) defines a developmental disability as a physical or mental impairment that begins before age 22 years that alters or substantially inhibits a person's capacity to do at least three of the following:

- take care of him or herself (dress, bathe, eat, and other daily tasks)
- speak and understand spoken language clearly
- learn
- walk or move around
- make decisions
- live independently
- earn and manage an income.

Examples of developmental disabilities include Attention Deficit Hyperactivity Disorder (ADHD), autism, fetal alcohol syndrome, learning disabilities, mental retardation, epilepsy, cerebral palsy, genetic disorders such as Down's Syndrome or Fragile X Syndrome, Pervasive Developmental Disorders (PDD) and speech and language disorders (ADD Mission Statement, n.d.). Children with developmental disabilities face multiple challenges because their needs cross many developmental boundaries. Families often have to coordinate multiple services that can include special health care needs, learning challenges, physical limitations, and cognitive challenges. However, there are many resources available to support children with developmental disabilities and their families through federal and state systems; they are reviewed later in this chapter. The next section explores the relationship between poverty and disability.

Poverty as a Cause of Disability

As discussed in Chapter 7, there is ample evidence to suggest that poverty has an adverse impact on the health and development of children (Bradshaw, 2002, 2003). Poverty increases the risks for poor developmental, educational, emotional, behavioral, health, and social outcomes for children (Msall, Bobis, & Field, 2006: Newacheck, Stein, Bauman, & Hung, 2003; Parish & Cloud, 2006). Children born into poverty are more likely to: (1) have impaired cognitive and language development; (2) experience poorer health; (3) be less successful in school; (4) experience psychological and behavioral issues; and (5) become disabled (Emerson, 2004). Children who live in single-parent households with incomes below the poverty line are at highest risk of experiencing developmental disability (Fujiura & Yamaki, 2000). Families living in poverty have fewer formal and informal resources and supports than other families. They have less time and money available to meet the additional needs of a child with a disability.

Numerous studies have demonstrated the increased risk of developmental disability for children living in poverty (Fujiura & Yamaki, 2000; Hogan, Msall, Rogers, & Avery, 1997; Newachek & Halfon, 2000). Poverty places children at risk of exposure to environmental hazards, such as lead and other environmental toxins, and substandard housing resulting in the presence of molds, cockroaches, rodents, and cold damp air, all of which can have negative consequences for the health and development of a child (Emerson, 2004). Guralnick (1998) suggested that poverty and its associated risk factors, such as exposure to alcohol and drugs, poor parenting skills, prematurity, low birthweight and exposure to environmental toxins, can compromise the health and development of young children as well. Low birthweight is strongly associated with developmental disability and the United States has one of the highest rates of low birthweight among the world's wealthiest countries (Leonard & Wen, 2002). Bodensteiner and Johnsen (2006) reported that children weighing 1,500g or less at birth are at extremely high risk of experiencing a cerebellar injury potentially resulting in some form of lifelong disability. It has been suggested that the United States has higher rates of low birthweight because of inadequate health insurance that results in poor prenatal care, high substance abuse rates, and poor nutrition.

Access to health care is an important determinant of good health, and lack of access heightens the risk of disability. Nearly half of children living in poverty lack health care insurance (Msall, Bobis, & Field, 2006). As a result, they receive less comprehensive and preventive health care, fewer educational resources, and fewer social supports than children who live in families with higher incomes (Lee, Sills, & Oh, 2002). Families living in poverty are less likely to have access to quality prenatal care, primary care, acute care, and specialized medicine

(Bartley, 2004). Pregnant mothers living in poverty are less likely to receive adequate and regular prenatal care, to have a healthy diet, or to exercise, and they are more likely to suffer from poor health, substance abuse, and exposure to environmental toxins (Bartley, 2004). Children with disabilities, therefore, are exposed to risk factors earlier and more frequently than children from higher-income homes. Conversely, children with disabilities (and without) living in higher-income families have access to more resources and have more choices available to help their parents cope with the additional challenges of parenting a child with a developmental disability (Scorgie, Wilgosh, & McDonald, 1998).

Children living in poverty also risk exposure to adverse social conditions that include maltreatment, understimulating environments, homelessness, parental separation, substance abuse in the home, and crime (Ammerman & Balderian, 1993; Crosse, Kaye, & Ratnofsky, n.d.; Shannon, 2006; Sobsey & Varnhagen, 1988; Sullivan & Knutson, 2000; Verdugo, Bermejo, & Fuertes, 1995). Again, the risk of disability is greatly increased when children, especially very young children, are exposed to such social conditions. When a child has a developmental disability, families experience additional financial strains that families of children without disabilities do not experience. Next, we explore this relationship.

The Cost of Developmental Disability

There is evidence to suggest that families that include a child with a developmental disability experience downward social mobility, that is, descending into (for the first time or further into) poverty associated with caring for and raising a child with a developmental disability (Leonard & Wen, 2002). This situation can add additional financial and social costs that can increase the likelihood of a family falling into poverty and/or decrease their chances of escaping poverty (Birenbaum, 2002). Taylor (2005) estimated that the cost of raising a child with a disability is three times higher than raising a child who does not have a disability.

Early intervention services for young children can substantially improve developmental outcomes for children experiencing delays in development (Guralnick, 1998). However, early intervention involves an array of professional services that can carry a high financial cost. Support for paying these costs includes a confusing list of federal, state, and local programs and private insurers (Brown, Perry, & Kurland, 1994; Kates, 1997, 1998; Striffler, Perry, & Kates, 1997). In their focus group study, Shannon, Grinde, and Cox (2003) demonstrated the financial struggles families can face with a young child with a developmental disability. Families in their study struggled to pay for needed early intervention services and paying for these services had a significant impact on the families' financial situations. For example, families reported spending retirement and college funds, declaring bankruptcy or quitting jobs to qualify for Medicaid. Some families rejected early intervention altogether.

Disability can bring financial consequences for families in several areas including: (1) medical expenses; (2) loss of income or earning potential for individuals and or caregivers; (3) elevated childcare costs and (4) additional community and other living expenses (Brashler, 2006; Parish & Cloud, 2006). Despite these concerns, families that include children with developmental disabilities are underserved in the health care, mental health, and welfare systems (Msall, Bobis, & Field, 2006).

Children with disabilities tend to experience multiple health and developmental issues that require treatment intervention and support. Several studies have reported on the increased need for specialized therapies that require weekly appointments (Birenbaum, 2002; Dewees, 2004). Medications can impose a significant out-of-pocket expense for families with health insurance and an unmanageable expense for families without insurance. Disability often requires families to purchase adaptive equipment and to make expensive modifications to their home (Parish & Cloud, 2006). These out-of pocket expenses have been estimated to be two to three times higher than expenses for families that do not include a child with a disability (Newachek & McManus, 1988). The costs of these additional needs can quickly mount and overwhelm slim family budgets.

The financial burdens associated with caring for a child with a disability has been linked to employment. Also troubling is the fact that families that include children with disabilities have reported the need to turn down job offers, overtime and even pay increases in order to continue to maintain Medicaid and Social Security Income (SSI) eligibility (Msall, Bobis, & Field 2006). Many poor working families are employed in service sector jobs that do not include health insurance benefits for hourly employees. Therefore, if their income exceeds the eligibility thresholds for Medicaid, they lose the health care coverage and cannot afford private insurance.

Passage of the PRWORA placed increased importance on nonmaternal childcare for poor families and TANF requires mothers to participate in job training programs and to work in order to receive assistance. Research on the impact of nonmaternal childcare highlights the importance of high-quality childcare for the health and development of young children (Lee, 2005). Good care is associated with successful behavioral adjustment, improved cognitive and learning skills, emotional stability, and language abilities. Conversely, poor care is linked to developmental delays in several domains including behavioral–emotional, language, and learning development (NICHD, 2002).

As has been discussed throughout this book, childcare expenditures are a significant proportion of working families' total budget. Additionally, unavailability of childcare is a major reason for one or more parents not working (Lee, 2005). Parish, Cloud, Huh and Henning (2005) reported that approximately 33% of families with at least one child with a disability indicated that they have been denied childcare because of their child's disability and that the childcare they have accessed was deemed of lower quality than typical center-based care. Families with incomes above the federal poverty line spend approximately 7% of their income on childcare, whereas childcare for poor working families averages nearly 35% of total income (Parish & Cloud, 2006). Childcare costs for children with disabilities are significantly higher than they are for children in general (Newachek & Halfon, 2000). So families that include a child with a disability have difficulty finding and accessing childcare, which affects their ability to work; the childcare they do find and access is poor and they pay much more for the care, which adds up to more than one-third of their total monthly budget.

Impact on Family Functioning

There is a significantly higher divorce rate in families that include children with disabilities than families that do not (Capper, 1996). Parenting can place enormous stress on a marital relationship. Stress is dramatically enhanced when a child has a disability. The dreams and hope for the future that accompany new parenthood are often dashed when a child is born with a disability. Discovering that a child has a developmental disability can occur the moment the child is born (or even prenatally), or it can occur over time as a child has difficulties or misses typical developmental milestones. Capper (1996, p. 1) described a range of emotions including the "anguish, guilt, anger, depression, anxiety, embarrassment, denial, grief, and hopelessness" she experienced as the extent of her daughter's disabilities became evident. Capper coped with her distress by becoming intensely involved in her daughter's care and by aggressively learning everything she could about her daughter's disabilities, needs, and the services available to provide support. Many parents living in poverty, however, do not have the same resources and skills, and may struggle more with coping with the psychological stress of parenting a child with a disability.

The increased stress associated with raising a child with a developmental disability and living in poverty can create an immense amount of stress on a family system. Families are forced to engage in a considerable number of health and developmental care activities that can create both emotional and physical stress (Capper, 1996) and they can quickly become overwhelmed. Gibson and Weisner (2002) described a process by which families have to weigh the "transaction costs" (e.g. time and resources) of each additional service need their child and family require. Families eventually reach a critical stage where any additional cost outweighs any potential benefit.

Pearson (1996) suggested that the added stress experienced by caregivers may explain the increased risk of child abuse that children with disabilities face. Specifically, stress factors include parental disability, mental/emotional problems present in a family member, family social isolation, involvement with the legal system, child alcohol or drug dependency, and gang activity/involvement (Sullivan & Knutson, 2000).

According to Lloyd and Rossman (2005), mothers living in poverty who are raising children with disabilities experience higher rates of mental health issues. Women who are poor and have a child with a disability experience significant time and resource demands. As a result, they have lower employment levels than other mothers (Meyers, Brady, & Seto, 2000). These families must manage unexpected financial burdens and frequent medical appointments including related health activities, such as occupational and physical therapy, speech and language appointments.

There is evidence to suggest that families that include a child with a developmental disability have fragile support systems (Shannon, 2004). When a child with a disability arrives in the home, many families report disruption in their social networks. Friends and family often sever ties, which serves to further isolate the family. Limited resources compound the impact, especially on single mothers. Lack of money for basic needs, such as food, clothing, medical care, and housing, can add to psychological and emotional stress (Lloyd & Rossman, 2005). Furthermore, childcare is difficult to find, and high-quality care next to impossible (Taylor, 2005). Families, especially single mothers, face a difficult dilemma—they need to work to support their families but they cannot find suitable daycare for their special-needs children.

Single mothers raising children with developmental disabilities often experience high levels of emotional and physical stress (Lloyd & Rossman, 2005). Additionally they are less likely to benefit from respite from their caregiving duties, which is essential for maintaining physical and mental health. As a consequence, single mothers raising children with developmental disabilities experience higher rates of mental health concerns, such as depression and anxiety, and they are more susceptible to high blood pressure, migraine headaches, and ulcers. Conversely, dual-parent households report having more choices available to them and thus have lower reported levels of mental and physical ailments (Scorgie, Wilgosh, & McDonald, 1998).

Federal and State Policy

There is considerable support for families that include children with disabilities. However, families have a difficult time comprehending the scope of programs and entitlements available to them. Moreover, they often receive poor and sometimes conflicting advice from government officials about eligibility (Taylor, 2005). The next section discusses a brief list of support systems available to support families.

The Developmental Disability System

At the federal level, the U.S. Department of Health and Human Services, Administration on Children and Families, Administration on Developmental Disabilities (ADD) is charged with managing the federal developmental disability system. Every state is mandated by ADD to construct and oversee three separate systems to provide advocacy, supports, and direct services to individuals with developmental disabilities, their families and organizations that provide direct services. First, each state must have a protection and advocacy system to safeguard and advocate the rights of individuals with developmental disabilities. The Protection and Advocacy Systems (P & A) and Client Assistance Programs (CAP) comprise a nationwide network of mandated, legally based, disability rights agencies. Information about P & A systems in individual states can be accessed at the National Association of Protection and Advocacy Systems (NAPAS) website (http://www.napas.org). P & A is intended to provide referral, information, and legal representation and advocacy to individuals with disabilities on disability-related issues in special education, employment, housing, assistive technology, access to mental health and/or developmental disability services, medical services, financial assistance, vocational rehabilitation, elimination of physical barriers in public places, freedom from abuse, neglect and unwarranted restraint and seclusion (NAPAS website). Second, ADD mandates that each state provide direct services and supports to individuals with disabilities that are guided by a state agency. The State Councils on Developmental Disabilities program provides financial support to each state to promote activities for a Developmental Disabilities Council in that state. Each council is mandated to develop and implement a statewide plan to increase independence, productivity, inclusion, and integration into the community for people with developmental disabilities, through systems change efforts, capacity building and advocacy. A list of State Councils can be accessed at http://www.acf.dhhs.gov/programs/add/states/ddcs.htm. Finally, ADD mandates that each state promote best practices in conjunction with universities in their state. Therefore, the Association of University Centers on Disabilities (AUCD) was created to promote policy, practice, research, and training for and about individuals with developmental and other related disabilities through a national network of University Centers for Excellence in Developmental Disabilities Education, Research and Service (UCEDD). A complete list of each state's UCEDDs may be found at http://www.aucd.org.

Children and their families are entitled to a host of services through the Individuals with Disabilities Education Act (IDEA). IDEA requires states to provide comprehensive programs for infants, toddlers and school-age children and their families. The legislation promotes family-centered service delivery for all children with disabilities. Another important piece of federal legislation affecting children with disabilities is the Rehabilitation Act of 1973 (Public Law 93-112). The act focuses on providing training and placement of people with disabilities in full-time, part-time, or supportive employment in competitive jobs. Training provided under the act emphasizes skills needed to live independently. Section 504 of the Rehabilitation Act protects the rights of people with disabilities in schools and other educational programs that are federally funded by ensuring access to educational facilities and programs, including colleges and universities (Capper, 1996).

Medicare, Medicaid, managed care, SCHIP, private insurance or Veterans Benefits may pay for some or all of the costs associated with disability, but people are often unfamiliar with coverage and the complexity of the eligibility criteria and subtleties of coverage. Income maintenance can also be provided from the Social Security Disability Insurance Program (SSDI) and Supplemental Security Income (SSI).

Medicaid, particularly through the Early and Periodic Screening, Diagnosis and Treatment (EPSDT) program, is the single largest payer of early intervention services (Glascoe, Foster, & Wolraich, 1997; Kates, 1997; Orloff, Rivera, Harris, & Rosenbaum, 1992). Other federal funding sources include Head Start, Maternal and Child Health (MCH) Title V, Mental Health and Mental Retardation (MH/MR), Mental Retardation and Developmental Disabilities (MR/DD), and Title XX, Women, Infants and Children (WIC) (Striffler et al., 1997). Also, state funding, such as the State Child Health Insurance Program (SCHIP), may be accessed by families and providers to pay for early intervention services (Kates, 1998).

SSI is a federal income assistance program managed and administered by the Social Security Administration (SSA) that can be a major financial support for families coping with a developmental disability. SSI is an income assistance program intended primarily for individuals aged 65 or older and people aged 18 or older who are blind or disabled. However, children younger than 18 with specific disabilities are also eligible (SSA, 2001). SSI eligibility is based both on meeting means-tested financial requirements and specific disability requirements. Eligibility criteria for a child with a developmental disability living in a single parent household include a monthly gross income less than $2,333 and assets/resources less than $2000. The child must have one or more mental or physical impairments that can be medically documented and result in "marked" and "severe" functional limitations. Additionally, these limitations must have lasted or be expected to last at least one year or end in death (SSA, 2006). SSA defines "marked" limitation as performing at a rate of less than 70% in the developmental domains of fine and gross motor skills; self-care activities of daily living; learning, persistence, concentration, and pace (e.g. completing tasks) and social-emotional skills. The designation "severe" refers to a rate of development of 50% or less and is considered an extreme delay (SSA, 2006).

The SSI program appears to be effective at relieving some of the financial burdens that families face. Lukemeyer, Meyers, and Smeeding (2000) demonstrated that families that include children with moderate to severe disabilities and receive SSI are significantly less likely to live in poverty than children who do not receive SSI. However, only 20% of low-income single-mother-headed households with at least one child with a disability were receiving SSI benefits in 1996 (Lee, Sills, & Oh, 2002). Additionally, only one in five mothers of children with severe disabilities was receiving SSI benefits. The culprit appears to be the PRWORA. Approximately 100,000 children with disabilities lost their eligibility for SSI benefits to welfare reform (American Academy of Pediatrics, Committee on Children with Disabilities, 2001a). From 1996 to 2002, nearly 22% of children who were eligible for SSI prior to 1996 lost their eligibility (Msall, Bobis, & Field, 2006).

Welfare reform impacted children with developmental disabilities in another negative way by limiting Medicaid eligibility. Traditionally, SSI eligibility automatically conferred Medicaid eligibility. The Balanced Budget Act of 1997 attempted to correct this issue by allowing children who lost SSI benefits following welfare reform to remain Medicaid-eligible. However, any applications occurring after the reforms were no longer automatically qualified for Medicaid if denied SSI. Individuals applying for Medicaid needed to meet separate eligibility criteria (American Academy of Pediatrics, Committee on Children with Disabilities, 2001a).

Implications for Policy and Practice

With comprehensive and effective intervention, developmental disabilities are often preventable. At the very least, the developmental consequences of many disabilities can be limited. For example, early intervention positively influences the health and development of young children experiencing developmental delays. Poverty is also preventable. The list of potential strategies for both assisting families that include children with disabilities living in poverty and preventing families from sliding into poverty is daunting. Because the needs of children with disabilities cross most service delivery arenas (e.g. behavioral, educational, health, and mental health) and the needs of families include employment, childcare, insurance, and other financial concerns, solutions must examine the potential for support from each system.

Families are required to serve many roles in order to meet the needs of their children who have disabilities. They must serve as a child advocate to make sure they receive the services for which they are eligible as primary caregivers (e.g. providing daily specialized health care needs or implementing behavioral plans), and as case manager to coordinate the delivery of services that cross service delivery boundaries. Serving all of these roles can quickly overwhelm any family, but the added stress of poverty can have devastating consequences.

Families need both formal and informal support in several areas including respite care, counseling, parent support groups, parenting education, and individuals to educate and advocate for parents regarding their child's disability and the programs available to them. Families need access to quality and affordable childcare so they can work. Families need health insurance so that they have access to prenatal, preventative, and specialized health care. Families need access to safe and affordable housing.

Raising a child with a disability costs more than raising a child without a disability. Therefore, families require a sufficient income that they can count on to meet all the specialized care needs that a child with a disability requires. While some support is available through the various federal and state disability-related programs described previously, they are not adequate in and of themselves. Professionals need to consider the tradeoffs between the intensity of services and the ultimate outcome or benefit for a child and family. More services do not necessarily translate into services that have a greater impact on the child and family. Professionals must work closely with families to strike a balance between the frequency or intensity of services, the cost of those services, and the ultimate impact on the child and family.

According to Lizanne Capper (1996, p. vii), "a parent of a child with multiple disabilities, whatever the disability, [is] looking for the same thing—support." Advocacy and support begin with understanding the law, family rights, and the services available to meet the needs of children with disabilities and their families. Advocacy also requires assertiveness. Assertiveness is not a given for parents of children with disabilities; many parents struggle with asserting themselves with providers and policymakers to advocate for their children (Shannon, 2004).

Many professions focus on alleviating poverty and the plight of those who experience it. Children with disabilities represent a significant proportion of the population of people living in poverty. Additionally, professionals encounter children with disabilities in nearly every setting in which they practice. Children with disabilities often have difficulty in school, experience mental health issues, are at higher risk for maltreatment, and have special health care needs. They need support from many different professionals and many different service delivery systems. Interdisciplinary practice and cooperation are essential to meeting the needs of these children and their families.

References

Administration on Developmental Disabilities Mission Statement. (n.d.). *About ADD*. Available HTML: http://www.acf.dhhs.gov/programs/add/addabout.html (accessed 7 January 2007).

Administration on Developmental Disabilities. (n.d.). *List of state developmental disabilities councils.* Available HTML: http://www.acf.dhhs.gov/programs/add/states/ddcs.htm (accessed 9 January 2007).

American Academy of Pediatrics, Committee on Children with Disabilities. (2001a). The continued importance of Supplemental Security Income (SSI) for children and adolescents with disabilities. *Pediatrics, 107*, 790–3.

American Academy of Pediatrics, Committee on Children with Disabilities. (2001b). Developmental surveillance and screening of infants and young children. *Pediatrics, 108*, 192–5.

American Academy of Pediatrics, Committee on Children with Disabilities. (2006). Identifying infants and young children with developmental disorders in the medical home: An algorithm for developmental surveillance and screening. *Pediatrics, 118*, 405–20.

Ammerman, R. & Balderian, N. (1993). *Maltreatment of children with disabilities*. Chicago: National Committee to Prevent Child Abuse.

Annie E. Casey Foundation. (2002). *Kids count data book: State profiles of child well-being.* Baltimore, MD: Author.

Association of University Centers on Disabilities. (n.d.). *List of university centers of excellence in developmental disabilities.* Available HTML: http://www.aucd.org (accessed 9 January 2007).

Bartley, M. (2004). *Health inequality*. Cambridge: Polity Press.

Birenbaum, A. (2002). Poverty, welfare reform, and disproportionate rates of disability among children. *Mental Retardation, 40*, 212–18.

Bodensteiner, J. & Johnsen, S. (2006). Magnetic resonance imaging findings in children surviving extremely premature delivery and extremely low birthweight with cerebral palsy. *Journal of Child Neurology, 21*, 743–7.

Bradshaw, J. (2002). Child poverty and child outcomes. *Children and Society, 16*, 131–40.

Bradshaw, J. (2003). Poor children. *Children and Society, 17*, 162–72.

Brashler, R. (2006). Social work practice and disability issues. In S. Gehlert & T. Browne (Eds.), *Handbook of health social work* (pp. 448–70). Hoboken, NJ: John Wiley.

Brown, C., Perry, D., & Kurland, S. (1994). Funding policies that affect children: What every early interventionist should know. *Infants and Young Children, 6*, 1–12.

Capper, L. (1996). *That's my child: Strategies for parents of children with disabilities*. Washington, DC: Child and Family Press.

Crosse, S., Kaye, E., & Ratnofsky, A. (n.d.). *A report on the maltreatment of children with disabilities.* Washington, DC: U.S. Department of Health and Human Services.

Dewees, M. (2004). Disability in the family: A case for reworking our commitments. *Journal of Social Work in Disability & Rehabilitation, 3*, 3–20.

Emerson, E. (2004). Poverty and children with intellectual disabilities in the world's richer countries. *Journal of Intellectual and Developmental Disability, 29*, 319–38.

Fujiura, G. & Yamaki, K. (2000). Trends in demography of childhood and poverty disability. *Exceptional Children, 66*, 187–99.

Gibson, C. & Weisner, T. (2002). Rational and ecocultural circumstances of program take-up among low-income working parents. *Human Organization, 61*, 154–66.

Glascoe, F., Foster, E., & Wolraich, M. (1997). An economic analysis of developmental detection methods. *Pediatrics, 99*, 830–8.

Guralnick, M. (1998). Effectiveness of early intervention for vulnerable children: A developmental perspective. *American Journal on Mental Retardation, 102*, 319–45.

Hanley, B. (2002). Intersection of the fields of child welfare and developmental disabilities. *Mental Retardation, 40*, 413–15.

Hebbeler, K., Wagner, M., Spiker, D., Scarborough, A., Simeonsson, R., & Collier, M. (2001). *A first look at the characteristics of children and families entering early intervention services.* Available HTML: http:// www.sri.com/neils/reports.html (accessed 28 November 2006).

Hogan, D., Msall, M., Rogers, M., & Avery, R. (1997). Improved disability population estimates of functional limitation among children aged 5–17. *Maternal and Child Health Journal, 1*, 203–16.

Kates, D. (1997). Funding context for early intervention. In S. Thurman, J. Cornwell, & S. Gottwald (Eds.), *Contexts of early intervention: Systems and settings* (pp. 39–54). Baltimore, MD: Brookes.

Kates, D. (1998). Constructing an interagency funding system for early intervention services. *Infants and Young Children, 11*, 73–81.

Lee, K. (2005). Effects of experimental center-based child care on developmental outcomes of young children living in poverty. *Social Service Review, 79*, 158–80.

Lee, S., Sills, M., & Oh, G. (2002). *Disabilities among children and mothers in low-income families* (IWPR Publication #D449). Washington, DC: Institute for Women's Policy Research.

Leonard, B., & Wen, X. (2002). The epidemiology of mental retardation: Challenges and opportunities in the new millennium. *Mental Retardation and Developmental Disabilities Research Reviews, 8*, 117–34.

Levy, J. (1995). Social work. In B. Thyer & N. Kropf (Eds.), *Developmental disabilities: Handbook for interdisciplinary practice* (pp. 234–47). Cambridge, MA: Brookline.

Lloyd, C. & Rosman, E. (2005). Exploring mental health outcomes for low-income mothers of children with special needs: Implications for policy and practice. *Infants and Young Children, 18*, 186–99.

Lukemeyer, A., Meyers, M., & Smeeding, T. (2000). Expensive children in poor families: Out-of-pocket expenditures for the care of disabled and chronically ill children in welfare families. *Journal of Marriage and the Family, 62*, 399–415.

Meyers, M., Brady, H., & Seto, E. (2000). *Expensive children in poor families: The intersection of childhood disabilities and welfare.* San Francisco: Institute of California.

Meyers, M., Lukemeyer, A., & Smeeding, T. (1998). The cost of caring. *Social Service Review, 72*, 209–33.

Msall, M., Bobis, F., & Field, S. (2006). Children with disabilities and supplemental Security Income: Guidelines for appropriate access in early childhood. *Infants and Young Children, 19*, 2–15.

National Association of Protection and Advocacy Systems. (n.d.). Mission statement. Available HTML: http://www.napas.org (accessed 14 December 2006).

National Institute of Child Health and Human Development (NICHD), Early Childcare Research Network. (2002). Child care structure, process, outcome: Direct and indirect effects of child-care quality on young children's development. *Psychological Science, 13*, 199–206.

Newacheck, P. & Halfon, N. (1998). Prevalence and impact of disabling chronic conditions in childhood. *American Journal of Public Health, 88*, 610–17.

Newacheck, P. & Halfon, N. (2000). Prevalence, impact, trends in childhood disability due to asthma. *Archives of Pediatrics and Adolescent Medicine, 154*, 287–93.

Newacheck, P. & McManus, M. (1988). Financing health care for disabled children. *Pediatrics, 81*, 385–94.

Newacheck, P., Stein, R., Bauman, L., & Hung, Y. (2003). Disparities in the prevalence of disability between black and white children. *Archives of Pediatrics and Adolescent Medicine, 157*, 244–8.

Orloff, T., Rivera, L., Harris, P., & Rosenbaum, S. (1992). *Medicaid and early intervention services: Building comprehensive programs for poor infants and toddlers.* Washington, DC: Children's Defense Fund.

Parish, S., Cloud, J., Huh, J., & Henning, A. (2005). Child care for low-income children with disabilities: A population-based analysis of cost and access. *Children and Youth Services Review, 27*, 905–18.

Parish, S. & Cloud, J. (2006). Financial well-being of young children with disabilities and their families. *Social Work, 51*, 223–32.

Pearson, S. (1996). Child abuse among children with disabilities. *Teaching Exceptional Children, Sept/Oct*, 34–7.

Peterson, C., Wall, S., Raikes, H., Kisker, E., Swanson, M., Jerald, J., *et al.* (2004). Early Head Start: Identifying and serving children with disabilities. *Topics in Early Childhood Special Education, 24*, 76–88.

Rounds, K., Weil, M., & Bishop, K. (1994). Practice with culturally diverse families of young children with developmental disabilities. *Families in Society, 75*, 3–15.

Scorgie, K., Wilgosh, L., & McDonald, L. (1998). Stress and coping in families of children with disabilities: An examination of recent literature. *Developmental Disabilities Bulletin, 26*, 22–42.

Shannon, P. (2004). Barriers to family-centered care in early intervention. *Social Work, 49*, 301–8.

Shannon, P. (2006). Children with disabilities in child welfare: Empowering the disenfranchised. In N. Boyd-Webb (Ed.), *Working with traumatized youth in child welfare* (Chapter 9). New York: Guilford Press.

Shannon, P., Grinde, L., & Cox A. (2003). Families' perceptions of ability to pay for early intervention services. *Journal of Early Intervention, 25*, 164–72.

Sobsey, D. & Varnhagen, C. (1988). *Sexual abuse, assault, and exploitation of Canadians with disabilities*. Ottawa: Health and Welfare Canada.

Social Security Administration (SSA). (2001). *Supplemental Security Income* (SSA Publication No. 05-11000). Washington DC: Author.

Social Security Administration (2006). *Understanding Supplemental Security Income(SSI)*. Available HTML: http://www.ssa.gov/notices/supplemental-security-income/text-understanding-ssi.htm (accessed 22 November 2006).

Striffler, N., Perry, D., & Kates, D. (1997). Planning and implementing a finance system for early intervention services. *Infants and Young Children, 10*, 57–65.

Sullivan, P. & Knutson, J. (2000). Maltreatment and disabilities: A population-based epidemiological study. *Child Abuse and Neglect, 24*, 1257–73.

Taylor, A. (2005). Hidden benefit. *Community Care, 1592*, 50–1.

U.S. Department of Education. (2001). *Twenty-third annual report to Congress on the implementation of the Individuals with Disabilities Education Act*. Washington, DC: Author.

Verdugo, M., Bermejo, B., & Fuertes, J. (1995). The maltreatment of intellectually handicapped children and adolescents. *Child Abuse and Neglect, 19*, 205–15.

Wise, P., Wampler, N., Chavkin, W., & Romero, D. (2002). Chronic illness among poor children enrolled in the Temporary Assistance for Needy Families program. *American Journal of Public Health, 92*, 1458–61.

Critical Thinking Questions

1   Think of all the ways in which children with disabilities were negatively impacted by the passage of welfare reform in 1996. How would you amend the current policy to address the needs of this vulnerable population?

2   The No Child Left Behind Act passed by Congress and signed by President Bush is supposed to make schools more responsive to the needs of all students, especially students living in poverty. Schools that do not show "improvement" can face loss of funding. Think of the ways this piece of legislation can impact schools with large numbers of poor children. What are the risk factors associated with poverty?

3   Think of all the ways that disabilities bring hardship to impoverished families. What kinds of policies would you create to address these hardships? What current policies would you change or eliminate to ease the burdens faced by poor families?

9 Foster Care and Families Apart
Poverty, Placement, and Potential

Carrie Jefferson Smith

The intersection of poverty and child welfare has long been acknowledged and debated, with particular emphasis on the vulnerability of poor children for placement in the foster care system (Billingsley & Giovannoni, 1972; Courtney & Dworsky, 2006). In 1909, a special commission on the care of dependent children advised President Theodore Roosevelt that, barring unusual circumstances, poverty alone should not be used as a reason for removing children from the home (Herman, 2005). Nevertheless, poor families are several times more likely to be separated from their children than families with adequate financial means (Barth, Wildfire, & Green, 2006). Families of color are at even greater risk of having their children placed in foster care than their White counterparts. These disparities are often exacerbated by substance abuse, mental illness, domestic or child abuse, homelessness, parental absence or incarceration, and/or segregated, oppressed, and resource-poor communities. As a result, children and families in the foster system often face a host of challenges that tear the family apart, causing serious emotional trauma, social dislocation, and ongoing economic hardship.

This chapter explores foster care in the context of poverty. After a brief historical overview, I present major issues that confront families, communities, and policymakers, with a primary focus on their impact on children's health, safety, and general well-being. Next, I offer recommendations to reduce the necessity for placements, to assist families toward reunification or other permanent alternatives, and to support families and communities to decrease recidivism of foster care placements.

Foster care in America has its roots in the work of Charles Loring Brace, who in the mid-1800s saw the need to establish a refuge for thousands of unsupervised children (many the offspring of new immigrants) roaming the streets of New York City. His intentions were both altruistic and regulatory: to provide for the needs of unparented children and to protect the public from roaming gangs of desperate youth who routinely engaged in nuisance or criminal behavior in order to survive. Under the auspices of the New York Children's Aid Society, Brace began the first outplacement organization.

Quickly replicated in cities across the country, these agencies sent thousands of children on "orphan trains" to homes throughout the Midwest (Trattner, 1999).

Children of color were generally excluded from these social welfare services since the institution of slavery operating in the South was expected to address the social welfare needs of the slave population (Chipungu, 1991). Even in New York City, which had abolished slavery in 1827, Blacks were not embraced by social service or child welfare agencies (Billingsley & Giovannoni, 1972). Only after funding policies were passed that benefited states financially for foster care placements were children of color brought into the child welfare system in large numbers (Smith & Devore, 2004).

The birth families that became involved in this early outplacing system were viewed as inferior to mainstream families. Many placed children were abused and exploited for their labor. Initially, placing agencies did little to protect birth parents' rights or monitor the children's progress. As awareness grew about the risk to children in an unregulated system, local, state, and federal policies developed to protect the child and parents' rights. Support systems also arose to address the needs of families into which children were placed (O'Connor, 2001). The Social Security Act of 1935 dramatically expanded foster care, providing for aid to dependent children and funding for child welfare services, spawning the current foster care system.

Poverty and Placement: Definitions, Demographics, and Statistics

From the outset, placing children in foster care has been closely connected with poverty. Despite practice principles and policies to avoid removing children from families solely because of poverty, most experts agree that poverty is a causative factor in the decision to place children in foster care. To understand how foster care relates to poverty, it is helpful to review contemporary definitions of key terms and to situate foster placements and outcomes in the context of privilege and power (see Chapter 1 for more detail).

Researchers distinguish two types of poverty: absolute and relative. *Absolute poverty* refers to minimal basic needs for survival or adequate food (calories), shelter, and clothing to protect against the elements. *Relative poverty* is a deprived standard of living compared to other members of society. Despite having basic needs met, people may be considered poor "if they possess fewer resources, opportunities, or goods than other citizens. Relative poverty (or deprivation) can be understood as inequality in the distribution of income, goods, or opportunities" (Karger & Stoesz, 2006, p. 111).

The U.S. government calculates an official *poverty threshold* based on income and family size and adjusts it periodically for inflation using the Consumer Price Index. According to the Census Bureau, an estimated 38.2 million people (18.3%) fell below the poverty threshold in 2005 (Webster & Bishaw, 2006). Approximately 17% of the U.S. child population (12 million children) are poor and about five million live in extreme poverty (less than one half the poverty threshold). The racial breakdown of indigent children in 2004 was 33% Black, 28% Latino, 10% White and 9% Asian (Fass & Cauthen, 2006).

The Purpose of Foster Care and the Role of Foster Parents

Although foster care is usually thought of in a family care framework, it encompasses other placement types, such as residential care and group home placements. Blumenthal's (1983) definition of foster care, which demonstrates both function and practice principles in child welfare (Pecora *et al.*, 2000, p. 296), is used in this chapter:

> the provision of planned, time-limited, substitute family care for children who cannot be adequately maintained at home, and the simultaneous provision of social services to these children and their families to help resolve the problems that led to the need for placement.

The function of foster care is to provide safe substitute care within the practice principles of timely problem resolution and reunification of families. If families cannot be reunited, alternative permanent arrangements are established to ensure child permanence, safety, and well-being.

The role of foster parents has changed greatly since Brace's fledgling system, when they were caretakers of unrelated children who would never return to their parents. Today, foster parents are required to be part of a team designed to enhance the return of children to their parents or to nonbiological parent permanency. In many jurisdictions, when people are assessed to become licensed caregivers, they are evaluated as "resource families" that can become either foster parents or adoptive families. And many contemporary foster parents are relatives of their foster children.

Current Statistics on Children in Foster Care

In 2001, approximately 8.9% of the U.S. population aged 0–17 years lived in foster care (Webster & Bishaw, 2006). The authoritative source for state and national foster care data is the Department of Health and Human Services (DHHS) Adoption and Foster Care Analysis and Reporting System (AFCARS), which collects, "case-level information on all children in foster care for whom state child welfare agencies have responsibility and on children who are adopted under the auspices of the state's public child welfare agency" (USDHHS, 2005, p. 2). Data estimates about foster children are presented in three categories: *point in time* (children in care on a specific day of the year); *entries* (children who entered care during a specific timeframe); and *exits* (children who exited care during a specific time period).

Currently, the U.S. foster care system serves some 800,000 children each year (US DHHS, 2006a). Because states receive funding awards or penalties based on compliance with Adoption Incentive Programs, they often submit updated information beyond their initial report three or more years later, which AFCARS allows in order to improve child foster care and adoption data. The AFCARS data for 30 September 2004 (including updates through 2006) indicate that there were about 517,000 children in foster care placements on that date.

According to the Administration for Families and Children's 2006 estimates, 47% of children in foster care are female and 53% male; 46% live in family foster care settings, 4% in pre-adoptive homes, 24% with paid or unpaid relatives, and 19% in group homes or other residential settings. The rest are in a supervised independent living arrangement (1%), reunited with their parents on a trial basis (4%) or classified as runaways (2%) (USDHHS, 2006a).

Children of color constitute about 58% of the national foster care population (USDHHS, 2006a). While scholarly debate focuses on the disproportionate representation of Black children in the foster care system, in reality White children outnumber Black children, and other ethnicities are counted among children of color. The specific estimates are that non-Hispanic Whites make up 40% of foster children, Black non-Hispanics 34%, and Hispanics 18%. Other children of color include Asian non-Hispanics (1%), Hawaiian/Pacific Islanders (0.2% or 1,057 children), Alaska Native and American Indian groups (2%), and mixed-race (3%). Ethnicity is unknown for the remaining 2% (USDHHS, 2006a). The disproportionate representation of children of color in foster care mirrors the proportion of this group living in poverty.

In addition, roughly 20,000 youth "age out" of foster care annually when they turn 18. Although they have not been adopted or reunited with their families, many of these adolescents are no longer eligible for foster care subsidies although they often lack the skills and resources to support themselves on their own.

Families in the Foster Care System

A child's presence in the foster care system automatically denotes that a finding of abuse or neglect has been made. This finding may stem from a suspicion of abuse that has resulted in an emergency/temporary placement while further investigation is underway or a court determination that abuse or neglect has occurred (including death or incapacity of a caregiver) and the child may not be safely reunited with the birth family until the conditions that resulted in the maltreatment have been resolved.

An estimated three million reports alleging child maltreatment were received by state and local child protective service (CPS) agencies for fiscal year 2004, according to the National Child Abuse and Neglect Data System (NCANDS). Approximately 872,000 children were determined to be victims of abuse or neglect (USDHHS, 2006b) and 305,000 entered foster care (USDHHS, 2006a), including nonvictims (usually siblings) removed during the ensuing child protection investigation (USDHHS, 2006b). More than 60% of child victims experienced neglect rather than direct abuse. Frequently, however, statistical data are inconsistent across different agencies and sources.

The 2004 Child Maltreatment report indicates a greater likelihood of placement among children who are: (1) prior victims of abuse or neglect, (2) disabled, (3) victims of multiple kinds of maltreatment, (4) non-White or (5) abused or neglected by their mothers (USHSS, 2006b). Though basic data on child abuse (types, victim's sex, race, age) and profile information about abusers are kept by states, family descriptive information is lacking. Parent demographic data are not routinely or systematically aggregated for state or national databases, and we generally know little about a family's needs regarding such issues as substance abuse, mental health, homelessness, or employment. In recognition of this knowledge gap, the PRWORA authorized an in-depth longitudinal study of families in the child welfare system. Managed by the Administration for Children and Families, the National Survey of Child and Adolescent Well-Being (NSCAW) runs through 2010 and will gather more comprehensive information about families in the system. Also, NSCAW is examining dynamic program, practice, and policy issues related to outcomes for children and families, and will help guide program, practice, and policy directions in child welfare.

Despite inadequate profile data about the parents, available information suggests they include higher than average numbers of poor, single, or incarcerated parents, the mentally ill (26%), physically limited (22%) and substance abusers (23%) (Macomber, 2006). Since Pelton (1989, p. 63) noted that foster care wards are mostly "poor children from impoverished families," other studies have confirmed poverty as a key risk factor for placement (Barth et al., 2006; Coulton et al., 1995). Almost half of all foster children come from homes eligible for welfare (U.S. Congress, 2004) and nearly half of identified incidents of child abuse or neglect occur in families receiving welfare (Pelton, 1994). Research has established the links among poverty, abuse/neglect, and foster placement. And poverty is associated with other challenges for families that raise the risk of their children entering foster care.

Family Challenges Associated with Poverty and Placement

By definition, impoverished families have fewer resources to resolve problems or provide for children. This puts poor children at greater risk of a finding of abuse or neglect, increasing the likelihood of foster care placement. This section briefly reviews the problematic outcomes for children separated from their families, then discusses special challenges poor families often face that may result in child removal. Finally, I summarize the cycle of poverty as it relates to foster care.

The negative impacts of parent–child separation are well known. Children often experience grief and trauma over being taken from a parent, even for a brief period and even if abused. Feelings of guilt and fear of punishment are common. Foster children have three to seven times more developmental delays, acute and chronic health conditions, and emotional adjustment problems than other poor children (Rosenfeld et al., 1997). Since their physical, emotional, mental health, and social needs are frequently neglected, foster wards are much more likely to remain poor as adults. Thus current research and practice caution against removing children from families unless absolutely necessary.

Single Parents, Father Absence, and Lack of Financial Support

Single parents are more likely to be poor and are at especially high risk of losing children to foster care. MedicineNet (2002) reported that offspring of single parents with annual incomes below $15,000 were 31 times more likely to be viewed by child protective service workers as endangered. A 2003 Urban Institute report (Malm, 2003) analyzing data from over two dozen states revealed that more than half the children in foster care came from mother-only households.

In an Illinois study that reflects national trends in the growth of single-parent homes, Goerge and Lee (2000) found that the number of children living in two-parent homes dropped from 73.1% in 1985 to 67.5% in 1995. Mother-only households increased by 13% (755,000 to 853,000); father-only homes grew from 47,000 to 98,000 (109% increase), and the number of children living with a nonparent grew by 67%, from 52,000 to 87,000. As a result, an increasing number of children are living in families with one caretaker and one income.

The income challenge for families in the foster system is exacerbated by absent fathers who do not provide financial support for their children. The proportion of cases involving noncustodial fathers in the child welfare system is estimated to be much higher than the numbers for children in general (28%) or poor children (29%); 80% of children who enter foster care do not have fathers living in the home, compared with 72% of all children served by child welfare agencies. Malm, Murray, and Geen (2006) found that although the paternity of absent fathers is known for more than 80% of foster and other children in the child welfare system, foster children are at particular risk for diminished relations with their fathers. Only 54% of foster children had had contact with noncustodial fathers in the previous year, compared with 66% of children served by the child welfare system and 72% of children in the general population. One study of four states found that not only were nonresident fathers rarely involved in case planning, but also nearly half were never contacted by the child welfare agency (Malm, Murray, & Geen, 2006).

Financial support from a noncustodial parent is essential to poor children, but a foster child is less likely to receive support from a noncustodial father (16%) than a child in the general population (42%). Such payments are used to repay the state while a child is in foster care and may enhance efforts to return the child to the birth family by providing financial resources to the home. Support may also reduce the risk of a child's removal from an indigent mother. We have little specific data on absent fathers; even less is known about noncustodial mothers.

Incarcerated Parents

Harrison and Beck (2002) estimate that more than 1.4 million parents are incarcerated in state and federal prisons. The majority are men (93%), but incarcerated women are more likely to be the primary caretakers of children so their children's living arrangements are more likely to be disrupted. Fathers are more often imprisoned for violent crimes (46%), mothers for drug offenses (35%). More than half (58%) of the children of incarcerated parents are 10 years old or younger (Mumola, 2000). The majority live with a grandparent (usually the mother's parents) when a parent goes to jail, but roughly 10% of women's and 2% of men's offspring are placed in foster care (Travis, McBride, & Soloman, 2005).

Incarceration creates serious challenges for families in a foster care context (Travis, McBride, & Soloman, 2005; Young & Smith, 2000). Communication and case planning with parents becomes difficult. Maintaining relationships with children is even more difficult, since jails and prisons are notoriously unfriendly in providing child-safe and appealing visitation spaces and timeframes. In addition, permanency time limits for children in foster care may eliminate any real opportunity for reunification because sentencing terms often exceed the government's established 12 months to permanency policy.

Even if an incarcerated parent is able to maintain good connections with her or his children and engage in effective case planning, a parent convicted of a felony may have great difficulty providing for children upon release. Felony status frequently restricts employment, housing, further education, even the right to vote, and public assistance through TANF is denied for life. These restrictions make it much harder for parents to get back on their feet and resume their parenting role once they get out of prison—and they "sentence" children to ongoing poverty and higher risk of another foster placement. Harsh drug policies with extremely long sentences for nonviolent drug offenses have had a disproportionate impact on people of color (mainly women) and poor neighborhoods.

Substance Abuse

Substance abuse may pose the greatest risk of foster placement for low-income families. According to Macomber (2006, p. 3), "As many as 78% of children in foster care have a parent with a history of substance abuse, and [up to] 94% of infants in foster care are born to women who abuse substances." The Child Welfare League of America (1996) has estimated that 48–80% of infants prenatally exposed to alcohol or drugs will need child welfare services before their first birthdays.

Beyond the serious threats of a felony conviction, incarceration and the hardships they cause for families with children, chemical dependency contributes to unemployment, poor health, child maltreatment, and other ills that make parent–foster child reunification difficult. A government study (USDHHS, 1999) found that children of addicted parents remained in foster care an average six months longer (11 months vs. 5 months) than children whose parents did not abuse drugs. They were also less likely to exit foster care within a year (55 vs. 70%). In addition, children of substance-abusing mothers experience a host of behavioral, emotional, and health-related difficulties (Young & Smith, 2000).

Physical and Mental Illness

Poor health and mental illness increase the risks of both foster care and poverty. Illnesses associated with substance abuse include major depression, schizophrenia, HIV/AIDS, hepatitis, and other physical and mental problems. Such conditions, which are costly to treat, are much more prevalent among the parents of children in foster care, and they are likely to inhibit effective parenting, leading to child placement. Without effective drug/medical treatment and followup, such illnesses exacerbate poverty, especially among families in the child welfare system, who often lack adequate health insurance.

Children in foster care have more physical and mental health needs than children in the general population. Although foster children have access to health care, they do not get the kind of care they require on a consistent basis. An USGAO (1995) report estimated that 12% had not received routine health care, 34% lacked immunizations, and only 10% had had services for developmental delays. Moreover, though more than three-quarters of the children were at high risk of HIV exposure, fewer than 10% had been tested (USGAO, 1995, p. 2). Children in relative foster care with relatives also tend to receive fewer health care services.

In recent years, many poor parents have resorted to relinquishing their children to foster care or juvenile justice care in order to get the medical or mental health services their children need (Bass, Shields, & Behrman, 2004). Some states have initiated waiver programs to enhance parents' abilities to provide for their children and thus reduce the need for foster care. Though the cost remains high (up to $12,900 per year per child), such waivers compare favorably with foster care costs ($30,000 per year) and juvenile justice placements ($70,000 per year) (Capriccioso, 2004).

Homelessness

Homelessness is perhaps the quintessential expression of poverty, and substance abuse, incarceration, and physical or mental illness put families at much higher risk of becoming homeless and entering the foster care system. Barbell and Freundlich (2001) estimated that 37% of America's homeless are families with children. Such families face a potential finding of neglect and mandated child placement—or may voluntarily give up their children to foster care (Shinn & Weitzman, 1996). A seminal study (Ooms, 1990) found that homelessness was a factor in more than 40% of foster care placements and the primary factor in at least 18% of cases.

Studies have repeatedly shown the connection between poverty and homelessness among former foster children. In a study of adolescents who had exited foster care in Illinois, Courtney and Dworsky (2006) found that at age 19.5 years, 45% had housing difficulties, and 40% lacked a high school diploma or GED, decreasing their chances of gainful employment. These poor youth are likely to "graduate" from foster care to welfare.

Minimum Wage Jobs: The Working Poor and Immigrant Families

The official poverty line does not include many families who struggle to pay their bills and provide for their children. Near-poverty families are often unable to make ends meet without support. This is important because welfare reform limits lifetime cash assistance, so virtually all welfare system families will be working.

To identify such families, the Urban Institute used a threshold of twice the poverty line, or about $38,000/year for a family of four (Ace, 2003). Using this figure, they suggested that about one-fourth of all working families with children and about one-third of nonelderly families with children are low-income; both groups face challenges paying for food, rent, and other staples of daily living (Ace, 2003). Minimum-wage families may be judged to "neglect" their children because they cannot afford necessities, such as proper clothing. Working mothers face the additional challenge of finding affordable childcare.

There is growing concern about immigrant children and their risk of foster care placement. An estimated one-fourth of all immigrant children live in poor families, compared with 16% of U.S.-born children. They face hardships including insufficient food, inadequate or overcrowded housing, and lack of health care (Zedlewski, 2000). But little data is available about immigrant foster children.

Kinship (Relative) Care and Multigenerational Families

Estimates of children in kinship care arrangements range from 124,153 (USDHHS, 2006a) to 542,000 (Macomber, Geen, & Main, 2003). Figures vary because of differing definitions of kinship care and different data-gathering techniques. The federal office that collects state data (AFCARS) counts only cases for which the state has legal custody of a child, whereas other systems collect data on all cases in the child welfare system.

Research indicates that child welfare agencies rely heavily on relatives in making foster care placements. Using 1997 National Survey of America's Families data, Geen (2003) found that despite variations among states, numbers of foster children living with kin and nonrelative foster parents were similar: About 230,000 children lived with nonrelated foster parents, and 200,000 children were placed in foster homes with relatives after a court determination of abuse or neglect. Half of children in formal kin care "live in low-income households compared with 24% of children living with non-kin foster parents" (Macomber, Geen, & Main, 2003, p. 1). These researchers also suggest that kinship care presents greater hardships for foster children than nonrelative care. One reason may be lack of financial support by government agencies.

Child welfare agencies have the option to formally or informally place children who come to their attention. Formal kinship placements always involve a court determination of child maltreatment. But state agencies may forgo the court process when seeking kin to provide care. Relatives may consent to take in a child before a court intervenes, "to avoid further entanglement with the child welfare system," or to keep a parent from losing custody of the child (Macomber, Geen, & Main, 2003, p. 1).

Formally licensed foster care relatives receive monthly reimbursements plus supportive services (e.g. health care, transportation) for their wards, but agencies do not provide equivalent services to informal (unlicensed) kinship providers. In 2002, 32% of children placed with relatives were cared for by someone who did not receive any form of payment (Macomber, 2006). Research indicates further that 76% of all children in kinship care (formal and informal) live in low-income homes and often do not get the financial assistance for which they are eligible (Macomber, Geen, & Main, 2003). This disparity particularly affects Black children, whose mothers are more likely to die from AIDS or receive drug-related prison terms than the general low-income population. Informal kin care can strain resources and increase poverty.

Most relative foster parents are grandmothers, and the economic issues related to women and poverty persist in their homes. These multigenerational families may face additional stress and economic hardship if the grandparent is also caring for a grandchild's dependent mentally or physically ill parent, especially if they have a low or fixed income.

Foster Care and the Cycle of Poverty and Placements

Though many youth who leave foster care function well, achieving stable families and successful careers, the majority face health, employment, and other challenges as adults. Once in foster care, poor children are unlikely to escape the deprivation of their birth families. This section summarizes negative outcomes for poor foster children, and explores their return to the social welfare or criminal justice systems.

The abuse or neglect that leads to placement often results in physical and mental health problems, developmental delays, educational difficulties, and behavioral problems (Freundlich & Wright, 2003). A 2003 report to Congress (USDHHS, 2006b) indicated that 27% of older foster youth "had a diagnosed disability." These issues are often compounded by negative experiences in foster care (e.g. grief and loss of connections with family, school, and community; separation anxiety; and inadequate attention to medical and psychological needs). Former foster wards may lack the ability to establish healthy bonds because of multiple placements or further neglect or abuse by foster caretakers (e.g. destitute kinship families). Psychological or physical problems often limit educational, employment, and housing options. Risk behaviors, such as drug use and unprotected sex, are also more common among these adolescents, exposing them to addiction, HIV infection, unplanned pregnancy, early childbirth, and single parenting.

Though state laws vary, children typically age out of foster care when they reach 18 or graduate from high school. At emancipation, financial support ends and they are on their own. While some youth have a formal plan of support, many do not. Teens may return to their birth families (and its problems) because they have nowhere else to go. Many end up homeless; Roman and Wolfe (1995) reported that about 3 in 10 homeless adults were formerly foster wards. Moreover, parents who spent time in foster care, and also experienced homelessness or housing instability, are almost twice as likely to have their children placed in foster care as parents who have been homeless but not in foster care. Some foster alumni join the military to seek a better life. Casey Family Programs (2005) reports that these young people are much more vulnerable to post-traumatic stress disorder and mental health problems than other military recruits.

Homelessness, unemployment and a lack of other resources or family support increase the prospect of former foster wards entering the social welfare system as adults. Without adequate health, parenting skills, or economic opportunities, these young people are also likely to become ill-equipped (and indigent) parents and to have their children placed in foster care, with negative outcomes for the next generation of children.

Finally, foster children are more likely to enter the juvenile justice and adult criminal justice systems than the general youth population (Bass *et al.*, 2004). This outcome may be related to having had an incarcerated parent and risky behaviors, such as engaging in drug dealing or prostitution to survive. A criminal justice background contributes to problems finding employment and accessing affordable health care. Even if they avoid future criminal behavior, this pattern reinforces intergenerational poverty and often causes foster "graduates" to rely on welfare programs.

Impacts of Specific Policies and Trends on Foster Care and Child Outcomes

Recent federal policies and national trends have had a significant impact on the foster care system and services to low-income families with children.

Since the passage of PRWORA (1996), states have more autonomy to decide what services or benefits to provide to their constituencies. Touting the need to empower the poor, this "welfare reform" law emphasizes personal responsibility for self and family, establishes work requirements and lifetime limits for cash payments, and strengthens child support enforcement. It also urges that extended families be the first option when children need out-of-home placement. As a result, poor families have exited welfare rolls in large numbers and it is likely that increased placements of poor children have placed a heavier burden on low-income kinship families.

The Adoption and Safe Families Act or ASFA (PL 105-89) (1997) was adopted to respond to the permanency needs of the growing population of children under the supervision and care of child welfare agencies. ASFA stresses the health and safety of children in the system as the main concern in permanency planning. The timeframe to permanency was reduced from 18 to 12 months so foster wards could be moved more quickly into permanent homes. ASFA has made family preservation more difficult for poor parents dealing with incarceration and/or substance abuse. The 12-month time limit for the state to hold the first permanency hearing and petition for termination of parental rights is inconsistent with drug treatment regimens (12 months of sobriety post treatment) and current practices of long prison sentences for drug offenses, denying most incarcerated parents adequate opportunities for reunification planning. In practice, the aggravated circumstances clause for "suspending reasonable efforts" and terminating parental rights under ASFA may be used to declare a child abandoned by a parent, when in reality extended drug sentences prevent reunification within 12 months. Incarcerated parents experience many difficulties trying to maintain contact with child welfare workers regarding permanency issues.

Also, ASFA emphasizes "concurrent planning" (simultaneous planning for family reunification and alternative arrangements) including termination of parental rights. A departure from traditional thinking in working with families, this policy sends a double message, implying that there is little hope for reunification. Such a message may be particularly unsettling in poor communities and to people of color, who often view government intervention in a fatalistic way and give up on having their children returned. Since families involved with the child welfare and criminal justice systems are disproportionately poor, they are at increased risk of losing their children permanently.

Termination of parental rights and freedom for adoption does not necessarily result in adoption, especially for children of color. Many children with incarcerated and substance-abusing parents who are eligible for adoption under ASFA will likely join the estimated pool of 117,000 children who wait an average of 27 months for adoption once they have become eligible (Children's Defense Fund, 2000). Older and special-needs children, especially minorities, may not exit foster care until they age out of the system.

In addition, general political trends since the mid-1980s have limited opportunities and services for impoverished families and children. "War on Drugs" legislation passed by politicians aiming to appear tough on crime not only imposed longer prison terms for drug offenses, but mandatory sentences took away judges' discretion to consider mitigating circumstances. Such policies have been more detrimental to women and children than to men, since women, especially poor women of color, are often exploited by intimate partners/dealers and intimidated or tricked into operating as "mules" to transport drugs. Mandatory drug penalties based on possession fail to take into account abuse or deception cases. As a result, more women lose their children to foster care, more taxpayer dollars are spent on prison costs, and less money is available for needed social services. Another trend that has negatively affected foster children is state legislation or worker bias that hinders gay and lesbian couples from becoming foster or adoptive parents. Such families may be able to provide loving homes and strong financial support to needy children, but may face legal or societal barriers to parenting.

Recommendations and Conclusion

Foster caregivers, child welfare professionals, and birth families form a complex system aimed at addressing the needs of vulnerable children. Collaboration among these groups is crucial for the future success of children and their families. Though the impact of recent policy legislation is not yet clear, research has provided key information about the impacts and outcomes of foster care. Here recommendations are offered that address specific issues for improving the life chances of indigent foster children. They are based on five "best practice" principles outlined by Dougherty (2001) and include: (1) a family focus that views foster care as a service for the entire family, not just the child or parent(s); (2) a child-centered orientation that places individual needs at the forefront of case planning; (3) community-based service delivery so children can remain connected with important people in their lives and live in familiar environments; (4) developmental appropriateness so the care and services children receive are responsive to age and physical, cognitive, behavioral, and emotional status; and (5) cultural competence so the strengths and values of all families are respected and accommodated. Recommendations to improve foster children's life chances include:

• *Improve cultural competence training and work to eradicate biased practices toward poor and minority populations.* Cultural competence training can interrupt practices that contribute to poor outcomes for low-income families, especially people of color, involved in the system. In the past, under state programs, local agencies applied services to various cultural and ethnic groups differently—often inequitably. Block granting allows for a resurgence of such problems, more so if service workers are poorly trained or supervised, so organizations need to train and evaluate workers on cultural sensitivity and issues of equity and equality, and take corrective actions as appropriate.

More agency-based and academic research is needed to better understand racial and class bias and to develop strategies to curtail practices that promote treatment, service, and outcome disparities in historically oppressed groups. The voices of foster children and their parents, foster parents, service providers, and communities affected by foster placement should help shape interventions; such key informants should collaborate in program/service implementation and receive appropriate compensation. In addition, ethical protocols should be ensured, and research outcomes should always be shared with community participants so all stakeholders benefit from the findings.

• *Apply a strengths-based approach to addressing family challenges and aim for family stability whenever possible.* Collaborative strategies in interventions with poor families that focus on their strengths and values have proved much more effective in resolving problems than a directive approach. In decisions about whether to remove a child, aim to build on resilience and adhere to "minimum adequate standards of care" principles, especially in resource-poor communities. Job training, affordable childcare, and special programs such as budget management, should be made available to poor families to assist them in providing for their children. Parents and adolescents can also benefit from parent training, as well as healthy lifestyle, relationship formation, and partner selection preparation. Such skills can help change unhealthy family patterns.

• *Provide adequate support to foster families, including informal kinship care arrangements.* Foster parents are entrusted with the care of our nation's most vulnerable children and are responsible for two-thirds of all foster child adoptions (Grimm & Darwall, 2005). But as a group, foster parents, particularly kinship caregivers, are poorer than families in the general population. When foster families lack adequate financial support or needed services, they cannot provide quality care or engage effectively in planning for good outcomes for their wards (e.g. reunification, adoption, independence). Child-only grants may not meet the needs of children in care, and low-income families, especially foster relatives, are frequently left to struggle on their own and to sink further into poverty. Moreover, little is known about how indigent kin and nonkin foster parents support themselves when there are no foster children in the home. Research is needed to gain this knowledge and to determine the gaps in support for the children they take in. Foster families may require additional financial assistance, job training, or budget management programs. Policies should be adopted to help meet specific needs.

• *Develop policies to help families maintain housing and related services when children are placed in foster care to facilitate reunification.* When children are removed from birth parents, these families often lose their eligibility for low-income housing. Some parents become homeless; many are no longer able to maintain an environment to which children may return. Families need assistance to secure affordable housing so that reunification plans can be implemented in a timely way.

• *Provide adequate medical and mental health services, as well as educational support.* Medical and psychological screenings, diagnosis, treatment, and followup are essential for all foster children, including HIV testing where appropriate (e.g., sexually abused children), in order to address current needs and reduce or prevent long-term medical and mental health issues that contribute to unemployment, addiction, and other problems. Policy changes are needed to provide adequate funding to implement and monitor programs to support assessments and followup. Similar funding is required to provide for the educational needs of children in foster care.

• *Promote policies and provide services to engage fathers and strengthen child support enforcement.* Such efforts, which could benefit thousands of foster children each year, may not only provide better financial support for placement and reunification, but may assist in building long-term emotional support and relationship stability for these youth. Moreover, with growing numbers of father-only households, research is needed to determine whether these homes differ from mother-only households and to assess how to best address impoverished children's needs.

• *Help incarcerated parents maintain connections with their children in foster care and monitor the children more closely.* Child welfare workers may need training to access information to engage incarcerated parents to establish realistic permanency plans under ASFA. They can assist families in navigating the criminal justice system in order to respond to the children's psychological needs, and help implement models for reconnecting people to the community after prison. Such models have shown success in reducing recidivism in incarceration, homelessness, and other negative outcomes that foster poverty. Special liaisons might be used to gather data, examine issues, and search for best practice information on the needs of children of incarcerated parents; they might also provide consultative support to workers monitoring the progress of these children.

• *Promote effective communication and collaboration between welfare and child welfare agencies.* Despite serving many of the same clients, these agencies have had little interaction historically (Macomber, Malm, Fender, & Bess, 2001). Research and cooperation in service delivery can help us better understand the links between poverty and child abuse or neglect and develop best practices for successful outcomes.

- *Develop better support services for adolescents during the transition from foster care to independence.* Aging out of care should not be a graduation to joblessness, prostitution, homelessness, incarceration, or other negative outcomes. Current approaches to prepare foster adolescents for adult responsibilities stress independence and self-sufficiency but do not address developmental issues that support better outcomes (see Propp, Ortega, & NewHart, 2003). Youth exiting social welfare programs need effective discharge planning, opportunities for ongoing support, and mentoring to prevent poverty and related problems. Also, programs should be developed to assist those who might benefit from remaining in foster care past age 18 (Courtney & Dworsky, 2006).

In summary, employing the practice wisdom of prevention is vital to address the challenges of poverty and their impact on foster care. Prevention programs may seem more costly up-front, but the long-term payoff for individuals, families, communities, and the nation is invaluable. Debates about the deserving and undeserving often overshadow the real problems caused by poverty, promote bias, and weaken will toward effective prevention and intervention strategies. Yet the economics of attempting to reconnect shattered bonds and spirits, shelter displaced, grief-stricken children, house the homeless, provide ongoing medical or drug treatment, fight crime, pay for prisons, and restore the lives of the formerly incarcerated reveal the incalculable cost of responding after the system is broken. To produce healthy, well-adjusted, productive citizens, the cycle of poverty and dependence perpetuated by the foster care system must be dismantled.

America's poor families are disproportionately represented in the foster care system, and this outcome is incongruent with expressed public policy and our values of fairness, equity, and social justice. Policy, program and practice areas must be addressed to enhance the prospects for each child and family that encounters the system. Foster placements are designed to be temporary arrangements. Services must insure that foster care will not perpetuate social conditions that tear families apart, maintain poverty, reinforce a cycle of dependence, and reduce the future potential of vulnerable children.

References

Ace, G. (2003). *Five questions for Gregory Ace.* Washington, DC: The Urban Institute.

Barbell, K. & Freundlich, M. (2001). *Foster care today.* Washington, DC: Casey Family Programs.

Barth, R. P., Wildfire, J., & Green, R. (2006). Placement into foster care and the interplay of urbanicity, child behavior problems, and poverty. *American Journal of Orthopsychiatry, 76,* 358–66.

Bass, S., Shields, M., & Behrman, R. (2004). Children, families, and foster care. *The Future of Children, 14,* 5–29.

Billingsley, A. & Giovannoni, J. (1972). *Children of the storm: Black children and American child welfare.* New York: Harcourt Brace Jovanovich.

Blumenthal, K. (1983). Making foster family care responsive. In B. McGowan & W. Meezan (Eds.), *Child welfare: Current dilemmas—future directions* (pp. 299–344). Itasca, IL: Peacock.

Capriccioso, R. (2004). *Foster care: No cure for mental illness.* Connect for Kids. Available HTML: http://www.connectforkids.org/node/571 (accessed 14 January 2007).

Casey Family Programs. (2005). *Assessing the effects of foster care: Mental health outcomes from the Casey National Alumni Study.* Seattle: Author.

Child Welfare League of America. (1996). *Alcohol and other drugs: A study of state child welfare agencies' policy and programmatic response*. Washington, DC: Author.

Children's Defense Fund. (2000). *The state of America's children* (Yearbook 2000). Washington, DC: Author.

Chipungu, S. (1991). A value-based policy framework. In J. Everett, S. Chipungu, & B. Leashore (Eds.), *Child welfare: An Afrocentric perspective* (pp. 290–305). New Brunswick, NJ: Rutgers University Press.

Coulton, C.J., Korbin, J.E., Su, M., and Chow, J. (1995). Community-level factors and child maltreatment rates. *Child Development*, 66, 1262–76.

Courtney, M. & Dworsky, A. (2006). Child welfare services involvement findings from the *Milwaukee TANF applicant study* (working paper). Available HTML: http://peerta.acf.hhs.gov/pdf/cps_involvement.pdf (accessed 20 December 2006).

Dougherty, S. (2001). *Toolbox # 2: Expanding the role of foster parents in achieving permanency*. Washington, DC: Child Welfare League of America.

Fass, S. & Cauthen, N. (2006). *Who are America's poor children? The official story*. National Center for Children in Poverty, Columbia University Malmin School of Public Health. Available HTML: http://www.nccp.org/pub_cpt05b.html.

Freundlich, M. & Wright, L. (2003). *Post-permanency services*. Seattle: Casey Family Programs.

Geen, R. (2003). *Kin foster parents as a percent of all foster parents*. Washington, DC: The Urban Institute.

Goerge, R. & Lee, B. (2000). *The state of the child*. Available HTML: http://www.chapinhall.org/article_abstract.aspx?ar=1286 (accessed 21 December 2006).

Grimm, B. & Darwall, J. (2005). Foster parents: Who are they? Reality vs. perception. *Youth Law News*, 26, 1–8.

Harrison, P. & Beck, A. (2002). *Prisoners in 2000* (Bulletin, NCJ 195189). Washington, DC: U.S. Department of Justice Statistics.

Herman, E. (2005). *The adoption history project*. Available HTML: http://darkwing.uoregon.edu/~adoption/timeline.html (accessed 8 January).

Karger, H. & Stoesz, D. (2006). *American social welfare policy: A pluralist approach*. Boston: Pearson Education.

Macomber, J. (2006). *An overview of selected data on children in vulnerable families*. Washington, DC: The Urban Institute.

Macomber, J., Geen, R., & Main, R. (2003). Kinship foster care: Custody, hardships, and services. Washington, DC: The Urban Institute. Available HTML: http://www.urban.org/url.cfm?ID=310893 (accessed 25 October 2007).

Macomber, J., Malm, K., Fender, L., & Bess, R. (2001). *Welfare reform and opportunities for collaboration between welfare and child welfare agencies*. Washington, DC: The Urban Institute.

Malm, K. (2003). *Getting non-custodial dads involved in the lives of foster children*. Washington, DC: The Urban Institute.

Malm, K., Murray, J., & Geen, R. (2006). *What about the dads? Child welfare agencies' efforts to identify, locate and involve non-resident fathers*. Washington, DC: The Urban Institute.

MedicineNet. (2002). *Is there an association between poverty and child abuse?* Available HTML: http://www.answers.com/topic/child-abuse (accessed 23 December 2006).

Mumola, C. (2000). *Special report: Incarcerated parents and their children*. Washington, DC: U.S. Department of Justice, Bureau of Justice Statistics.

O'Connor, S. (2001). *Orphan trains: The story of Charles Loring Brace and the children he saved and failed*. Boston: Houghton Mifflin.

Ooms, T. (1990). *The crisis in foster care: New directions for the 1990s*. Washington, DC: Family Impact Seminars.

Pecora, P., Whittaker, J., Maluccio, A., Barth, R., & Plotnick, R. (2000). *The child welfare challenge*. New York: Aldine De Gruyter.

Pelton, L. (1989). *For reasons of poverty*. New York: Praeger.

Pelton, L. (1994). The role of material factors in child abuse and neglect. In G. Melton & F. Barry (Eds.), *Protecting children from abuse and neglect* (pp. 131–81). New York: Guilford.

Propp, J., Ortega, J., & NewHart, F. (2003). Independence or interdependence: Rethinking the transition from "ward of the court" to adulthood. *Families in Society, 84*, 259–66.

Roman, N. & Wolfe, P. (1995). *Web of failure: The relationship between foster care and homelessness*. Washington, DC: National Alliance to End Homelessness.

Rosenfeld, A., Pilowsky, D., Fine, P., Thorpe, M., Fein, E., Simms, M., *et al.* (1997). Foster care: An update. *Journal of the American Academy of Child and Adolescent Psychiatry*, 36, 448–57.

Shinn, M. & Weitzman, B. (1996). Homeless families are different. In J. Baumohl (Ed.), *Homelessness in America* (pp. 109–22). Phoenix, AZ: Oryx.

Smith, C. & Devore, W. (2004). Black children in the child welfare and kinship system: From exclusion to over inclusion. *Children and Youth Services Review*, 26, 427–46.

Trattner, W. (1999). *From poor law to welfare state: A social history of welfare in America*. New York: Free Press.

Travis, J., McBride, E., & Soloman, A. (2005). *Families left behind: The hidden cost of incarceration and reentry*. Washington, DC: The Urban Institute.

U.S. Congress, House Committee on Ways and Means. (2004). *2004 Green Book*. Washington, DC: U.S. Government Printing Office.

U.S. Department of Health and Human Services. (1999). *Blending perspectives and building common ground: A report to Congress on substance abuse and child protection*. Washington, DC: U.S. Government Printing Office.

U.S. Department of Health and Human Services. (2005). *Foster care: Numbers and trends*. Available HTML: www.childwelfare.gov (accessed 30 November 2006).

U.S. Department of Health and Human Services. (2006a). *AFCARS: Preliminary FY 2005 estimates as of September 2005*. Available HTML: http://www.acf.hhs.gov/ programs/cb/stats_research/afcars/tar/report13.htm (accessed 25 October 2007).

U.S. Department of Health and Human Services. (2006b). *Child Maltreatment 2004*. Washington, DC: U.S. Government Printing Office.

U.S. General Accounting Office (1995). *Foster care: Health needs of many children are unknown and unmet*. Available HTML: http://www.gao.gov/archive/1995/he95114.pdf (accessed 11 Junuary 2007).

Webster, B. & Bishaw, A. (2006). *Income, earnings and poverty data from the 2005 American Community Survey*. Available HTML: http://www.census.gov/prod/2006pubs/acs-02.pdf (accessed 4 November 2006).

Young, D. & Smith, C. (2000). When moms are incarcerated: The needs of children, mothers, and caregivers. *Families in Society*, 81, 130–41.

Zedlewski, S. (2000). *Family economic well-being. Snapshots of American families: A view of the nation and 13-states from the national survey of American Families*. Washington, DC: The Urban Institute.

Critical Thinking Questions

1   It has been said that every child who enters the foster care system has the right to experience one single, stable foster care placement (rather than being bounced from placement to placement). What are your thoughts about how to achieve a single, stable foster care placement for each child?

2   Smith discusses the challenges faced by families whose children are placed in foster care and offers several recommendations to improve foster care in the United States. In your opinion, what can we expect from foster care? Is foster care successful if the child outcomes are equivalent to outcomes in the general population of poor children? Or are we morally responsible to enhance the future chances of foster children beyond their chances had they remained in their family of origin?

3   Youth "aging out" of foster care are an especially vulnerable group. There are relatively few services and programs to assist them in their transition to adulthood. Many children "aging out" of the system have difficulty finding living situations and supporting themselves and few are able to attend college. Often the services that do exist are inflexible because they tend to be defined by age rather than by service needs. In your opinion, how might their chances of success be improved?

10 Poverty and Education

Alfred L. Joseph and Tammy Anne Schwartz

It is 5.00 a.m. Lisa hears her single mother, Brenda, begin moving in the other room of their small apartment. Brenda is getting ready to head out to work as a waitress for $2.35 an hour. Her tips average $30.00 a day. According to the US government, $120.00 in food stamps should feed a family of four. Little does the government know that the food stamps last about a week. The rest of the month Brenda must rely on neighborhood-based social service agencies to feed her family. Where might the next batch of assistance come from?

Lisa, her two siblings and their mother are tired, because at 3.00 a.m. they were awakened by the sound of the apartment door opening and closing. An intruder had entered and Lisa was awake to hear it. After some terrifying moments, a dash to the only phone located near the front door and a wait, an army of local police appeared at the door and confirmed that somebody was aiming to harm them—someone from a family who deals drugs and lives two buildings away in the same complex. Lisa begs her mother to ask one of her teenaged uncles to move in. It would make her feel safer. Twelve years old and sleeping with fear—constantly. What will happen next she wonders?

On her way to school, Lisa passes a family sitting on the front steps of their apartment building. Their belongings are displayed like a dark closet for the rest of the neighbors to see. Men in suits yell, "Get your damn stuff out of here, lady! Next time you'll pay your rent, won'cha?!!" Her eyes intentionally avoid the eyes of the children and she quickens her pace to get past this scence as soon as possible. Though she dutifully continues to school, she really wants to run back home and beg her mother to make sure their rent is paid this month.

Lisa comes home from school where she is a fifth grader and enters her family's apartment in a government-subsidized housing complex. Due to the vagaries of life that is common to many people with little money, they have moved several times. Lisa tries to start her homework. She finds her mother on the only piece of funiture they have—a bed that doubles as a couch by day. Brenda is sitting and staring. She does not want to prepare dinner. She does not want to clean the apartment. She has been sitting for days in the emptiness while her three children attend school. Lisa's mother is depressed and Lisa knows it. Yes, a fifth grader who lives in constant chaos, fear and worry must grow the necessary radar for these moments, because when they come, Lisa must take on the role of the adult who cleans and makes dinner so that she and her younger siblings will be fed. When might the next day come that requires 12-year-old Lisa to become an adult?

As a child growing up in poverty, Lisa faces a litany of physical, emotional and psychological violations that leave her vulnerable. And then—well, then, there is school. The school environment, at least for children facing the daily material realities of poverty, can be an additional source of vulnerability rather than an intellectually engaging refuge from the unknowns of daily life.

Blaming the Victim

We pass through this world but once. Few tragedies can be more extensive than the stunting of life, few injustices deeper than the denial of an opportunity to strive or even to hope, by a limit imposed from without, but falsely identified as lying within.

(Gould, 1981, p. 28)

These words by the late Harvard paleontologist, Stephen Jay Gould, were directed at those who spent a great deal of time trying to find significant intellectual differences among people that would explain the vast discrepancies in wealth and power that exist in U.S. society. Since America's inception, there has been a tendency to look at the success or failure of people in almost total isolation. American mythology is replete with rags-to-riches stories that highlight the personal qualities of individuals, while downplaying the inherent privileges that come with class position or race. Familiarity with the language and culture are also dismissed as unimportant. If the desire, determination, and ability are there, all obstacles can be overcome. You have no one to blame but yourself. The message is crystal clear: success or failure is squarely upon the shoulders of the individual. Unfortunately, these ideas are not limited to the adult population. They permeate every aspect of U.S. society, including the nations' schools. Study hard, pay attention, obey all the rules, do your homework and you will find success. The work ethic that guarantees success in the outside world is applicable inside the classroom.

Over 30 years ago, William Ryan (1976), in his groundbreaking book *Blaming the Victim*, noted that in order to avoid serious discussions of the consequences of poverty, racism, and great social inequality, many people try mightily to find faults and defects, intellectual and otherwise, in the poor. This is particularly true, he believed, when it comes to children of color. In a chapter about poor children called, "Savage Discovery in the Schools," Ryan explained in some detail that the school experiences for poor children was very likely to be different from their more wealthy counterparts. This happened in a number of ways. For example, Ryan noted that teachers and other school personnel were more likely than not to entertain unflattering assumptions about poor children and their families, a disproportionate number of whom were Black and Latino. At best, teachers had lowered expectations for poor children and, at worst, many teachers believed that their students were intellectually or culturally deprived. Ryan took issue with how the "problem" of educating poor children was constructed. In responding to those who believed that middle-class students were better prepared for schooling than their poorer colleagues, Ryan (p. 37) wrote:

> It would not be unreasonable to present this proposition in its reversed form: The school is better prepared for the middle class child than for the lower class child. Indeed, we could be tempted to say further that the school experience is tailored for and stacked in favor of, the middle class child.

Writing almost 30 years later, Books (2004) echoes some of the same concerns about the treatment of poor children in schools. Though she calls for more research and reform to make schools better, she is apprehensive because these efforts tend to do little more than to focus on "alleged deficiencies." Books wants teachers to focus on, "what's wrong not with the poor but, but rather with a social system that provides a wealth of opportunities for some and constraints for others" (p. 2). It should really come as no surprise that poor children and their families are subjected to more scrutiny and criticism than the nonpoor since this is what the poor are subjected to in society.

Schools should be places where all children, no matter what their social class, race, or ethnicity, are nurtured and provided the opportunity to maximize their potential. Historically, students were to be treated "equally" and given the chance to succeed, their success limited only by how hard they were willing to work and sacrifice. Because of this view of schooling, education has occupied a unique place in American society. Lester Frank Ward, well-known author and scholar, summed up the popular perception of education as a force for equality. Though these words were written over 130 years ago, they still accurately describe this pervasive sentiment:

> Universal education is the power, which is destined to overthrow every species of hierarchy. It is destined to remove all artificial inequality and leave the natural inequalities to find their true level. With the artificial inequalities of caste, rank, title, blood, birth, race, color, sex, etc., will fall nearly all the oppression, abuse, prejudice, enmity, and injustice, that humanity is now subject to.
> (Ward, 1872, as cited in quoted in Bowles & Gintis, 1976, p. 26)

In his book, *American education*, Joel Spring (2000, p. 76), commenting on the common school model, writes that, "children from all social backgrounds enter the common school and receive a common education." Once they have completed their education, students are expected to line up at the "social starting line" and compete "for jobs and status." It is important to note that this view of schooling places the onus on the student for any success or failure that may come their way. This vision of schooling minimizes the impact of poverty, school policies, racism, cultural differences, and different learning styles.

Academic Tracking

One way poor children can have different school experiences is through the widespread and controversial practice of academic tracking: the segregation of students based on curriculum. Tracked students are offered different curricula, such as college preparatory, vocational and general, based on standardized test scores, previous grades, and teacher or counselor recommendations (Joseph & Broussard, 2001; Oakes, 1985). Tracking made its way into U.S. schools at the beginning of the twentieth century during a period of large-scale immigration in which many of the immigrants came from eastern Europe. They were poor, predominantly Roman Catholic and Jewish, and viewed with great suspicion. Their children were ushered into the common schools, but were given a different type of education than their wealthier native-born classmates. They would be in the same buildings but they would receive a very different type of educational experience. Presently, the vast majority of U.S. schools still sort students by curriculum type (Ansalone, 2003; Joseph & Broussard, 2001). Tracking critics, Oakes and Lipton (1999, p. 13) explain:

> Even within the same school, American students usually do not have a common experience. Educators divide students into ability-grouped classes, track them into programs that either prepare for college or provide general or vocational courses, and separate them into special programs for "gifted" or "learning disabled" students.

Labeling students and placing them in various academic tracks sends powerful messages to teachers and to the students themselves. Ireson and Hallam (1999) write that teachers in the lower-track classrooms are more likely to stress conformity and have lower expectations of students, while the work that is done in the classroom is more likely to be highly structured and unlikely to stress critical thinking skills. The schoolwork tends to be centered on learning basic skills, rote learning, and repetition. Unlike students in the higher-tracked classrooms, where students are encouraged to be more analytical and independent in their thinking, low-track students are rewarded more for obedience than creativity. And like anything in our society where poverty is concerned, the impact of this practice is more heavily borne by children of color. Lleras (2006, p. 11), reporting on research with elementary students, found that "Black and Hispanic students are more likely than white students to be placed in lower reading groups for instruction."

Special Education

Special education placement is similar to academic tracking. Educators define special education as "individualized education for children with special needs" (Smith & Luckasson, 1992, p. 6). According to federal regulations (34 Code of Federal Regulations, 300.14), special education refers to "specially designed instruction, at no cost to the parent, to meet the unique needs of a handicapped child, including classroom instruction, instruction in physical education, home instruction, and instruction in hospitals and institutions."

In 1975, the U.S. Congress passed the Individuals with Disabilities Education Act (IDEA; PL 94–142). Addressing the needs of the then estimated two million underserved school-age children with disabilities was an undeniably noble goal. For too long children with "special needs" were largely ignored by the nation's schools. The ones who were allowed into public schools were often segregated, isolating them from their peers. The results of this legislation led to more children graduating from high school and attending institutions of higher education, though the numbers are still much lower than for non-special-education students. What started out with so much promise has, in the eyes of some, turned into the opposite. Instead of helping children harness as much of their ability as possible, critics now believe special education has proven to be dysfunctional for many students. They accuse special education of offering some students neither the instruction nor the curriculum they need to successfully navigate the school system (Losen & Orfield, 2002; Tutwiler, 2007). This is especially troubling when one examines the plight of poor Black and Latino schoolchildren.

Overrepresentation of Black students in programs for students with mental and learning disabilities and for severe behavioral and emotional disorders has been a persistent concern for over 30 years. In 1968, Dunn cited Office of Education statistics to provide evidence of disproportionate representation of students with "low-status backgrounds," including minority group members, in mild mental retardation programs (MMR; originally called educable mentally retarded or EMR). In 1973, Mercer found that the percentage of Black students in MMR special education was three times the percentage of Black students in the population. Nine years after that, Finn (1982) examined national representation trends using data from the Office for Civil Rights (OCR) and reported that Black students were still disproportionately represented in special programs for both emotional disturbance (ED) and MMR. The trends Finn documented were also evident in 1978, 1980, 1982 and, 1984 OCR data (Chinn & Hughes, 1987) and in 1986 (Reschly & Wilson, 1990), 1990 (MacMillan & Reschly, 1998) and 1992 (Oswald, Coutinho, Best, & Singh, 1999). During the same period, Chinn and Hughes (1987) found that Black students were underrepresented in classes for gifted and talented students.

While there have been some discrepancies in findings over the years, most have been due to variations in the operational definitions of "disproportionate representation" used in the various studies. Disproportionate representation, "occurs when the percentage of minority students in special education exceeds the percentage of these students in the total population" (Zhang & Katsiyannis, 2002, p. 180). Given this definition, and despite continued OCR monitoring and repeated litigation, the overrepresentation trend has remained consistent over the years. Artiles, Harry, Reschly, & Chinn (2002, p. 4) have noted that the children most often impacted nationally are "Blacks, particularly males [placed in] mental retardation (MR) and emotional disturbance (ED) programs" and Carter (1996, p. 23) noted that these children are, "usually hyperactive children . . . who get trapped in dead-end special education classes, and lose all prospects of future academic interest or achievement."

If special education instruction was equivalent to regular classroom instruction, this trend might not be problematic. However, as Patton (1998, p. 25) emphasized, students erroneously placed in special education programs "fail to receive a quality and life-enhancing education." In fact, there is general agreement that despite arguments in support of placement in special programs (low student/teacher ratio, legislation to protect student rights, individualized curriculum, guaranteed program funding), students in special education programs experience poor outcomes (Blackorby & Wagner, 1996) and stigmatization (MacMillan & Reschly, 1998). Patterson (2005, p. 311) echoes these sentiments, claiming that the challenge of this crisis is critical to the future of large numbers of poor and minority children. They go to school to be helped, but instead they find services that are inadequate and that almost guarantee "poor educational and community outcomes."

There is much discussion and debate over what causes the overrepresentation of Blacks and others in special education classes. According to conventional wisdom, poverty is a primary culprit. Poverty does put children at a higher risk of disability (Losen & Orfield, 2002; Patterson, 2005; see Chapter 8), but other scholars, like O'Connor and Fernandez (2006), are concerned about the oversimplification of such a complex issue. While acknowledging that poverty plays a role, they believe:

> it is schools and not poverty that place minority students at heightened risk for special education placement . . . there is nothing about poverty in and of itself that places poor children at academic risk; it is a matter of how structures of opportunity and constraint come to bear on the educational chances of the poor to either expand or constrain their likelihood of achieving competitive educational outcomes.
>
> (p. 10)

In a culture quick to blame victims for their predicament, O'Connor and Fernandez (2006) take a more cautious view. Instead of limiting their focus to the "deficiencies" brought into the school by poor children, they turn a critical eye to the education process. They argue that we need to openly acknowledge the reality that schools are essentially White middle-class institutions. White middle-class children set the norms for patterns of speech, behavior, and developmental milestones. They write:

> In the United States, middle-class Whites provide the referent against which other children are evaluated, while U.S. schools privilege the cultural repertoire of the While middle class and are otherwise structured to advantage Whites. In this context, poor and minority youth are destined to "demonstrate" more academic and behavioral problems, which increase their likelihood of being referred for special education. On being referred for evaluation, students are likely to be found eligible for special services.
>
> (p. 8)

Other scholars are also beginning to expand their focus to include other factors that may be responsible for the disproportionate levels of special education placement among minority groups and the poor. Kearns, Ford, and Linney (2005) believe that racist assumptions about the inferiority of Black parenting, the intellectual inferiority of Black students, and the lack of cultural knowledge of other racial and ethnic groups can contribute to an inordinate number of placement referrals. They also believe that overreliance on standardized tests of questionable validity can disadvantage students when referrals are made. And, as they point out quite clearly, once a student is referred to special education for "evaluation and testing," it is almost a certainty that the student will be placed in a special education program. In fact, the high numbers of referrals that lead to placement have caused some to examine issues of bias and misidentification (Kearns, Ford, & Linney, 2005). The numbers seem to support their concerns. From data collected in the 1990s, we see that even though Black students make up only 16% of the public school population, they account for 32% of students identified with a mild mental disability (MMD), 24% of students identified as having a serious emotional disturbance (SED), and 18% of students with a specific learning disability (LD). Recent research confirms similar trends (Kearns, Ford, & Linney, 2005). This is a very serious problem that needs much more study. The impact of placement is not limited to the schoolhouse. Indeed, some believe it has a strong influence on whether a child will even stay in school or not. Heubert (2002) points out that minorities and students with disabilities are likely to perform poorly on so-called high-stakes tests. This often leads to grade retention, which increases the likelihood of dropping out of school. In turn, dropping out of school has a devastating impact on future earnings, increasing the likelihood of remaining in poverty throughout the life course.

Dropping Out

Why children "choose" to leave school prior to graduation is a question that has plagued professionals, parents, and politicians for a number of years. The reasons are probably many and complex. One of the leading experts on dropping out (Rumberger, 2006, p. 131) puts it this way:

> Understanding why students drop out of school is the key to addressing this major educational problem. Yet identifying the causes of dropping out is extremely difficult to do because, like many forms of educational achievement (e.g., test scores), it is heavily influenced by an array of proximal and distal factors related to both the individual student and to the family, school, and community setting in which the students lives.

One of the facts about students who drop out is indisputable: they are overwhelmingly poor and children of color (Spring, 2000; Swanson, 2006). Orfield (2006) believes that this is nothing short of a national emergency that has yet to be fully addressed by the educational establishment. He cites the fact that there is no national systematic way to count and track students who leave school early as evidence of the nation not fully coming to grips with the gravity of the dropping-out problem. Comprehensive statistics, likely because of funding issues, are kept on free lunches and test scores. But no one knows how many children simply disappear from school. Because there are no uniform measures, some school districts list students who have been incarcerated as "transfer students." What is most likely to happen is that students who have left school and who receive a GED or lesser certificates and credentials are not counted as having dropped out.

Many Americans would probably be surprised to learn that only about two-thirds (68%) of all high-school students who enter the ninth grade actually leave the twelfth grade with a regular high-school diploma. Even more disturbing are the graduation rates for children of color (Orfield, 2006). Losen (2006) reports that Black males have the lowest graduation rate at 42%. Native American males follow at 47%, Hispanic males at 48%, White males at 70% and Asian/Pacific Islanders males at 73%. In each ethnic category, the female counterparts have slightly higher graduate rates. This has rightly been described as a national emergency. Students leaving school without diplomas face a decidedly bleak future. Many of them will face a lifetime of sporadic and/or low-paid work. Some will fare worse: they will begin a revolving door relationship with the criminal justice system. The overwhelming majority of the nation's more than two million prisoners are high-school dropouts.

Phil is also a part of Brenda's life: they are a couple. They eventually have a son who they name Brian. Like many poor people Phil had less than an ideal school experience. He struggled to get through and if it were not for the efforts of loved ones, he whould have dropped out. He graduated by the skin of his teeth. No skills—just a piece of paper that insinuated, "Fine, we're through with you. Don't care if you can't read, can't do math. We've done what we can do. Want the paper that stamps you graduated? Fine. Here." Several years later, after receiving Oxycotin for pain related to tooth decay, Phil became addicted. Several years after that, he found himself serving time in prison for theft from his employer, his family and even his own son. While in prison he sent Brenda the following in a letter: "also what we talked about was people not even being able to read. I see it in here first hand."

Like many others before him who did not succeed academically, and later, for a variety of reasons, found themselves in prison, Phil discovered a part of himself that craved reading and other things academic. While in prison, he wrote eloquent letters, read many books about American history, and desired to know more about math. He shared that passion with his fellow inmates by offering to read to them—letters from home, books and legal documents. In that same letter to Brenda he wrote: "I see it [inmates' inability to read] here first hand. I read them their letters or documents, I really feel for them. I not only want to read it to them, I want to teach them how to do it. It would really be something to teach someone how to do that in here." Why does it take this long for folks like Phil to find a connection to school?

Wald and Losen (2007) speak of a "school-to-prison pipeline" in their research on the connections between school and prisons. The numbers are staggering and they are getting worse with no end in sight. High-school completion rates have been falling for quite some time. Wald and Losen (p. 34) report that, "high school completion rates for the decade between 1990 and 2000 fell in all but seven states, with poor and minority students faring far worse than their white, more affluent peers." Few people believe that the situation is improving. Ironically, many believe that this problem is being fueled partly by a piece of legislation designed to enhance the school experience for all children, but especially poor children.

No Child Left Behind

In 2002, just days after being sworn into office, President George W. Bush signed the No Child Left Behind Act (NCLB; PL 107–110). One goal of NCLB is to improve public education across the board, especially for poor children and children of color (Books, 2004). To achieve this goal, as well as several others, NCLB authorizes the federal government to play a larger role in holding schools accountable as they seek to improve academic achievement. High-stakes testing is one of the ways in which schools monitor student progress.

Critics claim that testing leads to more grade retention, which can lead to students making the decision to leave school early (Allensworth, 2006). Another criticism is that since funding will be tied to student achievement (i.e. test scores) schools will have little incentive to keep students whose scores could drag down averages that are probably already low. Losen (2006, p. 50) plainly states that, "NCLB's test-driven accountability could exacerbate resource inequality and make the dropout crisis even worse."

> Brain is now in the sixth grade. His mother, like many of the poor, are mere objects to the economy. They are brought into it when there is need for cheap labor and they are expelled when their labor is no longer required. Brenda is now out of work, and due to financial pressures, her marriage to Phil is now over. She lives in poverty: her family gets by on welfare and food stamps. Recently, Brain has been withdrawn at home. When questioned by an aunt, Brain begins to cry and with great pain tells his aunt, "I'm no good because I didn't pass my proficiency test." He is going to be retained in the sixth grade if he does not go to summer school. The unnecessary burden of shame based on a high-stakes test is painful to witness.
>
> Several years later, Brain struggles in school and has no interest in associating himself with anything academic. His mother now works the graveyard shift bathing the elderly at a nursing home. She is tired and has little energy to be his educational advocate and make a difference. The cycle continues.

NCLB is supposed to go a long way in transforming schools so that they may better serve all students, especially those millions of poor and minority children who have been so ill-served in the past. President Bush and his administration told us that we were to demand and expect success from students and teachers alike. Guided by the "high expectations" operating principle, NCLB was going to reward success and punish failure as documented by standardized tests. Books (2004) is less than enthusiastic about the prospects for success. She argues that the more likely outcome will be to shift dollars away from "failing" public schools to more "effective" private schools. Johnson and Johnson (2006) believe the only beneficiaries will be those who publish the standardized tests and those who offer tutoring services. Clearly, there is great skepticism about whether this legislation will meet the needs of children living in poverty. Although students in high-poverty schools are not achieving the academic success of their peers in low-poverty schools, hope does exist.

For the past 20 years, researchers have been examining the practices of high-performing, low-poverty schools (see Barone, 2006; Bell, 2001; Borman, 2005; Carter, 2000). In spite of the recent top-down, accountability-driven confines of NCLB, educational leaders, administrators, teachers, and visionaries have created some educational environments in which low-poverty students find success. Current research shows that high-performing, high-poverty schools are places with: (a) a focus on academic achievement; (b) clear curriculum choices; (c) frequent assessment of student progress and multiple opportunities for improvement; (d) an emphasis on nonfiction writing; and (e) collaborative scoring of student work (Reeves, 2003). Reeves coined the phrase "90/90/90 schools" to refer to schools where 90% or more of the students are eligible for free or reduced-price lunch, 90% are ethnic minorities and 90% or more meet state or district reading standards. The work being done by Reeves and others is promising. Reeves is concerned about the U.S. inclination to look for easy solutions to complex social problems; the more inexpensive the solution, the more it is preferred. Reeves warns that, "there are no magic potions to deliver improved student achievement. The best that researchers and policymakers can do is to examine the preponderance of the evidence and draw appropriate conclusions" (p. 19). We ignore his advice at great risk.

References

Allensworth, E. (2006). Graduation and dropout rates after implementation of high-stakes testing in Chicago's elementary schools: A close look at students most vulnerable to dropping out. In G. Orfield (Ed.), *Dropouts in America* (pp. 157–79). Cambridge, MA: Harvard Education Press.

Ansalone, G. (2003). Poverty, tracking, and the social construction of failure: International perspectives on tracking. *Journal of Children and Poverty, 9*, 3–20.

Artiles, A., Harry, B., Reschly, D., & Chinn, P. (2002). Over-identification of students of color in special education: A critical overview. *Multicultural Perspectives, 4*, 3–10.

Barone, D. (2006). *Narrowing the literacy gap: What works in high-poverty schools*. New York: Guilford Press.

Bell, J. (2001). High-performing, high-poverty schools. *Leadership, 31*, 8–11.

Blackorby, J. & Wagner, M. (1996). Longitudinal post school outcomes of youth with disabilities: Findings from the longitudinal transition study. *Exceptional Children, 62*, 399–414.

Books, S. (2004). *Poverty and schooling in the U.S.: Contexts and consequences*. Mahwah, NJ: Lawrence Erlbaum Associates.

Borman, G. (2005). National efforts to bring reform to high-poverty school: Outcomes and implications. *Review of Research in Education, 29,* 1–28.

Bowles, S. & Gintis, H. (1976). *Schooling capitalist America—Educational reform and the contradictions of economic life.* New York: Basic Books.

Carter, R. L. (1996). The unending struggle for equal educational opportunity. In E. Lagemann & L. Miller (Eds.), *Brown vs. Board of Education: The challenge for today's schools* (pp. 9–26). New York: Columbia University Teachers Press.

Carter, S. (2000). *No excuses: Lessons from 21 high-performing, high-poverty schools.* Washington, DC: Heritage Foundation.

Chinn, P. & Hughes, S. (1987). Representation of minority students in special education classes. *Remedial and Special Education, 8,* 41–6.

Code of Regulations – Title 34: Education, Part 300.14.

Dunn, L. (1968). Special education for the mildly mentally retarded: Is much of it justifiable? *Exceptional Children, 35,* 5–21.

Finn, J. (1982). Patterns in special education placement as revealed by the OCR Survey. In K. Heller, W. Holtzman, & S. Messick (Eds.), *Placing children in special education: A strategy for equity* (pp. 322–81). Washington, DC: National Academy Press.

Gould, S.J. (1993). *The mismeasure of man.* New York: W. W. Norton

Heubert, J. (2002). Disability, race, and high-stakes testing of students. In D. Losen & G. Orfield (Eds.), *Racial inequity in special education* (pp. 137–65). Cambridge, MA: Harvard Education Press.

Ireson, J. & Hallam, S. (1999). Raising standards: Is ability grouping the answer? *Oxford Review of Education, 25,* 343–58.

Johnson, D. & Johnson, B. (2006). *High stakes: Poverty, testing and failure in American schools.* Lanham, MD: Rowan and Littlefield.

Joseph, A. & Broussard, C. (2001). School social workers and structured inequality: A survey of attitudes and knowledge of tracking. *School Social Work Journal, 25,* 59–75.

Kearns, T., Ford, L., & Linney, J. (2005). African-American student representation in special education programs. *Journal of Negro Education, 74,* 297–310.

Lleras, C. (2006). Looking for roots of educational inequality: The role of ability grouping practices in elementary school. Paper presented at the American Sociological Association Annual Conference. Montreal, Canada.

Losen, D. (2006). Graduation rate accountability under the No Child Left Behind Act and the disparate impact on students of color. In G. Orfield (Ed.), *Dropouts in America* (pp. 41–56). Cambridge, MA: Harvard Education Press.

Losen, D. & Orfield, G. (2002). Introduction: Racial inequity in special education. In D. Losen & G. Orfield (Eds.), *Racial inequity in special education* (pp. xv–xxxvii). Cambridge, MA: Harvard Education Press.

MacMillan, D. & Reschly, D. (1998). Overrepresentation of minority students: The case for greater specificity of the variables examined. *Journal of Special Education, 32,* 15–24.

Mercer, J. (1973). *Labeling the mentally retarded.* Los Angeles: University of California Press.

Oakes, J. (1985). *Keeping track: How schools structure inequality.* New Haven, CT: Yale University Press.

Oakes, J. & Lipton, M. (1999). *Teaching to change the world.* Boston: McGraw-Hill.

O'Connor, C. & Fernandez, S. (2006). Race, class, and disproportionality: Re-evaluating the relationship between poverty and special education placement. *Educational Researcher, 35,* 6–11.

Orfield, G. (2006). Losing our future: Minority youth left out. In G. Orfield (Ed.), *Dropouts in America* (pp. 1–11). Cambridge, MA: Harvard Education Press.

Oswald, D., Coutinho, M., Best, A., & Singh, N. (1999). Ethnic representation in special education: The influence of school-related economic and demographic variables. *Journal of Special Education, 32,* (194–206).

PL 107–110, 107th Cong., No Child Left Behind. (The Elementary and Secondary Education Act).

PL 94 Congress, Individuals with Disabilities Education Act.

Patterson, K. (2005). Increasing positive outcomes for African-American males in special education with the use of guided notes. *Journal of Negro Education, 74,* 311–20.

Patton, J. (1998). The disproportionate representation of African-Americans in special education: Looking behind the curtain for understanding and solutions. *Journal of Special Education, 32,* 25–31.

Reeves, D. (2003). *High performance in high poverty school: 90/90/90 and beyond.* Available HTML: http://www.sabine.k12.la.us/online/leadershipacademy/high%20performance%2090%2090%2090%20and%20beyond.pdf.

Reschly, D. & Wilson, M. (1990). Cognitive processing vs. traditional intelligence: Diagnostic utility, intervention implications and treatment validity. *School Psychology Review, 19,* 443–58.

Rumberger, R. (2006). Why students drop out of school. In G. Orfield (Ed.), *Dropouts in America* (pp. 131–55). Cambridge, MA: Harvard Education Press.

Ryan, W. (1976). *Blaming the victim.* New York: Vintage Books.

Smith, D. & Luckasson, R. (1992). *Introduction to special education: Teaching in an age of challenge.* Boston: Allyn & Bacon.

Spring, J. (2000). *American education.* Boston: McGraw-Hill.

Swanson, C. (2006). Sketching a portrait of public high school graduation: Who graduates? Who doesn't? In G. Orfield (Ed.), *Dropouts in America* (pp. 13–40). Cambridge, MA: Harvard Education Press.

Tutwiler, S. (2007). How schools fails African American boys. In S. Book (Ed.), *Invisible children in the society and its schools* (pp. 141–56). Mahwah, NJ: Lawrence Erlbaum Associates.

Wald, J. & Losen, D. (2007). Out of sight: The journey through the school-to-prison pipeline. In S. Book (Ed.), *Invisible children in the society and its schools* (pp. 27–37). Mahwah, NJ: Lawrence Erlbaum Associates.

Zhang, D. & Katsiyannis, A. (2002). Minority representation in special education: A persistent challenge. *Remedial and Special Education, 23,* 180–87.

Critical Thinking Questions

1   How do schools reflect some of the tensions found in the greater society? Think about dropout rates, special education placements and tracking as you develop your answer.

2   Some have said that schools are a mere reflection of the greater society in which they exist. If this is true, can schools ever really serve all students in a society characterized by massive economic, social, and political inequality?

3   Can schools realistically be expected to provide upward mobility for all people? Why or why not?

11 Going It Alone
Single Motherhood and Poverty

C. Anne Broussard

Single parenthood has long been a popular focus for social commentators, politicians, and academics. At one time or another, it has been blamed for poverty, inherited welfare dependence and the "decline" of the family as indicated by high divorce, declining marriage, and increasing cohabitation rates. Single parents have been faulted for sexually transmitted diseases, substance abuse, food insecurity, violence and reduced family safety, child abuse and neglect, poor academic achievement, lower IQs, poor behavioral and cognitive outcomes for children, juvenile delinquency, childhood obesity, poor physical and mental health, and a host of other problems. Many of these claims have received attention in the scientific literature and relationships among variables often do exist. However, when scientists control for socioeconomic status, most of these relationships simply vanish (see Downey, 1995; Finn & Owings, 1994; Jeynes, 2002; McLanahan & Booth, 1989; Marks, 2006).

Published statistics tell us that there were approximately 3.8 million children in 2.3 million single-parent households in 1970, a number that grew to 49.4 million children in 12.9 million single parent homes in 2006 (U.S. Census Bureau, 2006). Various sources predict that more than 50% of children under age 18 today will spend part of their childhood in single-parent households, and since the proportion of two-parent families has been declining steadily since 1970, a large proportion of young parents also spent part of their childhood with single parents. Despite current attempts to promote marriage and to make divorce more difficult to obtain, single parenthood is a permanent part of the U.S. landscape.

Single-parent families are far more likely to be mother-headed than father-headed. In 2006, 10.4 million single-parent families (more than 8 of every 10) were headed by women, while only 2.5 million were headed by men (U.S. Census Bureau, 2007). That year, close to 30% of mother-only families were poor compared to 13.2% of father-only families and 4.9% of married couple households. The poverty rate is even higher (close to 40%) in Black and Hispanic single-parent families. Macrolevel structural influences that lead to poverty in mother-only families, and the effects of family poverty on children, are addressed elsewhere in this volume; therefore this chapter focuses on the consequences of poor single motherhood for the mothers themselves. Three facets of single motherhood are addressed: (1) Who are they and why are they poor? (2) What constitutes family in mother-only households? and (3) What are the consequences of single motherhood for the mothers themselves? The next section begins by putting a face on single-mother families.

Putting a Face on Single Mothers in Poverty

Who and Why?

In 2004, the majority of single mothers (46%) were divorced or legally separated, just under a third (30.5%) had never married, close to 2% were widowed and the remaining single-mother households represented a combination of grandmothers and other female relatives raising children, women raising non-related children, and married women with absent spouses. While more than half of single parents (57%) had one child, single mothers were slightly more likely than single fathers to have two or more children in the home. Over half (53.8%) the households were White, a quarter (26.8%) Black, 15% were Hispanic and the remaining percentage comprised a mixed category (U.S. Census Bureau, 2006).

Despite the high poverty rate, 8 of 10 single mothers were gainfully employed in 2004 and the majority worked full-time throughout the year. Mother-only families are distributed across the country, but rural states, especially in the south, tend to have higher concentrations of poor families (Lopoo, 2005). While several researchers (Brown & Lichter, 2004; Lichter & Jenson, 2002; Weber, Duncan, & Whitener, 2002) have confirmed that mother-only families in rural areas experience higher poverty rates than those in urban areas, Jolliffe's (2006) recent research suggests that the prevalence and depth of poverty in metropolitan areas might be more extreme (p. iii).

Single-parent families are likely to be poorer than two-parent families for several reasons that have been documented repeatedly in the scientific literature over the past 20 years. The median annual income for mother-only families with children under age six is roughly a quarter that of two-parent families, despite comparable family size of about two children per household. In fact, single mothers with dependent children have the highest poverty rate across *all* demographic groups. According to research (see Seccombe, 2000; U.S. Census Bureau 2007), mother-only families of all racial and ethnic groups are more likely to be poor because women have lower earning capacity, public assistance and childcare subsidies are inadequate, and laws governing child support from nonresidential fathers are not enforced. Moreover, their poverty tends to last a lifetime. Johnson and Favreault (2004) found that women who spent 10 or more years raising children alone were 55% more likely than their married counterparts to remain poor into old age.

The next section describes mother-only families by age group, beginning with teen mothers and ending with custodial grandmother families.

Teens

According to the Department of Health and Human Services (2006), the U.S. teen birthrate, which was highest in 1991 at 61.8 births per 1000 females aged

15–19, dropped gradually to 40.4 births per 1000 in 2005, a 35% decline for that age group. The decrease was more dramatic for younger teens aged 15–17, who experienced a 45% decline. The greatest decline occurred among Black teenagers, with a 59% reduction since 1991.

Nevertheless, close to a million 15–19-year-olds still become pregnant each year, and the U.S. adolescent pregnancy rate remains the highest among western industrialized countries. Why do adolescents continue to bear children at such a high rate? Past research points to many factors including an intergenerational effect. The children of adolescent mothers are significantly more likely to bear children as adolescents than children of older mothers (Barber, 2001; Campa & Eckenrode, 2006). Other important predictors include age at puberty (Newcomer & Udry, 1987), age at first sexual intercourse (Campa & Eckenrode, 2006; Miller, Benson, & Galbraith, 2001), less educationally enriched early home environments (Campa & Eckenrode, 2006), parenting skills (Whitman et al., 2001), substandard educational and career opportunities (Corcoran, 1999), and family poverty and living in a single-parent household (Campa & Eckenrode, 2006; Ellis et al., 2003).

Adults

Most single mothers are adults rather than teens. The "average" single mother is divorced and in her early 30s with one or two children. In 2004, well over a third (36.8%) of single mothers were age 40 and older, up from about a quarter 10 years earlier (Hamilton, Martin, & Ventura, 2006). General birthrates for individual groups in 2005 reveal that women in their early 20s experienced a slight increase to 102.2 birth per 1,000. Among 25 to 29-year-olds, the birthrate was 115.6 births per 1,000, while women aged 30 to 34 exhibited their highest rate since 1964 at 95.9 births per 1,000. Increases for other women in their 30s and 40s were less dramatic, though the rates were higher than they have been in a long time: 9.1 births per 1,000 for women 40 to 44 years and 0.6 births per 1,000 for women 45 to 49 years, the highest rates since 1968 and 1970, respectively (Hamilton, Martin, & Ventura, 2006).

Grandparents

The number of grandparents raising grandchildren has increased in recent years. In 2000, 5.8 million grandparents were residing with grandchildren under age 18 and about 42% were responsible for childcare (Simmons & Dye, 2003). Grandparents who live with and care for grandchildren regularly are called custodial grandparents, and if there is no parent present, the household is known as a "skipped generation household." While many are single, most custodial grandmothers are married women under age 65 (Fuller-Thomson & Minkler, 2000). They are significantly younger than co-residential or noncaregiving grandmothers, tend to live in the south, and to have lower levels of education (Fuller-Thomson & Minkler, Pruchno & McKenney, 2000). Moreover, grandparents often care for multiple grandchildren at a time (Caputo, 1999) and grandparent-headed households tend to last longer than six months (Bachman & Chase-Lansdale, 2005).

Custodial households are especially extensive among poor families and custodial grandparent incomes tend to be lower than noncustodial incomes (Fuller-Thomson & Minkler, 2000). In 2000, 56% of custodial grandparents held jobs and 19% lived in poverty (Simmons & Dye, 2003).

While custodial households can be found among all ethnic and racial groups, Black grandparents have been more likely than Whites or Hispanics to have responsibility for childcare (Simmons & Dye, 2003). Recent statistics show that about 4% of White, 6% of Hispanic and close to 10% of Black children reside in grandparent homes (Bachman & Chase-Lansdale, 2005).

Why are grandparent-headed households on the rise? The literature (Bachman & Chase-Lansdale, 2005; Hayslip & Kaminski, 2005; Ruiz, 2002) suggests that grandparent-led households often develop in response to urgent needs their children experience, such as single-parent relief, teen pregnancy, divorce, incarceration, child abuse or neglect, parental absence or abandonment, and serious health problems or death. Custodial grandparents are included here not only because many of them are single, but also because many are in the caretaking role because their children are single parents.

What Constitutes Family for Single Mothers?

Married versus Unmarried Parenthood

The proportion of children born to unmarried women aged 15 to 44 has increased dramatically during the past several decades from approximately 5% of all births in 1960 to 18% in 1980 to about 37% today (Hamilton, Martin, & Ventura, 2006). Unmarried birth trends differ by age, with older mothers accounting for a growing proportion of nonmarital childbearing at the same time that teen births have decreased dramatically. In 2005, unmarried births accounted for more than half of all births to women 20–24 years and almost 3 of every 10 births to women 25–29. Moreover, recent decades indicate a trend toward multiple children in the home.

While unmarried childbearing has been increasing among all racial and ethnic groups, Ventura *et al.* reported in 2001 that 69% of unmarried births were to Black mothers, compared to 42% to Hispanics and 22% to Whites. Poverty plays a large part in findings like these, since Black and Hispanic families are more likely to be poor than are White families (Trent & Crowder, 1997).

Cohabitation and Age at Marriage

Unlike decades past, marital status does not necessarily indicate the number of adults in the household. Often unmarried mothers reside with the fathers of their children (Wu, Bumpass, & Musick, 2001). In 2006, the Department of Health and Human Services reported that more than 60% of women aged 25–39 had cohabited at least once, an increase that averages more than 1% per year in the preceding decade. Researchers (Carlson, McLanahan, & England, 2004; Mincieli *et al.*, 2007) attribute about half of all births since the 1980s to cohabiting women.

Meanwhile, the median age at first marriage, now approximately 25 for women and 27 for men, has increased from the 1950 ages of 20 and 23, respectively. Many women today choose not to marry at all. According to Graefe and Lichter (2002), 82% of Whites, 62% of Hispanics and 59% of Blacks marry at some time after a nonmarital birth. Yet a study published in 2007 (Bzostek, Carlson, & McLanahan, 2007, p. 2) reported that at a year post-birth, 48% of couples live apart and by five years post-birth, 63% live apart. Moreover, Osborne and McLanahan (2007) found that many unmarried parents repartner (e.g. experience multiple relationships) within a few years of the birth.

The quality of cohabiters' relationships and housing costs play a part in the decision to marry (Sigle-Rushton & McLanahan, 2002). Cohabiting couples in one study were reluctant to marry near the time of the birth for financial reasons. Prior to marriage, they wanted to own a modest home, furniture, a car, and enough savings to purchase an engagement ring and pay for a wedding (Carlson, McLanahan, & England, 2004, p. 7). Couples that earned $25,000 or more in the previous year were more than twice as likely to marry within the year as couples that earned less.

The steady increase in cohabitation coupled with delayed age at marriage or the decision not to marry has changed the family life course. Researchers (Casper & Bianchi, 2002; Manning, 2002) have documented that most remarriages and new marriages now begin with cohabitation. Indeed, several studies (Manning, Longmore, & Giordano, 2007; Manning, 2002; Musick, 2006; Smock, Huang, Manning, & Bergstrom, 2006) assert that rather than cohabiting in response to pregnancy, since the 1990s as many as 50% of couples may be choosing to cohabit in order to bear children and as a possible step toward marriage.

It is clear from cohabitation research that a majority of young adults have been in cohabiting relationships or will enter into them before or in lieu of marriage and that cohabitation is a growing context for childbearing and childrearing.

Consequences for Single Mothers

In 1995, Bowen, Desimone, and McKay (p. 117) stated:

> single mothers in poverty may increasingly find themselves in a "catch 22" situation: They may earn just enough from employment to move them beyond the income threshold necessary to qualify for means-tested public assistance, but not enough to provide for an adequate level of subsistence or to free them from the grasp of poverty.

Unfortunately, this statement still rings with truth. Single mothers face many issues that are less marked for their partnered counterparts: issues that sustain financial instability and prevent them from exiting poverty. The next section addresses some of these issues.

Childcare Costs

Lack of reliable, affordable, safe, high-quality childcare, especially for special- needs children (see Chapter 8), presents a major challenge to low-income single mothers' sustained workforce participation. According to Matthews (2006, p. 2), in 2001 40% of poor single mothers spent upwards of 50% of their cash income for childcare and an additional 25% turned over between 40 and 50%. Indeed, the lower the household income, the higher the proportion that goes to childcare (Anderson & Levine, 2000). This enormous expense prompts up to two-thirds of poor single mothers to seek informal care from relatives and neighbors who are available during the long, irregular hours they are likely to work to get adequate income, especially in rural areas (Smith, 2006). Often individuals who provide informal services for low fees or for free are unlicensed, inexperienced and/or care for too many children at a time. Moreover, educational components, which have been shown to enhance development and school readiness (McCartney, Dearing, Taylor, & Bub, 2007), lack organization and may not be intentional or well-planned (Smith, 2006, p. 3).

Many single mothers are unable to find even poor-quality childcare, which keeps them out of the workforce altogether and forces them to apply for public assistance to ensure sufficient food, housing, and medical coverage. Han and Waldfogel (2001) found childcare costs had a significant negative effect on a mother's probability of working outside the home for all women, but especially for single mothers. They estimated that reduced childcare costs would increase single mothers' employment rate by up to 21%. Indeed, research has shown that subsidized childcare leads to higher likelihood of obtaining and keeping jobs and even to working longer hours (see Matthews, 2006).

Cohabitation versus Marriage

Cohabitation is hard to measure and ongoing research is inconclusive. Carlson, McLanahan, and England (2004) reported that cohabiters in their study tended to be poorer, less likely to be working, less well educated, more likely to abuse drugs and alcohol, and more likely to suffer from depression than married participants. Other research (Brown & Lichter, 2004; McLanahan, Donahue, & Haskins, 2005) suggests that cohabitation can be advantageous to single mothers because it can elevate their economic well-being above that of single mothers living alone (but still far below most married couples).

Nevertheless, federal and state policymakers are involved in an all-out marriage promotion campaign that highlights the negative consequences of cohabitation for families and children. The Bush administration has promoted programs aimed at improving relationship skills for poor couples, and surely all couples could use help building relationships. However, according to Edin, Kefalas, & Reed (2004, p. 8), the success of such programs depends upon more access to, "jobs that lead to financial security, and ... a rewarding life pathway." As is so often said, financial security is the key to alleviating most of the problems poor families face.

Age-Related Consequences

Teens

Research shows that young mothers, especially those under age 15, are at greater risk of birth complications like abnormal bleeding, anemia, eclampsia, hypertension, premature rupture of the uterine membrane and toxemia (Hayes, 1987; Jorgensen, 1993). They are less likely to get adequate prenatal care or to be properly nourished and more likely to experience premature or prolonged labor. Teen mothers are more susceptible to depression, low self-esteem, stress, feelings of helplessness, a sense of failure or despair, suicide attempts, and completed suicides than older mothers (Jorgensen, 1993). Finally, they have higher childbirth morbidity and mortality rates than older mothers (Hayes, 1987).

Decades of research (see Maynard, 1997) demonstrate that the economic consequences for teen mothers are extreme and lifelong, since they tend to complete fewer years of schooling. Older teens tend to make an earlier transition to adulthood, which makes them less likely than teens that remain at home to stay in school. Mollborn (2007) found that teen parents often cut their education short in order to pay for childcare, housing, food, and other necessities. Thus poor teens and teens that cannot continue to live at home leave school for jobs they hope will support them. Past research argues that lower-paying, less-skilled jobs reduce lifetime earnings and make teen mothers more likely to experience poverty, unemployment, and public assistance. Moreover, throughout their lives, their marriages tend to be less stable, they tend to have more children in a shoter time, and more unintended births (Hayes, 1987). Lifelong poverty means that approximately 75% of all children of single teen mothers spend their childhoods in poverty (Cherry, Dillon, & Rugh, 2001).

More current research suggests that the lifelong outlook for teen mothers may actually be better than the outlook for other poor teens. Zachry's (2005) research with young mothers who returned to school led her to conclude that motherhood prompted them to reevaluate the importance of completing school and suggests that adequate finances and a supportive school environment might improve young mothers' life course trajectory. Other research reinforces the conclusion that it is poverty in the mother's family of origin, and not teen motherhood, that is the issue. Using a national sample, economists Hotz, McElroy, and Sanders (2005), found that while teen mothers are less likely to receive a high school diploma, they are significantly more likely to obtain a GED. Furthermore, teen mothers tend to work more hours and achieve higher lifelong earnings than equally poor teens who delayed childbearing, ultimately leading to decreased chances of living in poverty and relying on public assistance.

Grandparents

Grandparents raising grandchildren are more likely to be poor and to face dangerous physical and emotional stress (Bachman & Chase-Lansdale, 2005; Ross & Aday, 2006; Waldrop & Weber, 2001). Their financial stress can skyrocket, largely due to interrupted labor force participation (Casper & Bryson, 1998) and increased health care costs for their adult children, grandchildren (Waldrop & Weber, 2001), themselves (Lee, Colditz, Berkman, & Kawachi, 2003), and possibly a partner. Recently, Goodman and Silverstein (2006) compared custodial grandmothers' poverty across ethnic groups. Despite similar educational levels,

Black custodial grandmothers experienced greater poverty than their White counterparts, while Hispanic grandmothers experienced the highest poverty rates and lowest educational levels.

Custodial grandmothers experience higher levels of psychological distress and depression than the general population (Fuller-Thomson & Minkler, 2000; Goodman & Silverstein). Younger grandmothers (Bachman & Chase-Lansdale, 2005), grandmothers who care for older children, and those who care for children with behavioral or emotional problems (Pruchno & McKenney, 2000) are especially at risk. The convoluted role responsibilities associated with being a parent to multiple generations, a grandparent, a friend to age-peers, and perhaps a spouse, leads to role ambiguity, role strain, and role confusion (Musil, Youngblut, Ahn, & Curry, 2002). Many resent their adult children for being unable to care for their grandchildren. Some feel entrapped in their unanticipated caregiving role (Kelley & Whitley, 2003) and mourn the losses that placed them in the role (Pinson-Millburn, Fabian, Schlossberg, & Pyle, 1996). They worry about their adult children (Pruchno & McKenney, 2002) and feel guilty for resenting them. Custodial grandparents *are* parents who must cope with their adult children's problems, including child abuse or neglect, incarceration, substance abuse, and death. Moreover, they fear compromised relationships with noncustodial grandchildren due to their inability to behave like grandparents and to spend enough time grandparenting (Emick & Hayslip, 1996; Hayslip, Shore, Henderson, and Lambert, 1998). Finally, they worry that their peer friendships suffer from lack of time and attention (Shore & Hayslip, 1994).

Some feel compelled to learn contemporary parenting skills (Hayslip & Kaminski, 2005). A majority face age-related physical limitations and health problems that jeopardize their ability to parent effectively on a daily basis (Kelley & Whitley, 2003; Minkler & Fuller-Thomson, 2001). Many report that daily childrearing activities have prevented them from participating in enjoyable activities alone or with peers and from following through on their old age plans (Jendrek, 1994). Hagestad (1988) calls transitions like this one from grandparenthood into parenthood "countertransitions" because they depend upon the actions of others rather than the individual's own plans.

While custodial grandparents are aware of these issues, they are unlikely to seek help for symptoms, which further jeopardizes their physical and mental health (Hayslip & Shore, 2000). While they are unlikely to seek medical care, they do worry about what would happen if they were to die or if failing health prevented them from providing childcare (Shore & Hayslip, 1994).

Despite the multiple negative consequences associated with custodial grandparenting, most think they would choose to do it anyway, citing being given a second chance at successful parenting and the pleasure associated with the closeness of the parenting relationship (Hayslip et al., 1998) as well as feeling more relaxed, wiser and involved with their grandchildren (Dolbin-MacNab, 2006), and feeling needed and productive (Emick & Hayslip, 1999) in providing a safe, caring home for their grandchildren.

Mental and Physical Health

While social scientists agree that poverty and poor mental health are related, a controversy about the direction of the relationship has been sustained for many years. Some scientists believe that poor women experience greater depression and poorer mental health because of preexisting difficulties. This is called the selection hypothesis. Others hold to a social causation hypothesis that asserts that poverty and its associated risks negatively affect mental health. Most research since the 1990s has supported the latter perspective that single mothers' exposure to higher levels of psychological distress puts them at high risk for mental health issues (Lehrer, Crittenden, & Norr, 2002; Press, Fagan, & Bernd, 2006).

What special risks do single mothers face? In addition to financial insecurity, they deal with food insecurity, discrimination, personal illness, and the poor health of relatives and children. They are more likely to live in unsafe neighborhoods that include violence, substandard housing, and serious environmental health risks, such as pollution from chemical plants. Single mothers are more likely than the general population to have experienced childhood adversity, unemployment, lack of social support, domestic violence, divorce, and separation (Brown & Moran, 1997; Hope, Power, and Rodgers, 1999).

Their stressors tend to be chronic and extreme. Single mothers report more threatening life events, more early childhood adversities and greater chronic stress and deprivation than the general population (Cairney, Boyle, Offord, & Racine, 2003). In 1998, Bassuk, Buckner, Perloff and Bassuk reported that 83% of poor mothers reported having been physically or sexually assaulted and more than a third suffered from post-traumatic stress disorder (PTSD). Cairney and colleagues found that the impact of life events on depression was stronger for single than for married women.

Consequently, single mothers are more likely than partnered mothers to experience mental disorders, including anxiety, depression, and substance use disorder (Crosier, Butterworth, & Rodgers, 2007; Wang, 2004; Hope et al. 1999; Targosz et al., 2003). The greater the financial hardship, the higher the likelihood of poor mental health (Brown & Moran, 1997). Seifert et al. (2000) found that more than 25% of women recently or currently on welfare met the diagnostic criteria for major depression. In research on welfare recipients with small children, Coiro (2001) found that 40% of poor Black mothers reported symptoms that met such diagnostic criteria, while Bassuk et al. (1998) found clinical depression among low-income women, whether homeless or in housing, to be twice the depression rate for women in the general population.

At the same time, they often lack the social support that could help to relieve the chronic pressure. When Cairney et al. (2003) compared single mothers to married mothers, they learned that single mothers reported less contact with family and friends, perceived less social support, and were less socially involved. Crosier et al. (2007) found perceived lack of social support, and financial hardship to be the most important factors contributing to poor mental health among single mothers.

Relationship history is also important. Afifi, Cox, and Enns (2006) compared married mothers to never-married, separated, divorced, and widowed mothers and found that married and never-married mothers were generally similar in their mental health profiles, but separated and divorced mothers were more likely to suffer from a number of disorders, including generalized anxiety and depression. While unmarried mother groups had similar incidences of PTSD, substance abuse and antisocial personality disorder, they were more likely than married mothers to develop these disorders. In their study, DeKlyen and colleagues (2006) included a measure for romantic involvement and found that married parents reported better mental health than all categories of unmarried parents and that nonromantic couples (whether cohabiting or not) reported poorer mental health than did romantic couples.

These relationships hold across age groups, as discussed previously, as well as across ethnic and racial groups and geographic locations. For example, 94% of Black custodial grandparents reported clinically significant stress levels (Ross & Aday, 2006) and custodial Hispanic grandmothers experienced lower well-being (Goodman & Silverstein, 2006). And in her study of over 500 poor, rural mothers, Turner (2006) reported significantly higher levels of lifetime major depressive disorder (37%) than exists in the general population (21%).

Single mothers' poor mental health indirectly affects their physical health over the long term (Wickrama *et al.*, 2006). Prolonged emotional stress has been associated with several physical conditions in single mothers, such as psoriasis, joint pain, hives (Carney & Freedland, 2000) and diabetes (Gavard, Lustman & Clouse, 1993). In addition, McIntyre *et al.* (2003) found that household food insecurity leads some single mothers to compromise their own nutritional intake in order to ensure an adequate diet for their children, a move that increases their morbidity over time.

Effects on Parenting Ability

Studies show that parenting is stressful and has a negative effect on adult well-being across social statuses (McLanahan & Adams, 1987; Polakow, 1993). Important single-parenting stressors include competing work and household roles (Simon, 1995), increased household chores (White, Booth, & Edwards, 1986), foregone education and careers and increased financial and time constraints (Ross, Mirowsky, & Goldsteen, 1990), coupled with childcare difficulties and poor health care access. Also, many health care professionals refuse Medicaid. In addition, some parents, especially rural mothers, must deal with lack of reliable transportation and long commuting distances to work, childcare or school, and lack of health care. Some mothers do not own cars and lack public transportation access, which can prevent them from entering the workforce, accessing health care, or getting to their children's schools for conferences. Another stressful rural issue that is less of a problem for urban parents is lack of anonymity. Rural parents often avoid mental health care because of high visibility in the community (Hoyt, Conger, Valde, & Weihs, 1997) and perceived stigma.

What does this mean for parenting ability? In addition to impairing personal emotional health, higher levels of depression are predictive of more punitive discipline, decreased nurturing and support, and less satisfaction with the parenting role (Ceballo & McLoyd, 2002). Conversely, mothers with strong emotional support tend to be warm and responsive (Marshall *et al.*, 2001), while strong instrumental support leads to decreased use of punitive discipline. It is important to note that all types of support are strained and diminished in poor neighborhoods (Ceballo & McLoyd, 2002).

Social and Community Support

While the effects of social support on psychological well-being are well documented, the source and type (instrumental vs. emotional) of support may make a difference for single mothers (Turner & Turner, 1999). Conflicting results make these relationships somewhat unclear. In 1989, Thompson and Ensminger found that while confiding in a friend reduced sadness and tension, confiding in a family member did not. Also, they reported that living with any other adult improved psychological well-being. In contrast, Jackson (1998) reported that family emotional support, but *not* living with a family member, reduced depression symptoms, while support from friends had no effect on symptoms. More recent research established that emotional support led to lower stress levels over time (Green & Rogers, 2001), but that instrumental support had no effect. And Turner (2006) found that support from both family and friends was associated with lower levels of depression.

Other research (Harknett, 2006; Henley, Danziger & Offer, 2005) has shown that support from family or friends, such as childcare or transportation, can be highly inconsistent and carries a price for single mothers, who are likely to need help at short notice or during irregular hours. Poor women tend to hold low-paying jobs with inflexible schedules, and few if any benefits. They rarely get time off for personal or family illness or other emergencies. Studies (Lein, Benjamin, McManus, & Roy, 2005; Moffitt & Cherlin, 2002) have noted that the informal support poor single mothers receive usually requires financial or other compensation. Reciprocation can be very important to poor, single mothers' friends and family members since they are likely to be similarly disadvantaged (Henley, Danziger, & Offer, 2005).

Custodial grandparents report that the lack of social support and social isolation associated with parenting represents a special burden for them (Ehrle, 2001; Hayslip *et al.*, 1998; Shore & Hayslip, 1994), especially when the grandchildren have emotional, behavioral, or learning problems (Emick & Hayslip, 1999). Musil (1998) reported that the more instrumental and emotional support custodial grandparents perceive, the lower their stress.

Conclusion

The research is clear. Poor single motherhood has lifelong implications for families. Poverty policy, despite multiple changes over the years, is such that many families tend to hover on the edge of poverty, unable to sustain their families independently and unable to qualify for government programs that might provide them with the supports they need to exit poverty once and for all. Single mothers have higher poverty rates than other family types for multiple reasons. They are likely to be divorced, to have been poor as children, and to have lower educational levels. They must attempt to find work in a labor force environment where gender and racial/ethnic inequities persist and where poor-quality educational experiences make it almost impossible to obtain jobs that will support a family. Moreover, they are more likely to have jobs without health benefits and where they are likely to be fired when illness strikes someone in the family. More often than not, single mothers are not in a financial position to pursue additional education that would enable them to get better-paying jobs with benefits packages. They are not likely to receive court-awarded child support payments regularly, or at all, and child support laws are not likely to be enforced. The cost of good, reliable childcare is likely to be prohibitive if unavailable. In contemporary families, an alternative family form—cohabitation—is on the rise. While cohabitation often brings more income into a household, it is not without problems for single mothers and available research suggests that it may not be ideal for the children.

What can be done about pervasive poverty among single-mother families? There are a number of short- and long-term solutions discussed in the literature. Short-term solutions include enforcing the child support laws passed in the 1980s, developing community supports that help individual families make ends meet, developing accessible centrally located community services, and providing childcare subsidies that enable poor single parent families to access quality childcare so that they can work free from worry over their children. Short-term solutions can be helpful but they tend not to enhance the ability to exit poverty for the long term. Alleviating poverty for single-mother families in the United States depends on long-term solutions. These are slow in coming because they involve substantial changes in the political and social structure of U.S. society: for example, changes in gender and racial/ethnic equity in the labor market, accessibility to quality health care coverage, affordable and accessible childcare and availability of quality education for all.

References

Afifi, T., Cox, B., & Enns, M. (2006). Mental health profiles among married, never-married and separated/divorced mothers in a nationally representative sample. *Social Psychiatry and Psychiatric Epidemiology, 41*, 122–49.

Anderson, P. & Levine, P. (2000). Child care and mothers' employment decisions. In D. Card & R. Blank (Eds.), *Finding jobs: Work and welfare reform* (pp. 420–60). New York: Russell Sage.

Bachman, H. & Chase-Lansdale, P. (2005). Custodial grandmothers' physical, mental, and economic well-being: comparisons of primary caregivers from low-income neighborhoods. *Family Relations, 54*, 475–87.

Barber, J. (2001). The intergenerational transmission of age at first birth among married and unmarried men and women. *Social Science Research, 30*, 219–47.

Bassuk, E., Buckner, J., Perloff, J., & Bassuk, S. (1998). Prevalence of mental health and substance use disorders among homeless and low-income housed mothers. *American Journal of Psychiatry, 155*, 1561–64.

Bowen, G., Desimone, L., & McKay, J. (1995). Poverty and the single mother family: A macroeconomic perspective. *Marriage and Family Review, 20,* 115–42.

Brown, G. & Moran, P. (1997). Single mothers, poverty and depression. *Psychological Medicine, 27,* 21–33.

Brown, J. & Lichter, D. (2004). Poverty, welfare and the livelihood strategies of nonmetropolitan single mothers. *Rural Sociology, 69,* 282–301.

Bzostek, S., Carlson, M., & McLanahan, S. (2007). *Repartnering after a nonmarital birth: Does mother know best?* (Working paper 2006-27-FF), Fragile Families and Child Well-Being Study, Center for Research on Child Well-Being. Available HTML: http://crcw.princeton.edu/publications/publications.asp (accessed 4 November 2006)

Cairney, J., Boyle, M., Offord, D., & Racine, Y. (2003). Stress, social support and depression in single and married mothers. *Social Psychiatry and Psychiatric Epidemiology, 38,* 442–9.

Campa, M. & Eckenrode, J. (2006). Pathways to intergenerational adolescent childbearing in a high-risk sample. *Journal of Marriage and Family, 68,* 558–72.

Caputo, R. (1999). Grandmothers and coresident grandchildren. *Families in Society, 80,* 120–6.

Carlson, M., McLanahan, S., & England, P. (2004). Union formation in fragile families. *Demography, 41,* 237–61.

Carney, R. & Freedland, K. (2000). Depression and medical illness. In L. Berkman & I. Kawachi (Eds.), *Social epidemiology* (pp. 191–212). New York: Oxford University Press.

Casper, L. & Bianchi, S. (2002). *Continuity and change in the American family.* Thousand Oaks, CA: Sage.

Casper, L. & Bryson, K. (1998, March). Co-resident grandparents and their grandchildren: Grandparent-maintained families (Working Paper #26). Washington, DC: U.S. Bureau of the Census.

Ceballo, R. & McLoyd, V. (2002). Support and parenting in poor, dangerous neighborhoods. *Child Development, 73,* 1310–21.

Cherry, A., Dillon, M., & Rugh, D. (2001). *Teenage pregnancy: A global view.* Westport, CT: Greenwood Press.

Coiro, M., (2001). Depressive symptoms among women receiving welfare. *Women and Health, 32,* 1–23.

Corcoran, J. (1999). Ecological factors associated with adolescent pregnancy: A review of the literature. *Adolescence, 34,* 603–19.

Crosier, T., Butterworth, P., & Rodgers, B. (2007). Mental health problems among single and partnered mothers. *Social Psychiatry and Psychiatric Epidemiology, 42,* 6–13.

Deklyen, M., Books-Gunn, J., McLanahan, S., and Knab, J. (2006). The mental health of married, cohabiting, and non-coresident parents with infants. *American Journal of Public Health, 96,* 1836–41.

Dolbin-MacNab, M. (2006). Just like raising your own? Grandmothers' perceptions of parenting a second time around. *Family Relations, 55,* 564–75.

Downey, D. (1995). Understanding academic achievement among children in step-households. *Social Forces, 73,* 875–94.

Edin, K., Kefalas, M., & Reed, J. (2004). A peek inside the black box: What marriage means for poor unmarried parents. *Journal of Marriage and the Family, 66,* 1007–14.

Ehrle, G. (2001). Grandchildren as moderator variables in the family: Social, psychological, and intellectual development of grandparents who are raising them. *Family Development and Intellectual Function, 12,* 223–41.

Ellis, B., Bates, J., Dodge, K., Fergusson, L., Horwood, L., Pettit, G., et al. (2003). Does father absence place daughters at special risk for early sexual activity and teenage pregnancy? *Child Development, 74,* 801–21.

Emick, M. & Hayslip, B. (1996). Custodial grandparenting: New roles for middle aged and older adults. *International Journal of Aging and Human Development, 43,* 135–54.

Emick, M. & Hayslip, B. (1999). Custodial grandparenting: Stresses, coping skills and relationships with grandchildren. *International Journal of Aging and Human Development, 48,* 35–62.

Finn, J. & Owings, M. (1994). Family structure and school performance in eighth grade. *Journal of Research and Development in Education, 27,* 176–87.

Fuller-Thomson, E. & Minkler, M. (2000). African American grandparents raising grandchildren: A national profile of demographic and health characteristics. *Health and Social Work, 25,* 109–17.

Gavard, J., Lustman, P., & Clouse, R. (1993). Prevalence of depression in adults with diabetes. *Diabetes Care, 16,* 1167–78.

Goodman, C. & Silverstein, M. (2006). Grandmothers raising grandchildren: Ethnic and racial differences in well-being among custodial and coparenting families. *Journal of Family Issues, 27,* 1605–26.

Graefe, D. & Lichter, D. (2002). Marriage among unwed mothers: Whites, Blacks and Hispanics compared. *Perspectives on Sexual and Reproductive Health, 34,* 286–93.

Green, B. & Rogers, A. (2001). Determinants of social support among low-income mothers: A longitudinal analysis. *American Journal of Community Psychology, 29,* 419–41.

Hagestad, G. (1988). Demographic change and the life course: Some emerging trends in the family realm. *Family Relations, 37,* 405–10.

Hamilton, B., Martin, J., & Ventura, S. (2006). Births: Preliminary data for 2005. National Center for Health Statistics. Health E-Stats. Available HTML: http://www.cdc.gov/nchs/products/pubs/pubd/hestats/prelimbirths05/prelimbirths05.htm (accessed 2 February 2007).

Han, W. & Waldfogel, J. (2001). Child care costs and women's employment: A comparison of single and married mothers with pre-school-aged children. *Social Science Quarterly, 82,* 552–68.

Harknett, K. (2006). The relationship between private safety nets and economic outcomes among single mothers. *Journal of Marriage and Family, 68,* 172–91.

Hayes, C. (1987). *Risking the future: Adolescent sexuality, pregnancy and childbearing,* Vol. 10. Washington, DC: National Academy Press.

Hayslip, B. & Kaminski, P. (2005). Grandparents raising their grandchildren. *Marriage and Family Review, 37,* 147–69.

Hayslip, B. & Shore, R. (2000). Custodial grandparenting and mental health services. *Journal of Mental Health and Aging, 6,* 367–84.

Hayslip, B., Shore, R., Henderson, C., & Lambert, P. (1998). Custodial grandparenting and the impact of grandchildren with problems on role satisfaction and role meaning. *Journal of Gerontology: Social Sciences, 53B,* S164–S173.

Henley, J., Danziger, S., & Offer, S. (2005). The contribution of social support to the material well-being of low-income families. *Journal of Marriage and Family, 67,* 122–40.

Hope, S., Power, C., & Rodgers, B. (1999). Does financial hardship account for elevated psychological distress in lone mothers? *Social Science and Medicine, 49,* 1637–49.

Hotz, V., McElroy, S., & Sanders, S. (2005). Teenage childbearing and its life cycle consequences. *Journal of Human Resources, 40,* 683–715.

Hoyt, D., Conger, R., Valde, J., & Weihs, K. (1997). Psychological distress and help seeking in rural America. *American Journal of Community Psychology, 25,* 449–70.

Jackson, A. (1998). The role of social support in parenting for low-income, single, Black mothers. *Social Service Review, 72,* 365–78.

Jendrek, M. (1994). Grandparents who parent their grandchildren: Circumstances and decisions. *The Gerontologist, 34,* 206–16.

Jeynes, W. (2002). *Divorce, family structure, and the academic success of children.* New York: Haworth.

Johnson, R. & Favreault, M. (2004). Economic status in later life among women who raised children outside of marriage. *Journals of Gerontology Series B: Psychological Sciences & Social Sciences, 59B,* S315–S323.

Jolliffe, D. (2006). *The cost of living and the geographic distribution of poverty* (Economic research report of the UD Department of Agriculture, Economic Research Service, #26). Available HTML: http://www.ers.usda.gov/Publications/ERR26/ (accessed 10 July 2007).

Jorgensen, S. (1993). Pregnancy and parenting. In T. Gullota, G. Adams, & R. Monemayer (Eds.), *Advances in adolescent development,* vol. 5 (pp. 103–40). Thousands Oaks, CA: Sage.

Kelley, S. & Whitley, D. (2003). Psychological distress and physical health problems in grandparents raising grandchildren: Development of an empirically based intervention model. In B. Hayslip, Jr. & J. Patrick (Eds.), *Working with custodial grandparents* (pp. 127–44). New York: Springer.

Lee, S., Colditz, G., Berkman, L., & Kawachi, I. (2003). Caregiving to children and grandchildren and risk of coronary heart disease. *American Journal of Public Health*, 93, 1939–44.

Lehrer, E., Crittenden, K., & Norr, K. (2002). Depression and economic self-sufficiency among inner-city minority mothers. *Social Science Research*, 31, 285–309.

Lein, L., Benjamin, A., McManus, M., & Roy, K. (2005). Economic roulette: When is a job not a job? *Community, Work and Family*, 8, 359–78.

Lichter, D. & Jensen, L. (2002). Rural America in transition: Poverty and welfare at the turn of the twenty-first century. In B. Weber, G. Duncan, & L. Whitener (Eds.), *Rural dimensions of welfare reform* (pp. 77–110). Kalamazoo, MI: W. E. Upjohn Institute for Employment Research.

Lopoo, L. (2005). *Poverty and fertility in the American south* (UKCPR Discussion Paper Series #2005-01). Syracuse NY: Center for Policy Research, Syracuse University.

Manning, W. (2002). The implications of cohabitation for children's well-being. In A. Booth & A. Crouter (Eds.), *Just living together: Implications for children, families and public policy* (pp. 121–52). Mahwah, NH: Lawrence Erlbaum.

Manning, W., Longmore, M., & Giordano, P. (2007). The changing institution of marriage: Adolescents' expectations to cohabit and to marry. *Journal of Marriage and the Family*, 69, 559–75.

Marks, G. (2006). Family size, family type and student achievement. Cross-national differences and the role of socioeconomic and school factors. *Journal of Comparative Family Studies*, 37, 1–24.

Marshall, N., Noonan, A., McCartney, K., et al. (2001). It takes an urban village. *Journal of Family Issues*, 22, 163–82.

Matthews, H. (2006). *Child care assistance helps families work: A review of the effects of subsidy receipt on employment*. Available HTML: http://www.clasp.org/publications/ccassistance_employment .pdf (accessed 1 October 2007).

Maynard, R. (Ed.). (1997). *Kids having kids*. Washington, DC: Urban Institute Press.

McCartney, K., Dearing, E., Taylor, B., & Bub, K. (2007). Quality child care supports the achievement of low-income children. *Journal of Applied Developmental Psychology*, 28, 411–26.

McIntyre, L., Glanville, N., Raine, K., et al. (2003). Do low income lone mothers compromise their nutrition to feed their children? *Canadian Medical Association Journal*, 168, 686–91.

McLanahan, S. & Adams, J. (1987). Parenthood and psychological well-being. *Annual Review of Sociology*, 5, 237–57.

McLanahan, S. & Booth, K. (1989). Mother-only families: Problems, prospects, and politics. *Journal of Marriage and the Family*, 51, 557–80.

McLanahan, S., Donahue, E., & Haskins, R. (2005). Introducing the issue. *The Future of Children-Marriage and Child Wellbeing*, 15, 3–12.

Miller, B., Benson, B., & Galbraith, K. (2001). Family relationships and adolescent pregnancy risk: A research synthesis. *Developmental Review*, 21, 1–38.

Mincieli, L., Manlove, J., McGarrett, M., Moore, K., & Ryan, S. (2007). *The relation context of births outside of marriage: The rise of cohabitation* (Research Brief #2007–13). Washington, DC: Child Trends.

Minkler, M. & Fuller-Thomson, E. (2001). Physical and mental health status of American grandparents providing extensive child care to their grandchildren. *Journal of the American Medical Women's Association*, 56, 199–205.

Moffitt, R. & Cherlin, A. (2002). *Disadvantage among families remaining on welfare* (Working Paper). Madison, WI: Joint Center for Poverty Research.

Mollborn, S. (2007). Making the best of a bad situation: Material resources and teenage parenthood. *Journal of Marriage and Family*, 69, 92–104.

Musick, K. (2006). *Cohabitation, nonmarital childbearing, and the marriage process* (CCPR Working Paper # 010-06). Los Angeles: Center for Population Research, University of California–Los Angeles.

Musil, C. (1998). Health, stress, coping, and social support in grandmother caregivers. *Health Care for Women International*, 19, 101–14.

Musil, C., Youngblut, J., Ahn, S., & Curry, V. (2002). Parenting stress: A comparison of grandmother caretakers and mothers. *Journal of Mental Health and Aging*, 8, 197–210.

Newcombe, S., & Udry, R. (1987). Parental marital status effects on adolescent sexual behavior. *Journal of Marriage and the Family*, 49, 235–40.

Osborne, C. & McLanahan, S. (2007). *Partnership instability and child well-being* (Working Paper 2004-16-FF), Fragile Families and Child Well–Being Study, Center for Research on Child Well-Being. Available HTML: http://crcw.princeton.edu/publications/publications.asp (accessed 31 October 2007).

Pinson-Millburn, M., Fabian, E., Schlossberg, N., & Pyle, M. (1996). Grandparents raising grandchildren. *Journal of Counseling and Development, 74*, 548–54.

Polakow, V. 1993. *Single mothers and their children in the other America*. Chicago: University of Chicago Press.

Press, J., Fagan, J., & Bernd, E. (2006). Child care, work and depressive symptoms among low-income mothers. *Journal of Family Issues, 27*, 609–32.

Pruchno, R. & McKenney, D. (2000). Living with grandchildren: The effects of custodial and coresident households on the mental health of grandmothers. *Journal of Mental Health and Aging, 6*, 269–89.

Pruchno, R. & McKenney, D. (2002). Psychological well-being of Black and White grandmothers raising grandchildren: Examination of a two-factor model. *Journal of Gerontology: Psychological Sciences, 57B*, P444–52.

Ross, C., Mirkowski, J., & Goldsteen, K. (1990). The impact of the family on health: The decade in review. *Journal of Marriage and the Family, 52*, 1059–78.

Ross, M. & Aday, L. (2006). Stress and coping in African American grandparents who are raising their grandchildren. *Journal of Family Issues, 27*, 912–32.

Ruiz, D. S. (2002). The increase in incarcerations among women and its impact on the grandmother caregiver: Some racial considerations. *Journal of Sociology and Social Welfare, 29*, 179–97.

Seccombe, K. (2000). Families in poverty in the 1990s: Trends, causes, consequences and lessons learned. *Journal of Marriage and the Family, 62*, 1094–113.

Seifert, K., Bowman, P., Heflin, C., Danziger, S., & Williams, D. (2000). Social and environmental predictors of maternal depression in current and recent welfare recipients. *American Journal of Orthopsychiatry, 70*, 510–22.

Shore, R. & Hayslip, B. (1994). Custodial grandparenting: Implications for children's development. In A. Gottfried & A. Gottfried (Eds.), *Redefining families: Implications for children's development* (pp. 171–218). New York: Plenum.

Sigle-Ruston, W. & McLanahan, S. (2002). The living arrangements of new unmarried mothers. *Demography, 29*, 415–33.

Simmons, T. & Dye, J. (2003). *Grandparents living with grandchildren, 2000* (Census 2000 Brief, # C2KBR-31). Washington, DC: U.S. Census Bureau.

Simon, R. (1995). Gender, multiple roles, role meanings and mental health. *Journal of Health and Social Behavior, 36*, 182–94.

Smith, K. (2006). *Rural families choose home-based child care for their preschool-aged children* (Policy Brief #3). Durham, NH: Carsey Institute, University of New Hampshire.

Smock, P., Huang, P., Manning, W., & Bergstrom, C. (2006). *Heterosexual cohabitation in the United States* (Research Report 09-606). Ann Arbor, MI: Population Studies Center, Institute for Social Research.

Targosz, S., Bebbington, P., Lewis, G., et al. (2003). Lone mothers, social exclusion and depression. *Psychological Medicine, 33*, 715–22.

Thompson, M. & Ensminger, M. (1989). Psychological well-being among mothers with school age children: Evolving family structures. *Social Forces, 67*, 715–30.

Trent, K. & Crowder, K. (1997). Adolescent birth intentions, social disadvantage, and behavioral outcomes. *Journal of Marriage and the Family, 59*, 523–35.

Turner, H. (2006). Stress, social resources and depression among never-married and divorced rural mothers. *Rural Sociology, 71*, 479–504.

Turner, R. & Turner, J. (1999). Social integration and support. In C. Aneshensel & J. Phelan (Eds.), *Handbook of the sociology of mental health* (pp. 301–19). New York: Kluwer Academic/Plenum.

U.S. Census Bureau. (2006). *Current population survey, 2006 annual social and economic supplement.* Washington, DC: Author.

U.S. Census Bureau (2007). *Income, poverty, and health insurance coverage in the United States: 2006* (Report P60, #233). Washington, DC: Author.

U.S. Department of Health and Human Services. (2006). *Fertility, family planning and the health of U.S. women: Data from the 2002 National Survey of Family Growth* (Series 23025). National Center for Health Statistics, Hyattsville, MD. Available HTML: http://www.cdc.gov/nchs/press room/06facts/births05.htm (accessed 4 July 2007).

Ventura, S., Martin, J., Curtin, S., Menacker, F., & Hamilton, B. (2001). Births: Final data for 1999. *National Vital Statistics Reports, 49*(1). Hyattsville, MD: National Center for Health Statistics.

Waldrop, D. & Weber, J. (2001). From grandparent to caregiver: The stress and satisfaction of raising grandchildren. *Families in Society, 82,* 461–72.

Wang, J. (2004) The difference between single and married mothers in the 12-month prevalence of major depressive syndrome, associated factors and mental health service utilization. *Social Psychiatry and Psychiatric Epidemiology, 39,* 26–32.

Weber, B., Duncan, G., & Whitener, L. (2002). *Rural dimensions of welfare reform.* Kalamazoo, MI: W. E. Upjohn Institute for Employment Research.

White, L., Booth, A., & Edwards, J. (1986). Children and marital happiness: Why the negative correlation. *Journal of Family Issues, 7,* 131–47.

Whitman, T., Borkowski, J., Keogh, D., Weed, K., & O'Callaghan, M. (2001). *Interwoven lives: Adolescent mothers and their children.* Mahwah, NJ: Erlbaum.

Wickrama, K., Lorenz, F., Conger, R., Elder, G., Abraham, W., & Fang, S. (2006). Changes in family financial circumstances and the physical health of married and recently divorced mothers. *Social Science & Medicine, 63,* 123–36.

Wu, L., Bumpass, L., & Musick, K. (2001). Historical and life course trajectories of nonmarital childbearing. In L. Wu & B. Wolfe (Eds.), *Out of wedlock: Causes and consequences of nonmarital fertility* (pp. 3–48). New York: Sage.

Zachry, E. (2005). Getting my education: Teen mothers' experiences in school before and after motherhood. *Teachers College Record, 107,* 2566–98.

Critical Thinking Questions

1   Given what you learned in this chapter about constraints for poor single mothers, suggest ways health and social services providers might work together to help rural women. Do you have different suggestions for urban women?

2   Several chapters have mentioned the marriage promotion agenda. Do you believe that policies that encourage marriage help poor women and their children lead better lives, or are marriage promotion supporters over-promising the benefits of this agenda?

3   Imagine that you are a single parent living on $1,766.67 per month (based on the poverty guidelines for a family of four from Table 1.1) and that you have a number of difficult decisions to make in order to live within your financial means. How would you prioritize your expenses: food, housing, health care, utilities, clothing for you and your children, childcare, school supplies, transportation? Can you think of any other expenses that you might incur? What about entertainment?

12 Old and Poor
America's Hidden Problem

L. Rene Bergeron

Gladys, 82 years old, lives alone:

> I'm not poor. When I was 25, had three kids, and lived in the woods of Vermont I was poor. Winters were hard; my husband drank whatever he earned. My older son and I would catch woodchucks, skin them and can them. Sometimes that was all we had to eat. That was poor. Now I have a roof over my head, I am warm in the winter; I can go to a food pantry once a week. I get a check every month. No, I'm not poor.

"But," I counter, "your health is at risk because you cannot afford your medication. You do not have enough money to have the in-home help that you need. You run out of food every month. You don't think that makes you poor?"

> No. Not when I think back to what my life was like. No. I am old; this is a part of old age. No one wants to waste good resources on the old. We are preparing to die. I do the best I can do. Mothers with children are poor. Not old people like me.

Frank, 83 years old, lives with his wife, Isabel, who is 78 years old:

> I never thought I would end up like this. Never. I worked hard all of my life. Paid my taxes, raised a family. Now I can't afford to live in my own home. I have to put it on the market because I can't afford the taxes, my wife's medication, heating oil, my car, and food. The back stairs need fixing. I can't find someone willing to come to do a small job like that. So, I will take less than market price if I have to because we cannot afford another winter in this house. I shouldn't have to make choices like this. I served my country in war. I held a job since I was 13 years old. I have never been on welfare. I shouldn't have to give up my home. The maddening thing is that no one in this town seems to care. No one wants to consider the choices we old people have to make because of inflation, property taxes, and illness. No one would think of me as poor. But a person with economic security would not be making the choices I am making!

Poverty is both a matter of perspective and reality. How an individual views his or her life situation as being poor is affected by personal perceptions of self-worth and how society views his or her worth. Ageism, discrimination based only on age, greatly influences how the old are viewed by society. This view is reflected in public policy. How the old view themselves is reflected by their attitude toward entitlement. An individual's life experiences also provide a measure for his or her perception of poverty. Gladys's previous experiences with poverty allow her to feel better off than how others might perceive her situation. Because her children are independent and she has no spouse, she is freed from considering their needs along with her own, which also influences her perception. Also, her view of self and old age affects her vision of what she deserves from society. Based on these factors, Gladys feels she is better off than in other periods of her life, thus she asks for very little from the society she interfaces with daily, even though she is at the poverty level.

Frank, on the other hand, is used to having some control over his life. Through consistent employment, he raised his family in a home he purchased. He enjoyed living a comfortable life with his wife and managed the early years of his retirement with some security. But situations beyond his control (e.g. rising taxes, home repairs, the cost of heating oil, his wife's illness and her need for therapy, coupled with her monthly medication) have depleted most of their life savings and forced him to sell his home. Thus he is bitter about the lack of assistance he receives from society. His perception of need is very different from Gladys's. Though selling his home will provide him with some financial security, his perspective is mitigated by his lack of control over the events leading to the sale and his fear that sacrificing his home may not be enough. He does not view himself as a person who should use resources designed for the poor, such as weatherization programs or supplementary heating programs. Therefore he refuses to apply for these resources. Additionally, the community and public policy programs may recognize Gladys's poverty, but not acknowledge Frank's situation because of his resources and the fact that he is not at poverty level.

This chapter provides a profile of old age and the older American family, a definition of elderly poverty, and an examination of how poverty affects the elderly. How individual perceptions and the lack of coordinated public policy programs impact solutions aimed at ending poverty among the aged will be interwoven throughout.

Who Are the Old?

The United States is a nation ambivalent about old age; therefore there is no universal agreement about the chronological age for determining when people enter the old age developmental stage. Individual states, various agencies and organizations, and retirement programs use ages between 50 and 75 years to determine when their old age programs and services go into effect. However, the U.S. Census defines 65 years plus as old age. In this chapter old age is defined as persons 65 years and older living in the United States, and the terms "older American," "aged" and "elderly" refer to persons in that age category, unless otherwise specified.

The growth of the older population in the United States has been dramatic. In 1900, only 3.1 million people were old. In 2000, that number shifted to 35 million and it is projected to grow to 72 million, representing nearly 20% of the U.S. population, by 2030 (He, Sengupta, Velkoff, & DeBarros, 2005). Females outnumber older males beginning at about age 35 when males, due to mortality rates, lose the 5% margin found at birth (He *et al.*). Within the total population the difference is relatively small, 96 males per 100 females, but this difference changes dramatically at 65 years of age with 69.8 males per 100 females. The most dramatic difference is in the oldest-of-the-old (85 years and older) category with 40.7 males per 100 females (Gist & Hetzel, 2004). This has grave implications for older women because more often they are left alone due to widowhood, live longer with more frailties, require higher rates of institutionalized care, and live in poverty in greater numbers than do males (He *et al.*).

In 2000, foreign-born elderly comprised about 11% of the total U.S. population and 10% of the over-65 population. About 62% of these foreign-born elders came to the United States prior to 1970. Non-English-speaking elderly made up 13% of this older population, with the primary non-English language being Spanish. Another 6% spoke English very well in addition to their native language (Gist & Hetzel, 2004). Higher poverty is more likely for elders without English proficiency because they tend to lack both education and the ability to secure better employment.

What Constitutes Family for Older Americans?

Older families may be comprised of family of origin, family by marriage, family of siblings, close friends, and intimate partners. McGoldrick (1982) asserts that families must be defined within an ethnic context in order to fully understand experiences and perception of life situations. The dominant view of the intact nuclear family, a White Anglo-Saxon Protestant (WASP) concept, is not the view held by other groups. For example, Black families consist of kinship networks, Italians consider three or four generations that include close friends and godparents, and Chinese families consider descendants and ancestors in their families (McGoldrick, 1982).

Family expectations also change within ethnic groups. When I worked with older patients in a medical setting, I learned that Greek families expected that the daughter, especially an unmarried daughter, would provide live-in care for aged parents with an emphasis on avoiding institutional care, while French Canadians were not as opposed to intuitional care should the elder's son support it. Mackin (1997) reported that Blacks, Hispanic, and Asian older Americans were more likely to live with an adult child than were non-Hispanic Whites (See Table 12.1).

Rural couples depend on each other, especially when children leave the area for education or other economic opportunities. As rural people age, especially women left without spouses, siblings take on a more significant role and children are expected to provide assistance, especially between mother and daughter (Kivett, 2001).

Table 12.1 Elderly (65+) Living with Children or Other Relatives

	Married Elders (%)	Unmarried Elders (%)
Whites	20	22
Blacks	44	41
Hispanics	48	38
Asians	63	51

Source: Figures from Mackin (1997). Results controlled for economic differences. Data based on samples of people 65 and older from the 1987 American Housing Survey and the 1984 Survey of Income and Program Participation.

Family composition changes over time. Approximately 28% of the elderly population lived alone in 2000, with 7.5 million women compared to 2.4 million men living alone (Gist & Hetzel, 2004). However, living alone does not mean that one does not consider oneself to be a part of a family system. Although it is common in U.S. culture for adult children to move away from their parents, sometimes living thousands of miles away, they stay in touch. The same is true for extended family and friends. And although different ethnic groups view parental caregiving differently, U.S. adult children and other family members do not tend to abandon their elderly.

After widowhood, remarriage—especially for elderly men—is not uncommon, thus reconfiguring past family systems and creating complex systems of stepchildren and other relatives. In fact, 71% of older men as compared to 41% of older women were married in 2003. Even in the oldest-of-the-old category, 56% of men were married compared to 13% of women (He et al., 2005). Remarriage has vast implications for older couples who divorce. Divorce in late life without remarriage may contribute to an elder's isolation and may bring serious financial insecurity. Financial settlements in old age do not allow the recuperation of losses through continued employment opportunities. Some older people may decide to live together rather than marry to avoid the complexity of merging finances or losing various benefits.

Heterosexual couples are not the only type of aged family household. Because gay marriages and civil unions are largely unrecognized in this country, society is often blind to how many older people form homosexual unions. In 2002, Cahill and South estimated that one to three million persons considered themselves lesbian, gay, bisexual, and transgendered, with an expectation that by 2030 this figure could rise as high as four to six million. Yet there is little research on the implications for this age group, especially regarding their financial security as they age.

Another family system of the aged is siblings who live together either because of never marrying, or because of widowhood. Sometimes friends will live together forming strong nonrelated family ties to lessen financial hardships and isolation.

Lastly, there is the grandparents-raising-grandchildren family system. Approximately 2,400,000 grandparents were raising grandchildren in the United States in

2001 (Minkler & Fuller-Thomson, 2005, p. S82). This population is disproportionately female and is prominently Black. The reason for this rising family structure is
a combination of factors that includes single parents' needs as well as parental drug
abuse and incarceration, unemployment, terminal or incapacitating illness or death,
and child abuse, neglect, and abandonment (Minkler & Fuller-Thomson, 2005).

Thus older Americans have a variety of nontraditional households that are complex and that may promote or impede financial security. Further, their problems may
go unrecognized by public policy programs, thus limiting access to financial services.

Who Are the Poor?

Before discussing the elderly poor, it is important to address the wealth of older
Americans. It is in part because of this wealth that poverty among the aged is a
hidden issue in the United States.

The Average Older American

Today's older Americans are better educated, better housed and better-off financially than in previous years. The median income for 65 and older householders
was $23,798 in 2006.

This figure, once adjusted for inflation, is about twice what it was in 1967 (He *et
al.*, 2005, p. 100). Often, income is enhanced by an older person's home being paid
off, or by living in controlled rent districts. Additionally, older people remain in the
workforce after retirement and these earnings contribute to their financial security
(He *et al.*; Gist & Hetzel, 2004). Approximately 74% of working men and 69% of
working women plan for their retirement (He *et al.*) and many save and invest earnings prior to their retirement years (Whitman & Purcell, 2006).

In 2001, the personal money income (PMI) of persons 65 and older was broken down into four major categories: asset income (overall 16% of PMI), pensions (overall 18% of PMI), part-time earnings (overall 24% of PMI), Social
Security (overall 39% of PMI), and 3% originates from other sources (He *et al.*,
2005, p. 95); 10% of older Americans had incomes of $50,000 or more
(Whitman & Purcell, 2006). Even these figures do not adequately show the
financial security of older people because they do not include assets beyond
income or the total household income of a family. In 2004, older Americans with
a total annual income of more than $26,575 had 16.7% coming from their assets
(Whitman & Purcell) indicating at least a partial reliance on asset income.

Retirement in America has changed over the years to include earlier retirements, multiple retirements with benefits attached to each, employment after
retirement, a shift from a focus on men to the inclusion of women in retirement
packages, and a moving away from depending on Social Security as the only
income source in retirement (Hardy, 2002). These changes have made a large
difference in the poverty levels of older Americans. Consequently there has been
a dramatic decrease in overall poverty from one in three in 1960 to one in 10 in
2006 (Whitman & Purcell, 2006).

The above figures provide a robust picture of relative financial security for older Americans, making it difficult for the general public to see the older population as one in need. Additionally, societal and personal ageist attitudes allow policymakers to wear protective blinders against the tenuous financial security of people like Frank in the opening case example. These blinders prevent actions to alleviate some of the poorest conditions of the elderly, such as homelessness. Lastly, there are five major programs available to the elderly and there is considerable general misconception that these programs are sufficient to meet their needs. One, Social Security benefits are tied to employment. Although some employers (e.g. self-employed people) may opt out of offering benefits, few do and more than 95% of all workers pay into the system. In order to collect Social Security benefits one needs to pay into the system for 40 quarters and then meet age or disability requirements (Mold, Fryer, & Thomas, 2004). Two, SSI is available to the aged, blind, or disabled who have limited income and resources. These individuals may also be eligible for Social Security Disability or Retirement benefits (Mold, et al., p. 601). Three, Medicare health insurance is linked to Social Security, and those who do not qualify for Social Security cannot receive Medicare. Four, Medicaid, health insurance for U.S. citizens and qualified aliens, is limited to the poor or near poor, and is run by states with federal government support, with varying qualifiers and services depending on the individual state in which one resides (Mold et al.). Five, several types of governmental, private non-profit and for-profit subsidized housing programs exist for families, the disabled, and the aged who meet eligibility requirements, including monthly and asset income limitation. These five programs have all contributed to making general poverty among older people a thing of the past. Yet a considerable proportion of the elderly population is very much alive and not so well in the American landscape.

Older Americans Susceptible to Poverty

In general, people are considered poor when they do not have the resources to meet basic food, clothing, health, and housing needs, thereby living in a substandard situation. Formally, however, persons are considered to be living in poverty if their income (before taxes) is below a government-designated level that is set on an annual basis. The formula for the poverty level considers the income necessary to obtain and sustain adequate nutrition and minimum housing. The poverty level is standard for the entire United States and does not consider cost variations found in different geographic locations, although it is adjusted based on household size. In 2006, the poverty level was set at $9,800 for a one-person family unit and at $13,200 for a two-person family unit (Federal Register, 2006).

Poverty rates increase in the older age groups of the elderly. In 2003, the overall poverty rate among the elderly was 10.2% (about 3.6 million) (He et al., 2005; Hall & Brown, 2005). Of that percentage, 2.6% lived below 50% of the poverty level (Hall & Brown). Poverty rates become disproportionate the older one becomes. For example, in 2003 the poverty rate for persons 65–74 years of age was 9%, but this figure rose to 12% for the aged 75 years and older (He et al.).

The Gender Issue

For women, poverty statistics are more dramatic. Although both men and women plan for retirement, women remain at a disadvantage because of their high employment in the service industry, interruption of work due to family obligations, and less advantageous retirement packages to couple with their Social Security benefits. He *et al.* (2005, p. 93) reported that in 1999 women "aged 65 and over received, on average, $8,224 as pension income as from an annuity and/or an employment-based pension plan, compared with $14,046 paid to their male counterparts." The same trend exists for Social Security benefits. Figures for 1999 showed women, on average, received $697 per month compared to the $905 men received (He *et al.*, p. 93). Additionally, certain groups, such as rural women, follow traditional marriage roles (e.g. homemaking, depending solely on the earnings and pension of their spouse), leaving them even more vulnerable (Kivett, 2001). Therefore women like Gladys, who have grown old being poor, will most surely remain poor even if they qualify for various social programs.

In 2003, 7% of older men lived in poverty, while 13% of older women did so (He *et al.*, 2005). Non-Hispanic Whites living alone had poverty rates of 17%, while the rate for Black and Hispanic women living alone was 40% (He *et al.*, 2005). Institutional sexism is demonstrated in the above poverty figures. Thus older women, especially minority women, are more likely victims of poverty than men. This phenomenon has been called "double jeopardy" because aging women must confront the effects of ageism and sexism, both of which contribute to their being poor. Minority women face even greater challenges than White women because of racism, which reduces their educational and occupational opportunities. Therefore, it is clear that women suffer more from poverty than men, single women suffer more than married women, women living alone suffer more than those living with family, and minority women living alone are in the greatest jeopardy.

Widowhood

Although the financial situation of elderly widowed women has greatly improved since the 1970s, when nearly "37% of new widows became poor after widowhood" (Sevak, Weir, & Willis, 2003/4, p. 31), to 12–15% in 1990 (Sevak, *et al.*), it still remains an important indicator of poverty for women. McGarry and Schoent (2005, p. 58) note that over the past 30 years poverty rates are still three to four times higher for elderly widows than for married older women. While part of this results from pension structures, a large part may be a result of women living longer than men and being caregivers to their ill spouses, or having provided care for an aged relative in their middle-age years, or providing care to grandchildren in their later years. Because of inadequate health care coverage in this country for acute and chronic conditions, personal savings and assets become an important means by which health care costs are met. The surviving spouse is then left in a tenuous living situation (McGarry & Schoent). Also, poverty is linked negatively to longevity among men—the poorer the male, the younger he dies. Thus women married to poor men lose their spouses earlier than nonpoor women, have a shorter time span to use the husband's retirement funds, and have a history of poverty that has not provided them with the means to break the cycle (McGarry & Schoent). Those of lower-income status rely on Social Security as their sole retirement pension, with perhaps some assistance from SSI, much more so than women of higher-income status. That is risky, because upon the death of a spouse Social Security benefits are reduced by one-third and this reduction may be just enough to move one from being near-poor to being below poverty. Surviving spouses could find that they fall into poverty if the spouse who dies had been working part-time, or carried the couple's various pension plans (McGarry & Schoent). Thus the situation Gladys faces in her old age is very typical, given her poverty history.

The Near-Poor

The overall 10.2% of older people in poverty takes on an additional 6.7% of the older population if consideration is given to those at the near-poverty level. Nearly poor people are those whose income is at or just slightly above the poverty line set by the federal government. Whitman and Purcell (2006) reported that 9.8% of the older population had incomes below the poverty level in 2004. However, if the near-poor are taken into account, then 38% of Americans 65 years and older had family incomes less than *twice* the poverty level (p. 53). Having incomes slightly above the poverty line often disqualifies them for programs that would assist their marginalized living conditions. These people live their lives making difficult choices that affect nutrition, medical care, housing, and leisure activity on a daily basis.

Older Rural People

The experience of aging is different in rural America than in metropolitan areas. Nonmetropolitan counties cover about 80% of the U.S. land mass, yet only 20% of the overall population lives there. About 15% of that population is over 65 as compared to about 11% in metropolitan areas (Roff & Klemmack, 2003). Rural elders tend to be White, male, married, depend on Social Security as their only pension, and to have lower educational attainment. Some 7.8 million older Americans live in nonmetropolitan areas although numbers vary depending on the region. These areas also have disproportionately poor elders and near-poor elders: 12% poor and 29% near-poor rural elders compared to 9.5% poor and 13.4% near-poor metropolitan elders. Ethnic groups have higher rates of poverty in rural America than their city-dwelling counterparts, including American Indians and Aleut Eskimos (28.5% of rural elders versus 6.5% of urban elders) (Roff & Klemmack). According to Golant (2006: 38), "more than one out of every three rural elderly Black residents age 75 or older is impoverished" compared to about one in five of their urban counterparts (Roff & Kemmack). Among Hispanics, the proportions of poor rural and urban residents were nearly equal in 2002 (22.1% in rural areas versus 21.8% in urban areas (Roff & Klemmack).

Other Considerations

Poverty among elders is complex and there are several conditions that may promote some groups to withstand the events that may promote poverty and others who because of their conditions fall into poverty.

Lack of Opportunity to Live with Others

Living with others greatly reduces the chance that an elder will feel the full effects of poverty. Mackin (1997) reported that if those over 65 years of age did not live with their adult children or other relatives, poverty would increase by almost 42% among the elderly population. Therefore, older people who do not have this opportunity have a greater chance of living in poverty. In 2000, approximately every tenth middle-aged person had one family member who was 85 years or older to whom he or she provided some type of caregiving. By 2050, this ratio is projected to be 30% (He et al., 2005). Unless baby boomers, especially women, plan carefully for financial security beyond their 70s, they may not have the various safety nets that provide a cushion against poverty-producing situations. Such situations include lack of support from adult children; and expending more than they can afford in the provision of care to aging relatives. This, and the reality that various assistance programs may provide less assistance as numbers of elderly "boomers" increase, can further impede their own financial security.

Grandparents Raising Grandchildren

The grandparents-raising-grandchildren family system, particularly those households where no parent is present, is especially susceptible to poverty (Mills, Gomez-Smith, & DeLeon, 2005). In 1997, 2.5 million households headed by grandparents housed 3.9 million children under the age of 18, and 1.3 million of these children did not have parents in that household (Smith, Beltran, Butts, & Kingson, 2000), with about 51% of the children age six or younger (Mills, et al.). In grandparent-headed households where at least one biological parents is present, the figure jumps from 3.9 to 5.6 million children (Smith et al.). About 13.5% of Black children, 6.5% of Hispanic children, and 4.1% of White children live in grandparent-headed households (Smith, et al.) and the Black grandparents are more likely to be "unemployed, live below the poverty line and have more grandchildren for whom they provide care" (Mills et al., p. 195). Several policies enacted by the federal government support and encourage children being placed in the foster care of their grandparents. For example, the Indian Child Welfare Act of 1978, the 1980 Adoption Assistance and Child Welfare Act, and the 1997 Adoption and Safe Families Act all have contributed to the reduction of children in traditional placements in order to secure care with relatives, including grandparents (Smith et al.)

Like caregivers to aged parents, grandparents caring for their grandchildren tend to neglect their own health and needs. Additionally, high stress in the provision of care compromises the health and psychological well-being of the grandparents. For example, if children have seen a lot of trauma, or come from violent and substance abusing households, or have been victims of abuse and neglect—as they typically have—then they are apt to need higher levels of care and have higher incidence of behavioral problems, increasing the responsibilities and expenses for the grandparents (Mills *et al.*, 2005). These households respond to stress through adaptation, such as by moving to more affordable housing or cutting back on expenses, returning to the workforce, or going into the welfare system (Mills *et al.*). It is probable that 60% of grandparents raising grandchildren will fall into poverty compared to those not raising grandchildren, even though 48% of them are employed in some way (Smith *et al.*, 2000).

Unfortunately for this group of care providers, the welfare system is less user-friendly and lacks national consistency. For years, the most familiar program that provided cash payment for children was AFDC. This federal program began with assistance to parents only, but by 1965 expanded to include Medicaid—the state medical assistance program for the poor—and moved beyond parent-only grants to include other relatives providing primary care (Hegar & Scannapieco, 2000). When PRWORA was enacted in 1996 without consideration for children in foster care with nonparental relatives (Hegar & Scannapieco; Smith *et al.*, 2000), TANF block grants replaced AFDC cash assistance. TANF carried new stipulations, time limits, and work requirements (Mills *et al.*, 2005; Smith *et al.*, 2000) and provided flexibility in setting program requirements to individual states, which led to considerable program inconsistency among states (Hegar & Scannapieco). TANF was not designed with the notion that the child's family unit may be grandparents raising grandchildren, with financial situations that are very different from parents raising children.

Additionally, grandparent households are not licensed or fully licensed foster care homes because they may not believe that the childcaring arrangement is permanent, or they do not want to further strain relationships with the biological parents by applying for programs that limit parental rights, or they do not want involvement with legal custody issues (e.g. guardianship proceedings that such arrangements might invoke) (Smith *et al.*, 2000). The foster care license affects cash payments for the care of the child. Furthermore, elders raising their grandchildren may face problematic housing issues for several reasons, including homes too small to accommodate grandchildren, housing/retirement communities that do not allow resident children, and subsidized housing with occupancy limitations. Some grandparents may risk losing their housing when temporary childcare becomes permanent.

Financially secure elders raising grandchildren face many challenges and need much support, but near-poverty or impoverished elders have enormous challenges, many of which go unmet by the formal agencies meant to provide for both the elderly and child populations.

Ability to Exit Poverty

Older people do not have the capacity to move out of poverty, as do younger people. Wu (2001) reports that for people 65 years and older who remained in poverty for four consecutive years, the ability to exit that situation was virtually lost. Factors relating to making the escape from poverty nearly impossible are an accumulation of health care costs, cost-of-living rises with inadequate adjustments to monthly income, and a lesser probability of being employed as one ages into one's 70s and 80s. Interestingly, cost-of-living increases in Social Security benefits do not necessarily alleviate poverty, because typically as one governmental program increases benefits, another program is decreased to match that gain. For example, a cost-of-living increase in benefits may result in an automatic increase in subsidized rent, or an automatic decrease in food stamps.

What Are the Effects of Poverty?

This section addresses four primary effects of poverty on the old: food insecurity, inadequate housing, barriers to health care, and abuse and neglect.

Food Insecurity

Food insecurity is the direct result of poverty and affects every age group. Food insecurity means that access to food is unstable and inconsistent, while hunger refers to the lack of available food (Hall & Brown, 2005). Of the two, hunger is more severe. In 2003, the United States had 12.6 million households, or 36 million people, who were "food insecure or hungry" (Hall & Brown, p. 329). U.S. census data collected in 2005 for the U.S. Department of Agriculture showed that 3.4 million elders (6.0% of elderly households) suffered from food insecurity and 650,000 elders (1.7% of elderly households) were hungry (Hall & Brown). These figures underreport the problem among impoverished elders because of their isolation and removal from mainstream society. Food insecure and hungry elders are in lower numbers nationwide than younger age groups, but in 2001, 11% of those using food pantries were elderly, and in 2004, of those requesting emergency food assistance, 12% were elderly (Hall & Brown).

The ramifications of food insecurity are enormous for elders with compromised physical health, as poor nutrition reduces sense of well-being, contributes to malnutrition, and leads to poor health conditions, depression and confusion (Hall & Brown). In fact, hunger can lead to death by starvation.

Inadequate Housing

Geographic location affects housing costs; housing may be affordable in one state and literally move one into homelessness in another. Many older people hope to "age in place," meaning that their first choice is to remain in the same home they have occupied through much of their life. This ability is affected by income, physical ability, the cost of living, being a victim of financial exploitation, providing care to other family members, and how many people reside within that space.

Libson (2006) reported that among the elderly with the lowest income, 38% pay more than 50% of their annual income in rent. Government programs supporting affordable senior housing are complicated and involve both the nonprofit and for-profit sectors, with varying income/asset requirements and age and disability requirements. Elderly supportive housing programs are not being expanded by the government to meet the growing population of elders, or the poverty needs of elders. Additionally, while expansion of affordable units is problematic, so is the lack of money reserves to repair or modernize units built in 1959–74 (Libson). Thus many units are not well-maintained and, if not tended to soon, may not be viable in the future. Also, many units built from 1960 through the 1980s were built with contracts the federal government made with private owners to provide rental subsidizes to low-income people. These contracts are now coming to term, leaving the private owners with the option to forgo renewal for low-income renters. Various voucher programs (e.g. Enhanced Vouchers, Housing Choice Vouchers, Project-Based Vouchers) that assist in increasing low-income housing availability to the elderly are not being promoted with any enthusiasm by the Bush administration, thus leaving their future use by the private sector housing market and housing authorities uncertain (Libson). But it is not just the current administration that has made housing such a sad issue for the old. In 1981, the federal government spent approximately $30 billion per year subsidizing low-cost housing; by 1988 that figure had fallen below $7 billion per year (Gibeau, 2001, p. 23). In addition to adding more affordable housing in this country, there is an imperative need to retain and repair all existing sources of current affordable housing, and to develop a "united national policy on housing" (p. 23).

The market price of housing and the affluence of a community have a direct correlation to whether low-cost housing, especially those with supportive services, will be available to the elderly, or whether they will eventually lose their homes. Other factors directly affecting the permanency of housing are exposure to house fires and natural disasters. Hurricanes, floods, tornadoes, ice storms, and mudslides all affect housing loss and have a direct link to homelessness. Unlike the younger population, it is near impossible for older people to recover from home loss whether they own or rent.

There are far fewer homeless elders than homeless families. And most certainly, for all their problems, programs like Social Security and SSI have been instrumental in keeping the elderly housed, as has Medicaid for securing long-term chronic care in nursing homes. However, as noted earlier, as the elderly population grows and current housing units age without proper repairs, and with a paucity of future units being built, homeless elders will become more visible to both service providers and the public. It is difficult to tease out the elderly statistics from the "600,000 people who are homeless on any given night" but Gibeau (p. 23) estimates that 10–15% are older adults. Gibeau reports on a one-night survey count, conducted in three different years, of Boston's homeless shelters, with sobering findings concerning the old. In 1993, 439 older adults were counted. This figure jumped to 554 in 1997 and climbed another 10% in 1999. Nearly 33% of the homeless elderly in the 1997 count had coexisting health and functional impairments, which included behavioral health issues and substance abuse, particularly alcohol. The 1997 survey also noted that there had been an 85% increase of newly homeless since the 1993 survey (p. 24).

Killion (2000, p. 349) found in her study of homeless Black women that elderly women who were homeless cited reasons such as adverse moves caused by death, illness, loss of a family member's job, substance abuse, or demolition of housing units.

The near-poor and those elders in poverty are extremely vulnerable to substandard housing, crowded housing, and lack of housing, with little chance of securing new housing unless there is a coordinated effort to provide for this age group.

Barriers to Health Care

Health care remains a puzzle of sorts in the United States. The two primary pieces are health care coverage and health care access. These are complex issues for older Americans. There is not enough room in this chapter to give a full explanation. However, because of the implications for poor people, it is important to discuss two major programs for the elderly: Medicare and Medicaid.

Medicare

Medicare is the closest health insurance policy that the United States has to a national health care insurance program. Established in 1965, it provides for both in-hospital (Part A) and outpatient (Part B) care for individuals who have worked for the required 40 quarters under the SS system. However, misconceptions exist about exactly what the Medicare program covers. In reality, there are huge gaps in coverage. Medicare does not cover most chronic conditions found in the elderly population, nor does it cover long-term chronic care provided by group homes, assisted living facilities, or nursing homes. Mental health coverage is marginal. It does not cover extended hospital stays and has only begun to implement a prescription drug program (Part D) voted by Congress in 2003 (McGarry & Schoent, 2005). Medicare also has rather sizeable deductibles and requires that individuals sign up and pay premiums for the outpatient and prescription coverage. For example, although Part A does not have a premium, it does have deductibles. Using figures from 2003, the hospital admission deduction was $840. In a continuous hospital stay, the co-pay for hospital stays beyond 60 days was $210 per day and if such stays exceeded 90 days, that co-pay rose to $420 per day. If hospitalization went beyond 150 days, Medicare stopped paying entirely (McGarry & Schoent). In order to "break" a continuous hospital stay or out-patient service to "renew" Medicare coverage, one needs to be out of a health care facility for a period of time, sometimes a difficult feat for those with unstable medical conditions.

Medicare outpatient care is elected by the individual and includes a premium. In addition to the premium, again using figures from 2003, the outpatient deductible was $100 with a subsequent 20% co-pay for services (McGarry & Schoent, 2005) (see USDHHS (2007) for current programs, premiums, and deductibles at http://www.medicare.gov/publications/pubs/pdf/10050.pdf). An interesting exercise for the reader to ascertain how complex the Medicare program has become is to visit this site and scroll through its many programs. It is also important to remember that essentially there is no private primary health insurance coverage for elders who do not qualify for Medicare (Mold *et al.*, 2004), unless they qualify for Medicaid. Therefore, a person wishing to purchase Medicare coverage would pay $3,792 per year for Part A, $704.40 for Part B, and $934 per year for Plan A Medigap (Mold *et al.*), in addition to the respective deductibles and out-of-pocket expenses.

Supplemental Insurance and Medicaid

Given the premiums and deductibles, many older Americans have supplementary coverage either through insurance programs that are part of retirement packages, or private insurance policies that they purchase independently, or, if their financial status is low enough to meet individual state guidelines, through Medicaid (the insurance for the poor). Therefore, poor people may have some advantage over those who do not meet state Medicaid guidelines in that they will qualify for no-cost or low-cost supplementary health coverage, which will interact with Medicare or will act as a primary insurance in the absence of Medicare. Medicaid combined with Medicare tends to provide good coverage for people as long as there are health care providers who will accept the state Medicaid reimbursement plan, and as long as people sign up for it. In 1996, fewer than 50% of elders living below the poverty line were enrolled in Medicaid (Mold *et al.*, 2004, p. 602). There are many reasons for this under-enrollment: people like Gladys do not define themselves as poor enough to apply, people like Frank find it very stigmatizing to accept "welfare," and some people have no awareness of the program. Other factors restricting application to Medicaid include lack of transportation to the appropriate offices, fear of authority, being overwhelmed by the application process, or not being able to supply the documentation necessary to process the application.

Problems with Medicare and Medicaid

Even with Medicare and Medicaid, there are still services that are not covered—services requiring out-of-pocket expenses. These costs accumulate over years of illness, but the out-of-pocket expenses are most dramatic in the last year of providing care to a terminally ill person. McGarry and Schoent (2005) report that the average expenditure during this time is about $5,684, a relatively large amount for those on a fixed income or with limited savings. Other costs worth mentioning are chronic care for those without private long-term insurance or Medicaid. In 2003, the average per year cost for a nursing home was $66,000. Additionally, the average out-of-pocket expenses for prescription drugs for Medicare beneficiaries was $1,000 annually and for those needing treatment drugs, tens of thousands of dollars per year (p. 60). The rising prescription costs left many elderly with a choice of buying food or medicine. It is too early in the life of Medicare's prescription drug program to understand the implications it may have in reducing poverty caused by prescription needs, but there is hope.

Clearly, access to health care belongs to those with adequate insurance coverage. A person like Frank, who had never been poor in his life, may find he enters poverty because he cannot afford care for his wife's long-term illness due to their assets. Thus, both insurance coverage and lack of insurance coverage can prevent poverty or induce poverty.

Access and Availability

Health care is far more complex than just whether a person has coverage. Access to health care among the poor remains very problematic. Medicare and Medicaid reimbursement rates and the distribution timing of reimbursements to health care providers may limit whether providers will accept a person with this type of coverage. Thus recipients may find that in order to receive services they must pay out-of-pocket anyway. Additionally, as this country moves toward more for-profit health care providers, people may be turned away if they have large balances or too little coverage.

Service availability in reasonable proximity to home reflects having available quality services, sophisticated services, and the needed type of service. Poor people, especially the elderly poor, typically do not have their own transportation, which creates a serious access barrier. Public transportation may be too difficult to get to, not handicapped-accessible, or simply nonexistent. These problems tend to be even more prevalent in rural areas (Novak, 2006). Other barriers include lack of knowledge (Novak) or lack of trust in the care provider. Disregard for cultural beliefs by health care providers may further impede elders from seeking health care services.

Poverty creates hard choices for older people. Should they buy medicine or food or pay the rent? Chronic illness may take an otherwise viable financial situation and create financial risk for poverty or near poverty.

Elder Abuse, Neglect, and Financial Exploitation

Elder abuse is not just an issue for poor elders because it cuts across all socioeconomic classes. However, the combination of abuse, neglect, and financial exploitation impact the poverty status of elders. One of the greatest assets older people have to minimize the effects of poverty or near-poverty is assistance from family members, but it may also be a drawback to some because elder abuse is perpetrated primarily by family members. Approximately 700,000 to two million elders are abused or neglected annually in the United States (Jordan, 2001). Often this abuse occurs because an impoverished or substance-abusing family member needs resources held by the elder, such as housing, food, or money. Thus need creates dependency by the family member on the elder (Schiamberg & Gans, 2000; Bergeron, 2004). If an elder is financially compromised to begin with, this dependency by a family member will further the elder's financial insecurity and may result in homelessness. Elders with assets and high money income are at high risk for financial exploitation that could compromise their life savings, home, and access to their monthly income, consequently moving them into poverty. The likelihood of this happening increases with the level of commitment an elder feels to his or her family, or if the elder suffers from a physical frailty like dementia that inhibits his or her rational choice, or if the behavior of the perpetrator induces fear in the elder.

Elder neglect also implies self-neglect by elders as they choose how they want to live, a reflection of the principle of self-determination. For example, an elder may choose not to receive medical care for religious or cultural reasons. Elders in poverty may self-neglect, not because of self-determination, but because of a lack of resources. For example, an elder in poverty may choose not to receive medical care because of inadequate health insurance and financial resources. This type of self-neglect forces elders to choose among the necessities of food, health care, and housing, thus creating or exacerbating poor health conditions, or creating a potential for homelessness.

Conclusion

The elderly poor is a complex group because of rich family diversity, varied backgrounds, educational and occupational backgrounds, their own view of their worth and place within the society, and the complicated programs designed to assist them. The charge for professionals on all levels is to pay close attention to this group and not to assume that past successes in reducing poverty among the old will continue unless purposeful action and attention are given both to maintenance of programs and creation of more responsive programs. Communities must look at this invisible group and not assume that they have services that meet or exceed their needs. Some of the best solutions to minimize the effects of poverty for the old may be to include expanding the supports found within families to neighborhoods and small communities. Finally, policymakers must consider the diversity in family structures and value these structures along with the elderly persons to create, evaluate, and maintain policies that continue to build on the great advancement made from the days of almshouses.

References

Bergeron, L. (2004). Elder abuse: Clinical assessment and obligation to report. In K. Kendall-Tackett (Ed.), Health consequences of abuse in the family (pp. 109–28). Washington, DC: American Psychological Association.

Cahill, S. & South, K. (2002). Policy issues affecting lesbian, gay, bisexual, and transgender people in retirement. Generations, Summer, 49–54.

Federal Register. (2006, 24 Jan.). 71, 3848–9.

Gibeau, J. (2001). Home free: An evolving journey in eradicating elder homelessness. Topics in Geriatric Rehabilitation, 17, 22–52.

Gist, Y. & Hetzel, L. (2004). We the people: Aging in the United States. Census 2000 Special Reports. U.S. Department of Commerce, U.S. Census Bureau. Washington, DC: Government Printing Office. Available HTML: http://www.census.gov/prod/2006pubs/p23-209.pdf (accessed 14 June 2007).

Golant, S. (2006). Supportive housing for frail, low-income older adults: Identifying need and allocating resources. Generations, 29, 37–43.

Hall, B. & Brown, J. (2005). Food security among older adults in the United States. Topics in Clinical Nutrition, 20, 329–38.

Hardy, M. (2002). The transformation of retirement in twentieth-century American: From discontent to satisfaction. *Generations, 26*, 9–16.

He, W., Sengupta, M., Velkoff, V., & DeBarros, K., (2005). U.S. Census Bureau, Current Population Reports: *65+ in the United States: 2005.* Washington, DC: U.S. Government Printing Office. Available HTML: http://www.census.gov/prod/2006pubs/p23-209.pdf (accessed 14 June 2007).

Hegar, R. & Scannapieco, M. (2000). Grandma's babies: The problem of welfare eligibility for children raised by relatives. *Journal of Sociology and Social Welfare, 27*, 153–71.

Jordan, L. (2001). Elder and domestic violence: Overlapping issues and legal remedies. *American Journal of Family Law, 15*, 147–56.

Killion, C. (2000). Extending the extended family for homeless and marginally housed African American women. *Public Health Nursing, 17*, 346–54.

Kivett, V. (2001). Rural older women. In J. Coyle (Ed.), *Handbook on Women and Aging* (pp. 3–13). Westport, CT: Greenwood Press.

Libson, N. (2006). The sad state of affordable housing for older people. *Generations, 29*, 9–15.

Mackin, J. (1997). Living arrangements vary for the elderly. *Human Ecology, 25*, 2.

McGarry, K. & Schoent, R. (2005). Medicare gaps and widow poverty. *Social Security Bulletin, 66*, 58–74.

McGoldrick, M. (1982). Ethnicity and family therapy: An overview. In M. McGoldrick, J. Pearch, & J. Giordano, (Eds.), *Ethnicity and family therapy* (pp. 3–30). New York: Guilford Press.

Medicare and You. (2007). *Official Handbook.* Department of Health and McGary, McGoldnick Human Services. Centers for Medicare and Medicaid. Baltimore, MD: CMS Publication No 10050. Available HTML: http://www.medicare.gov/publications/pubs/pdf/10050.pdf (accessed 14 June 2007).

Mills, T., Gomez-Smith, Z., & DeLeon, J. (2005). Skipped generation families: Sources of psychological distress among grandmothers of grandchildren who live in homes where neither parent is present. *Marriage & Family Review, 37*, 191–212.

Minkler, M. & Fuller-Thomson, E. (2005). African American grandparents raising grandchildren: A national study using the census 2000 American Community Survey. *Journal of Gerontology, 60B*, S82–S92.

Mold, J., Fryer, G., & Thomas, C. (2004). Who are the uninsured elderly in the United States? *Journal of American Geriatrics Society, 52*, 601–6.

Novak, M. (2006). *Issues in aging.* Boston: Allyn & Bacon.

Roff, L. & Klemmack, D. (2003). The demographics of aging in rural perspective. *Journal of Gerontological Social Work, 41*, 19–35.

Schiamberg, L. & Gans, D. (2000). Elder abuse by adult children: An applied ecological framework for understanding contextual risk factors and the intergenerational character of quality of life. *International Journal of Aging and Human Development, 50*, 329–59.

Sevak, P., Weir, D., & Willis, R. (2003/2004). *Social Security Bulletin, 65*, 31–44.

Smith, C., Beltran, A., Butts, D., & Kingson, E. (2000). Grand parents raising grandchildren: Emerging program and policy issues for the 21st century. *Journal of Gerontological Social Work, 34*, 81–94.

Whitman, D. & Purcell, P. (2006). Income and poverty among older Americans. *Benefits Quarterly,* Fourth Quarter, 48–61.

Wu, K. (2001). Older persons find it hardest to exit poverty. *Research Report (Pub ID: DD61).* Washington, DC: AARP Policy Institute.

Critical Thinking Questions

1   Given the changing nature of the American labor market (stagnating wages, fewer employers providing health benefits, bankruptcies that destroy pensions, etc.), what changes should be made to the U.S. Social Security system?
2   It is often said that social problems are embedded in societal structures. What are the main structural issues we should be concerned with as our society ages?
3   How does the intersection of gender, class, and race compound the problems faced by the elderly in our country?

Part III
Rethinking Family Poverty

13 Poverty, Stress, Resilience

Using the MRM Model for Understanding and Abating Poverty-Related Family Stress

Charles B. Hennon, W. Sean Newsome, Gary W. Peterson, Stephan M. Wilson, M. Elise Radina, and Bruno Hildenbrand

In this chapter, we seek to provide strategies for managing poverty-related family stressors. We explore the magnitude, resources, and meaning (MRM) model as a heuristic scheme of how families function as well as a guide for professional inquiry. In addition, we explore the model as a guide for community-based and grassroots interventions aimed at family capacity-building to manage poverty-related family stressors. This strategy looks to energize social movements that foster poverty-focused holistic, comprehensive, and sustainable improvement agendas. Throughout the chapter, we advance a resiliency, and empowerment approach that considers poor families to have expertise pertaining to their own personal issues surrounding poverty.

Family Poverty

We define poverty broadly and generally (see Hennon & Wilson, 2008; Wagstaff, 2002), using official federal guidelines. Flexibility in our definition enable us to include families coping with chronic poverty, temporary poverty, or those moving in and out of poverty. Poverty for some families is relatively short-term (i.e. less than two years) and is often associated with a potential harmful and/or negative event (e.g. divorce, ill health, or unemployment). Chronically poor families are those consistently poor over five years, and they are often associated with persistent difficulties, including disability or a female-headed household with many children (Rank & Hirschl, 2002; Wood, 2003).

In defining family, scholars note that it depends on "whom you ask, when, under what circumstances, and why" (Briar-Lawson, Lawson, Hennon, & Jones, 2001, p. 30). The judgment of who comprises a specific family is often individually and culturally constructed through interaction within a localized culture. Understanding the localized cultural definition of family gives insight into family values, meanings, and functioning, including who is or is not available to participate in the fight against poverty. More importantly, cultural understanding assists with assessing the strengths, weaknesses, needs, challenges, and stresses poor families encounter (Burks & Martin, 1985).

In the United States, poverty has been identified as a family stressor since the Great Depression (Crane & Heaton, 2008; Voydanoff & Majka, 1988). Currently, about 10% of families are officially classified as poor. Over 15% of families with children under age 18 and close to 38% of female-headed families with children under age 18 live in poverty (U.S. Census Bureau, 2005). It is important to note that these figures do not include families who move in and out of poverty, those at risk of moving into poverty, or the working poor (Belle & Doucet, 2003; Shipler, 2004; U.S. Department of Labor, 2002).

Given these considerations, it is clear that escaping poverty is difficult for many families, including those with employed family members (Williams & Williams-Morris, 2000). About one-third of employed people receive below-poverty wages. Of these, about one-third are solely responsible for the family's income and yet are persistent low-wage earners (Carnevale & Rose, 2001). Acs, Ross Phillips, and McKenzie (2001) found that one in six working-age Americans live in low-income households with at least one employed person. Barriers against achieving higher incomes include discrimination, lack of employment opportunities, and few jobs that offer meaningful, decent, and productive work (Belle & Doucet, 2003).

In addition to the barriers that might stand in the way of exiting poverty, research has found that urbanization is linked with poverty and family stress. The United Nations Population Fund (UNPF, 2007) projects that close to 3.3 billion people will live in urban areas by 2008 and 5 billion by 2030. Smaller cities will experience most of the urban growth, and many, due to lack of proper planning, fewer resources, and inadequately staffed governments, will face the threat of overwhelming poverty (UNPF). For many families in urban areas, threats of overwhelming poverty can result in inadequate clothing, housing, diet, social service and health care access, and other basic requirements. Child Trends (2002) suggested that some family types could be more at risk than others, with ethnic minorities, recent immigrants, unmarried and single-parent families, those headed by persons without high school diplomas, rural residents, and those living in chaotic environments and low-income/adverse neighborhoods most affected.

It appears that the impact of poverty on family functioning and human growth and development, "is as much involved with the culture or general context of poverty as it is with the economics of poverty" (Wood, 2003, p. 707), which is mediated, in part, through environmental deprivation. Heclo (1997, p. 143) referred to these sociocultural and environmental dimensions of poverty as, "a condition of misery, hopelessness, and dependency." This is true regardless of family type (e.g. single-parent, parent/child age, religious and ethnic identifications, immigration status, and rural/urban residence) (Crane & Heaton, 2008; Radina, Wilson, & Hennon, in press; United Nations Development Program, 2001, 2006; UNPF, 2007; U.S. Census, 2005; Wood, 2003). As a result, interventions must explore the importance of family capacity-building and promote strategies that foster inclusive and sustainable improvement agendas focused on decreasing family poverty and related issues.

MRM Model of Family Stress

The MRM model of family stress process (magnitude, resources, meaning) is a family action (research, needs assessment, intervention, evaluation) schema that incorporates ecological and relational perspectives (Briar-Lawson *et al.*, 2001), including how individuals subjectively and interpersonally make sense of their situations. MRM has a dynamic and processual orientation. Because stress and responses are conceptualized as mediated by cognitive appraisals and transactions with others and the environment, the MRM model includes a symbolic interactionist and phenomenological viewpoint. Stress and distress arise from the adaptational response of the family to the environment as appraised or defined. This is a transaction and stress is a relational and multi-faceted concept; stress results from the relationship among environmental demands, situation appraisal as affected by resources and constraints, and family actions in response to the situation. MRM recognizes that socioeconomic and physical environments, or social ecologies, are important attributes of the stress process.

The MRM model uses the family as the unit of analysis, thus focusing on family-level process in terms of "meaning-making" and stress management responses. Family-level can be difficult to conceptualize and operationalize. The model's intent is to focus on emergent family qualities that arise from interaction, negotiation, and acceptance because of harmonious agreements, passive acceptance, adherence to legitimate authority norms, or power use. Family dynamics ensue and affect the response to poverty-related stress. Individual humans bring their attributes to the family process. Characteristics that can describe the family emerge from interaction. Patterson suggested that family-level means at least two people; however, one person may be the driving force behind family action and stress response and thus directs resource use. This is a family-level response. While this could be true of families characterized by religious or other norms that give headship to one person, it is particularity characteristic of lone-parent families with young children or lone-person families (e.g. an elderly woman).

The model recognizes that individuals are usually embedded in larger networks and contextual factors cannot be ignored. While individual-level interventions are often appropriate, they can be conceptualized as resources available for the total family. Interventions that target individuals are often fragmented and do not consider in a holistic way the individual as a member of a family.

The MRM is a heuristic instrument and not a deterministic model of how families function. The model reconfigures the three basic factors of the ABC–X family stress model as dimensions, while incorporating relevant conceptualizations from additional family and human stress process models, such as the family adjustment and adaptation response model (Boss, 2002; Hennon & Peterson, 2007; Hill, 1949; Patterson, 2002). Also, the MRM figure (see Fig. 13.1) is a device for illustrating, conceptually, the dimensions, along with factors commonly considered to establish family stress levels. Each family varies along these parameters and in combination they can be envisaged as forming a social-psychological space (internal social ecology) in which families function. Where the family is located along all three dimensions simultaneously establishes the stress level and thus felt distress. In Fig. 13.1, LS represents a family with a low stress level and low felt distress (resilience), while SS illustrates a family experiencing severe stress and elevated distress or vulnerability levels.

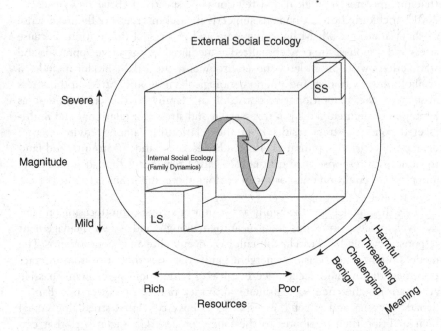

Figure 13.1 The MRM Model of Family Stress.

The theoretical perspective attributes the "cause" of stress to what emerges in a family when demands exceed capabilities. When the demands–capabilities imbalance persists and increases, family members often manifest distress symptoms (e.g. health-related problems, depression, and irritability). The interplay of resources and resource shortfalls with stressor magnitude and how family members appraise stressors modulates the degree of family stress. The combination of stressor magnitude, useable resources, accepted appraisals, and stress management strategies join into what is conceptually considered the current state of family stress and distress. Individual, family, and community resources available, along with the accepted situation appraisal and actions undertaken, structure the stress management strategy the family employs (Abery, 2006; Hennon & Peterson, 2007; Peterson & Hennon, 2005).

The stress management strategy used depends upon many elements, including intuition, personal attributes, family worldview, and internal family milieu. Other contributing factors include the extra-familial social ecology that might offer mechanisms for avoiding or reducing stressors, alternative definitions and meanings for the situation, and resource availability. Sometimes responding to stress can be a "kludge," or a cobbled-together response that is not well thought-out but still works, or a response that is ineffective and even exacerbates stress and problematic family dynamics. Ideally, perhaps, the strategy is achieved through encouraging diverse family opinions (e.g. creativity), endorsing consideration and debate of the relative merits of these opinions, and using an effective mechanism endorsed by a family member for settling upon a response. Stress management strategies can be classified as *impressive* (necessary and sufficient for managing daily life), *important* (helpful but not ideal), *irrelevant* (no positive or negative effect), *iterative* (no value added to what is already in operation), or *irresponsible* (damaging to family life). While stress management can be an individual problem-solving or avoidance activity (instrumental, change-orientated, and problem-focused versus palliative, accepted, or denied), the MRM model emphasizes the potential for family (or sub-systems like parents) negotiated action strategies to identify stressors and their family impairment potential, rationally taking stock of available resources, and thus realistically furnishing a management strategy that does not overwhelm resources, current and future family functioning, or quality of life.

Stress (a state) is the pressure to change current family functioning that arises from an imbalance between the demands inflicted upon a family and the family's capability for responding to demands. Some demands are normative (developmental) in that they are expected transitions and changes over the family and individual life course, while others are nonnormative (situational). They are unexpected and uncommon to most families. Demands also include internal ecology issues, like unresolved family tensions and dysfunctional interaction patterns, as well as onerous tasks or common daily hassles.

Distress is the emotional, psychological, social, and physical response to stress. Stressors are demands (events, conditions, changes) that exert pressure or strain on family systems and indicate a need for structural adjustments in interactional patterns (Boss, 2002; Hennon & Peterson, 2007). Adjustments could include family boundaries, family paradigm and goals, number and types of individual roles, family interaction dynamics, and relationship quality. Elevated demand, stress, strain, and distress levels do not equal maladjustment or dysfunction.

Resilience refers to how families (and/or their members) are able to buffer the potential effects of stressors and rebound from stress and adversity, or thrive despite adverse circumstances (McCubbin & McCubbin, 1988). It includes family strengths. Family hardships are often grave during stressful, challenging times, and can elevate family stress or even produce crisis (a state of disequilibrium and disorganization). Sometimes clarity, or even an epiphany, can come from chaos. That is, a family can find hope and willpower to survive, and flourish in ways that promote current and future resiliency. This capacity is sometimes termed regenerative power or elasticity.

Patterson (2002) distinguished resilience as a process from resiliency as an outcome. Resilience is "the process by which families are able to adapt and function competently following exposure to significant adversity and crisis," while resiliency is "the capacity of a family to successfully manage their life circumstances" (p. 352). Family resiliency includes many aspects.[1] Family capacity, which can be enhanced by access to resources, is another term for resiliency (Abery, 2006). Capacities include the meanings the family attributes to situational demands and the relative ability to meet them; available or acquirable resources; and stress management strategies the family uses in attempting balance between

demands and resources. Family capacity-building is a family-centered intervention goal (Briar-Lawson *et al.*, 2001).

Fig. 13.1 is a graphic representation of the MRM model. The circle represents
the external social ecology of a family, including community (and larger), neighborhood, extended family, and other characteristics or conditions. The arrows
signify that the internal social ecology of the family is dynamic. For example,
families can tap into their resiliency capabilities to adapt and function competently (resilience). The vertical parameter is the current magnitude of all stressors experienced. Families in poverty seldom deal with single stressors. The felt
magnitude of accumulated stressors can vary from mild to severe. Attempts to
alleviate a stressor can exacerbate others, while effective stress management can
alleviate or mediate a stressor and lower the magnitude of overall stress. The coping tactics of an individual family member (e.g. alcohol consumption, with-
drawal) can be dysfunctional for other members, thus influencing the overall
stress level. The immediate and residual impact of stressors (both objectively and
subjectively) on families can vary. Related demands and hardships also vary in
intensity and duration, and can pile up over time. Some stressors are acute and
of short duration; others are chronic and long-lasting. Some stressors require a
great deal of adjustment; others are minor irritations (Burks & Martin, 1985).
The magnitude parameter thus reflects that a family's current stressor situation
could vary from virtually no impact to an overwhelming impact. It also reflects
that families deal simultaneously with multiple stressors and related hardships,
and it is the totality of these that indicates stressor magnitude.

The horizontal parameter is the stock of resources potentially available for
managing experienced stressors. Some families are resource-rich, others resource-
poor. Resources are any informational, material, emotional, social, or human capital assets or capabilities that can buffer potential or actual stressors, manage felt
distress, buttress perceptual and ego defenses, negotiate a family definition of the
situation, and devise problem-solving behaviors. Resources thus include financial
means, material goods, useful objects, physical and social conditions (e.g. quality
housing, adequate employment, decent health insurance), community assets,
practical help, important knowledge, and a sustainable social/emotional support
network. Resources embody individual, relational, family, and extra-family capital. Some resources are more useful than others, depending upon the situation.

Some families might have a variety of adequate resources available, while others could be "well-off" in some areas (e.g. a safe neighborhood) and less so in others (e.g., money in a savings account). Resources remain only potentials unless
families consider and use them. Further, resources are finite and can be depleted,
including those that could be useful for other stressor conditions or stress management strategies. Families can fail to recognize this aspect of resource allocation, or horde resources to conserve them and ration their use (Hobfoll, 1989).
Such hording strategies may or may not prove beneficial; not using enough of an
available resource can worsen a situation, perhaps leading to crisis.

A resource shortfall exists when necessary or useful resources are not at the
family's disposal. The MRM interpretation maintains that all families have

strengths upon which they can build, in contrast to deficit model perspectives that result in families being blamed for deficiencies (Briar-Lawson *et al.*, 2001; Hennon & Peterson, 2007, McCubbin & McCubbin, 1988, Orthner, Jones-Sanpei, and Williamson, 2004; Walsh, 2002). Ineffective stress management responses can thus be interpreted as resulting from insufficient, but possibly only temporary, resource shortages rather than as relatively permanent traits. The role of interventions, as guided by this interpretation, is to provide material goods and information and to assist in culturally relevant skill-building.

The MRM emphasizes family potential and points to empowerment models where goals include helping families learn ways to overcome barriers and enhance the quality of life. The key is to use appropriate advocacy, family life education, and service delivery systems to enhance family functioning by employing family expert-ise along with empirically based professional knowledge that builds resource capa-bilities. Such approaches can foster family resiliency and empower families to tackle and overcome poverty-related stressors. Empowerment approaches also reduce the risk of family dependency on agencies and organizations. An important aspect of empowerment is transformative learning, or new family awareness that they can deal with situations in ways not yet considered (Radina *et al.*, in press).

The depth parameter is the meaning assigned to the current situation (Boss, 2002). Family members, individually and collectively, appraise the immediate situation and give it definition and meaning. Some people see situations as chal-lenges or opportunities: life as normal. Others take aggressive (blaming others or fate), defensive (don't blame me), negative (nothing can be done), avoidance (don't talk about it or plan any action), or denial (nothing is wrong) psycholog-ical stances. Each personal or family appraisal is unique, but can be conceptual-ized into a typology that reflects a gradation from benign to harmful. Benign appraisals indicate a satisfactory, nonperilous situation. Challenges are situation appraisals of events or issues that can be dealt with and moved beyond, perhaps through creative problem-solving or applying existing family rules (Gubrium & Holstein, 2000). If dealt with effectively, no harm will come to the family.

Threatening situation appraisals exist when the situation is defined as having the potential to cause family harm or loss (e.g. financial, emotional, social, health, life, morale), but the harm or loss has not yet occurred. If dealt with appropriately, the threat can be avoided or damage reduced; if not, harm will come to the family. Sometimes, the family believes the situation has already harmed them or loss has already occurred (e.g. a person's health has been compromised, money lost, or social prestige damaged). In such harmful appraised situations, the task might be to minimize future harm or try to recoup some of the loss and develop new family functioning methods.

Appraisals are not static and can vary over time: (1) as families reappraise specific stressors and the magnitude of accumulated stressors; (2) as resources are tapped, depleted, or replenished; and (3) as the efficacy of stress management strategies are measured for success. MRM attempts to capture the general appraisal negotiated by the family about the current state of family affairs. The family functions and considers future life in this arbitraged reality, which includes the family paradigm or natural attitude that influences both internal relations and transactions with the external social ecology.

The MRM model, consistent with symbolic interaction theory, argues that each person, through socialization and social interaction, "makes meaning" of social situations. Each "self" is a product of social interaction, and the self is involved in defining the meaning and how to respond to a given family situation. The definition of the situation, or the perceptions and appraisals accepted, has real consequences. A situation defined as hopeless leads to a different response than one defined as a minor hassle. People also take the role of the other and determine what is expected of self and other in terms of role-enactment or role-making. Thus one's identity as a socially situated family member can influence how to think about a particular stressor or accumulated stress, and how to respond (Gubrium & Holstein, 2000; Hennon & Peterson, 2004; Sandstrom, Martin, and Fine, 2003). Each family member's self as presented in socially situated interaction contributes to the emergent family-level definition of the situation and its effect on how to respond.

An Insider's View of Poverty and Family Stress

MRM suggests an insider's perspective is important for authentic understanding of how poverty-related stress is understood and lived by families. Research and interventions should employ qualitative and phenomenological participatory poverty assessments that incorporate the perspectives of economically impoverished people and other stakeholders (World Health Organization and World Bank, 2002). These approaches offer emic and eidetic understanding of the "lived" world as understood by participants most affected by poverty and economic distress (Hildenbrand 2005; Hildenbrand & Hennon, in press; Radina, Hennon, & Gibbons, in press; Shipler, 2004). Individuals and families experience life in general, and any specific phenomenon, as having a recognized past and present, and an anticipated future. What matters within the MRM framework is not so much the status of the poor or the fact of poverty, but rather what the family "makes" of it: that is, the taken-for-granted world of family life and the language used to live within it and describe it to self and others.

Within the purview of the MRM model, concern is with how family relationships and identities are interactionally constituted and sustained under the stress of poverty. Each family member's identity is influenced by his or her family paradigm, or by other "local cultures" and "going concerns" (Gubrium & Holstein, 2000). These cultures are coordinators of shared constructs and expectations about family life and the world. Going concerns are "relatively stable, routinized, ongoing patterns of action and interaction" and a "way of being who and what we are in relation to the immediate scheme of things" (Gubrium & Holstein, p. 102). To be understood is the process of how language is used in social interaction and how this use creates a meaningful world and self-identity under the stress of poverty. In experiencing life as a process, people might or might not use terms like resources and appraisals, or poor or stressed, to identify themselves.

With the use of the MRM model, scrutiny is given to how families come to define situations and family life (Giorgi & Giorgi, 2003; Gubrium & Holstein, 1993; Hildenbrand & Hennon, in press; Radina, Hennon, & Gibbons, in press; Shipler, 2004). Understanding this brings to light the ways by which families give meaning to the life they are living, and how everyday reality is intersubjectively structured, relative to a family living in poverty in this case (Giorgi & Giorgi, 2003). How people construct their identities around such issues as being poor (e.g. blame, sense of failure, victim, survivor) and their relationships with their children, lovers, spouses, parents, friends, communities, and so forth, are regarded as important. The inner world of the family, as revealed by the family, is paramount for establishing what poor families experience and could find useful (Giorgi & Giorgi, 2003; Hildenbrand & Hennon, in press). Such investigations discover how poor and near-poor families "make sense" of their lifeworlds, their social position as "poor" or "stressed" within these worlds, and what they believe could be empowering to facilitate movement to a different life.

The MRM aims to gain insight into what families believe are requirements for living a better life, which gives researchers better insight into what is considered a stressor, how it is defined and why, the consideration of what is or is not a useful resource, reluctance or willingness to seek help and from where, and how families as a group or individual members in harmony or conflict strive to deal with daily life and solve the problems of living. The professional's task is to understand the distinctions and correspondence between living a family life full of poverty induced stress and living in a more satisfactory way. Professional insight about how the two are linked can lead to praxis (i.e. action consequential of reflection) that helps empower families to recognize what is missing for growth to a state of more adequate family functioning. The MRM model of family action theory and research seeks "potential" and strives to ascertain a set of activities that, if implemented, allows families to improve their quality of life (cf. McElwee, 2007; National Wraparound Initiative, n.d.). Professionals in collaboration with families can conceptually construct a "world" different from the current poverty-stressed daily life—one that can then be a goal to achieve. Such transformation in living is not necessarily a stable process. Family life can still be problematic and fraught with relapse, and families can doubt their ability to sustain any change. Professionals and others can assist by supportive actions and "ways of constructively criticizing" that stabilize the new family dynamics (McElwee, 2007).

Adjustments and Adaptations

Under stressful conditions, people tend to search for information about the situation and reduce ambiguity. An insider's perspective helps researchers learn how people undertake this search. Sometimes when people gain knowledge about a stressor, they seek and activate different resources that better match the demands and hardships of the stressor situation. In some cases, this results from an active search for resources, or it might be due to interventions by family members, friends, faith-based organizations, schools, social service agencies, or family life education. Over time, families can move in their placement on the resource dimension. Sometimes families can tap new and appropriate resources; other times they drain available resources.

The meaning of the situation can also change as families gain additional knowledge, assess and use resources, and reappraise the situation. Over time, the meanings of families, lives or specific situations can become more negative or more positive. The MRM model reflects how families make more immediate adjustments and longer-term adaptations while they more or less successfully manage poverty-related stressful and/or crisis situations. It also points to how education and service delivery can help families avoid or reduce stressors, make better use of resources, and reappraise situations in more functional ways.

The MRM model recognizes that families and situations are not static; family members' (individually and together) placement within the sociopsychological space can change from minute to minute and from day to day. Knowledge of stressor magnitude and related hardships can change to awareness of more or less impact, and stress management strategies can be created and modified. The family process includes both shorter-term adjustments to current and new stressors and more permanent adaptations that persist over time. Adaptations become the going concerns based on experience that give a sense of predictability to daily life (Gubrium & Holstein, 1993, 2000). Families expect that future life will fit within the schema of the familiar life of the past. Adjustments and adaptations formulate daily family life. Barriers to more adaptive responses include that habitus (a system of durable and transposable dispositions that form the principle of generating and structuring practices and representations of the lifeworld) and self-conception do not automatically change. Thus families can get "stuck" in their poverty-related stress unless an internal or external impulse comes into play, and stress-related cyclical processes could continue to spiral and accelerate to problematic levels (Hildenbrand & Hennon, in press; Peterson & Hennon, 2005).

Implications for Family-Centered Intervention Action Agendas

If theories of poverty-related family stress, empowerment, and resiliency are realistic, the aim should be to demonstrate how they could be applied to real life. Families feel supported when they have adequate resources and receive appropriate services (Briar-Lawson *et al.*, 2001). There are many ways to support poverty-stressed families. Policy initiatives that address nurturance and socialization, family formation and membership, economic support, and protection of vulnerable members are one avenue to build family capacity (Patterson, 2002). Transfers and other subventions (e.g. welfare, food stamps; school vouchers; business incubators, with programs designed to speed up the development and growth of companies, and loans; low-cost health care; subsidized housing; Head Start) are also useful (Corey & Corey, 2007; Crane & Heaton, 2008). Community development, vocational training, and job creation are important targets for intervention, as are working for social justice, establishing English-as-a-second-language programs, developing community resource centers that offer "one-stop" service delivery, facilitating home–school relations, creating affordable childcare and health systems, and working to reduce discrimination and increase acceptance of diverse families. Culturally competent human service agencies and family life education also support families (Radina Hennon, & Gibbons, in press). It is important to note that some low-income families, as they devise "survival tactics," turn to formal service delivery agencies only as a last resort (Edin & Lein, 1997). Edin and Lein found that over 75% of low-income, lone-parent families obtained resources from social network and about 50% turned to supplementary employment, while only about 25% used private or public social services.

Impoverished families cannot be forced to comply with policy and practice initiatives, nor can these "fix" families. Ignoring family diversity leads to ineffective intervention and support or resistance to comply with interventions (Briar-Lawson et al., 2001). Investing in families and communities is a strategic development action for building family capacity and resiliency. Experience shows individuals are best served by professionals who "understand the family, social milieu and personal dynamics of their individual client" thus empowering and serving the individual and the family as a whole (Hildebrand, Phenice, Gray & Hines, 2000, p. 4). Professionals must develop families as partners and concentrate on families first—especially those in crisis—while also working for community development. Professionals are obliged to ask families what they need, want, and desire. Families are the experts in knowing what helps and what hurts (Briar-Lawson et al., 2001; Corey & Corey, 2007).

Other methods for supporting low-income families include advocacy, volunteer work, and localized action. Assisting one family at a time could be part of this schema of support (Briar-Lawson et al., 2001; Heclo, 1997; Wood, 2003). Fig. 13.2 illustrates a Familywatch advocacy/action agenda that ranges from supporting one family at a time to international policy and practice. Familywatch integrates diverse people with diverse knowledge and skill sets to "watch out for and over" families in or at risk for poverty (Briar-Lawson et al., 2001). This approach indicts policymakers, helping professions, family advocates, average citizens, and those most affected by poverty to form partnerships to advance family-centered approaches to ameliorate family poverty conditions, to help restore family functioning, and to work to eliminate future family suffering due to poverty. As a result, while governments and formal organizations can create resources and services, so can professionals and average citizens.

Familywatch is comparable to Neighborhood Watch or Habitat for Humanity in that low skills are necessary, while higher skills are appreciated. Motivation to help and support families is the basic necessity. Program participants can advocate for families in terms of legislative action, community policy, and services. These participants can also organize to provide a range of resources and services, such as home repairs, trash clean-up, technology donation, cooperative childcare, tutoring, help for substance abusers, domestic-abuse shelters, and fundraising and media campaigns that highlight family plights and strengths. Clothing/food collection and distribution, low-cost public transportation, after school programming, car-pool organization, door-to-door transportation to medical facilities and

International Policy Initiatives [HIV/AIDS, malarial, environmental concerns, technology transfer, refugees, human development, etc. Donation of money or skills to help organizations]

National Policy Initiatives

State/Regional Policy Initiatives

Community Policy Initiatives [Pressure groups, testimony, write/talk with policymakers, research and program evaluation, fundraising]

Community Development Action [Job creation, housing, health care, schooling, home–school relations, technology, English-as-second-language lessons; vocational training; understanding of laws and social norms, grant writing and fundraising]

Advocacy for families and resiliency to poverty, perhaps due to humanitarian, gender, social justice, religious or other moral/value reasons. [Use media, networks, organizations, agencies, school, religious organizations, etc. as stage and action base]

Joining/forming grassroots organizations, social movements, action teams, globalization from below, scapes to offer resources and services (social action) on behalf of poor families. Encouraging the involvement of natural helpers and family-centered wraparound programs. [Food banks, free stores, tool and technology lending banks, substance-abuse awareness and abatement programs, health clinics, transportation, childcare, legal and financial assistance, micro loans, mobilization of groups and action teams, encouragement of foster care and child support payments, fundraising/grant writing]

Supporting one family at a time via instrumental, emotional, informational resources and services including possible professional practice (legal, health, therapy, financial, educational), skills (plumbing, carpentry, vehicle repair and maintenance, tutoring, computer literacy), and informal support (help with substance abuse, domestic violence, childcare, temporary housing) to build family capacity to embolden empowerment and resiliency and not dependency. Being a natural helper.

Figure 13.2 Familywatch Advocacy/Action Agenda Pyramid.

social service agencies are also very important services needed by many. In addition to the tangible benefits listed above, information about nutrition, financial management, education, and micro-loans is also a valuable resource. All of these activities, it is hoped, will bring about an increase in enterpreneurship activities that will lead to greater human/social capital development. Participants with professional-level skills can offer low-cost or free legal and other help like medical, dental, or counseling. Working together provides a synergy benefit beyond the contributions of any one person, while each contribution is valuable and appreciated. Community action, which begins with asking what needs strengthening and what needs to be fixed, is important, as is working individually with families.

Conclusion

The MRM is a family action research and intervention model that considers that family stress often results from resource shortfalls. It indicates how families can: (1) be empowered when provided appropriate resources by both formal and informal service and education delivery systems; (2) better understand the stress process and adaptational outcomes; (3) best use available resources; (4) build capacity for more optimal responses to stressors; (5) maintain positive views toward life and current situations; (6) build support networks and grassroots action teams; (7) develop relevant acculturation strategies; (8) develop effective/more optimal stress management strategies; and (9) consider a different world in which they might live and how to achieve it. Informal support networks, as well as formal service and family life education delivery modalities, can overcome resource shortfalls while they bestow required resources so that families feel supported. Such delivery systems, sometimes called wraparound services, should be family-centered, timely, holistic, culturally sensitive, and relevant (Briar-Lawson *et al.*, 2001; Radina, Wilson & Hennon, in press; Unger, Cuevas & Woolfolk, 2007). Familywatch approaches grounded in the MRM model can be beneficial, as they focus on assisting one family at a time, improving neighborhoods and communities, and advocating for supportive policies and practices at local, national, and international levels.

Using the MRM model for intervention design enhances the development of culturally specific family-centered service delivery and can help to reduce family stress through two pathways. First, delivery of and access to adequate and appropriate resources may address a family's balance of stressors, resources, and meanings to promote resilience in the face of poverty. Appropriately equipped families can more effectively and efficiently manage stress. This would be primary intervention. The second pathway for intervention is for situations in which family stress is reaching critical levels, but has not yet overwhelmed family functioning and ability to respond to stressor demands. This would be secondary intervention. When families have reached a point of crisis and chaos, adequate family functioning must be restored. This is tertiary intervention. The introduction of interventions at critical points can empower families and prevent or reduce stress, enhance resiliency, and encouragement optimal outcomes.

Note

1   Given the ever present nature of family stress when faced with poverty, an important
question is why do some families seem more capable of enduring in the face of stress
and crisis? Research indicates that certain family strengths are integral components of
healthy family functioning and resiliency. The following family strengths appear to
enable families to be resilient when confronted with stress (adapted from McCubbin
& McCubbin, 1988):

- Accord, or relationships among family members that allow the resolution of
conflict and the reduction of chronic strain.
- Celebration and traditions, or acknowledgment of special events, religious and
other occasions, and family markers such as birthdays and anniversaries; honor-
ing holidays and important family experiences and events, often carried through
generations.
- Communication, or sharing beliefs and emotions among family members,
especially when information is exchanged in a style that indicates caring and
concern for each other.
- Financial management, or sound decision-making and skill, that permits meeting short- and long-term contingencies in a way that contributes to family
satisfaction.
- Hardiness, or the capacity to cope with or manage stress, that gives a sense
of family control over life (efficacy), displays family commitment, shows
confidence that the family will survive and smoothes the way for individual
and family growth, learning and challenges to each other for maximum self and
family actualization.
- Health, or the emotional, psychological and physical well-being of all family
members, and the continuation of wellness.
- Leisure activities, or preferences individually or conjointly held by family members
for spending free time.
- Personality, or the acceptance of individual traits, behavioral tendencies, outlook on life (paradigm), degrees of interdependency and being dependable.
- Support network, or the positive aspects of relationships with kin, friends, community members and others (formal and informal support networks).
- Time and routines, or creating a sense of continuity and stability in family life
via family meals, chores, bedtimes, weekly schedules, family togetherness, and
other ordinary and routine activities.

References

Abery, B. (2006). Family adjustment and adaptation with children with Down Syndrome. *Focus on Exceptional Children, 38*, 1–20.

Acs, G., Ross Phillips, K., & McKenzie, D. (2001). Playing by the rules, but losing the game: Americans in low-income working families. In M. Miller (Ed.), *Low-wage workers in the new economy* (pp. 21–44). Washington, DC: The Urban Institute.

Belle, D. & Doucet, J. (2003). Poverty, inequality, and discrimination as sources of depression among U.S. women. *Psychology of Women Quarterly, 27*, 101–13.

Boss, P. (2002). *Family stress management* (2nd ed.). Mountain View, CA: Sage.

Briar-Lawson, K., Lawson, H., Hennon, C., & Jones, A. (2001). *Family-centered policies and practices: International implications.* New York: Columbia University Press.

Burks, N. & Martin, B. (1985). Everyday problems and life change events: Ongoing versus acute sources of stress. *Journal of Human Stress, 11*, 27–35.

Carnevale, A. & Rose, S. (2001). Low earners: Who are they? Do they have a way out? In M. Miller (Ed.), *Low-wage workers in the new economy* (pp. 45–66). Washington, DC: The Urban Institute.

Child Trends. (2002). *Charting parenthood: A statistical portrait of fathers and mothers in America.* Washington, DC: Author.

Corey, M. & Corey, G. (2007). *Becoming a helper* (5th ed.). Belmont, CA: Thomson Brooks/Cole.

Crane, D. & Heaton, T. (Eds.). (2008). *Handbook of families and poverty.* Newbury Park, CA: Sage.

Edin, K. & Lein, L. (1997). *Making ends meet: How single mothers survive welfare and low-wage work.* New York: Russell Sage.

Giorgi, A. & Giorgi, B. (2003). Phenomenology. In J.A. Smith (Ed.), *Qualitative psychology: A practical guide to research methods* (pp. 25–50). Thousand Oaks, CA: Sage.

Gubrium, J. & Holstein, J. (1993). Phenomenology, ethnomethodology, and family discourse. In P. Boss, W. Doherty, R. LaRossa, W. Schumm, & S. Steinmetz (Eds.), *Sourcebook of family theories and methods: A contextual approach* (pp. 651–72). New York: Plenum Press.

Gubrium, J., & Holstein, J. (2000). The self in a world of going concerns. *Symbolic Interaction, 23,* 95–115.

Heclo, H. (1997). Values underpinning poverty programs for children. *The Future of Children, 7,* 141–8.

Hennon, C. & Peterson, G. (2004, July). *Adolescents' identity and family processes: A conceptual and empirical model.* Paper presented at the Second International Conference on New Directions in the Humanities, Prato, Italy.

Hennon, C. & Peterson, G. (2007). Estrés parental: Modelos teóricos y revisión de la literatura [Parenting stress: Theoretical models and a literature review]. In R. Esteinou (Ed.), *Fortalezas y desafíos de las familias en dos contextos: Estados Unidos de América y México* (pp. 167–221) [Strengths and challenges of families in two contexts: The United States of America and Mexico]. México, DF: Centro de Investigaciones y Estudios Superiores en Antropología Social (CIESAS) y Sistema Nacional para el Desarrollo Integral de la Familia (DIF).

Hennon, C. & Wilson, S. (Eds.). (2008). *Families in global context.* New York: Routledge.

Hildebrand, V., Phenice, L., Gray, M., & Hines, R. (2000). *Knowing and serving diverse families* (2nd ed.). Upper Saddle River, NJ: Merrill.

Hildenbrand, B. (2005). *Fallrekonstruktive Familienforschung. Anleitungen für die Praxis* [Case reconstruction in family research. Guidance for practice]. Wiesbaden: VS Verlag für Sozialwissenschaften.

Hildenbrand, B. & Hennon, C. (2008). Beyond the concept of "getting big or getting out": Entrepreneurship strategies to survive as a farm family. *International Journal of Entrepreneurship and Small Business.*

Hill, R. (1949). *Families under stress.* Westport, CT: Greenwood.

Hobfoll, S. (1989). Conversation of resources: A new attempt at conceptualizing stress. *American Psychologist, 44,* 513–24.

McCubbin, H. & McCubbin, M. (1988). Typologies of resilient families: Emerging roles of social class and ethnicity. *Family Relations, 37,* 247–54.

McElwee, G. (2007). In search of Montsalvatch: Making sense of interviewing farmers. Manuscript submitted for publication review.

National Wraparound Initiative. (n.d.). *National wraparound initiative.* Available HTML: http://www.rtc.pdx.edu/nwi (accessed 7 September 2007).

Orthner, D., Jones-Sanpei, H., & Williamson, S. (2004). The resilience and strengths of low-income families. *Family Relations, 53,* 159–67.

Patterson, J. (2002). Integrating family resiliency and family stress theory. *Journal of Marriage and the Family, 64,* 349–60.

Peterson, G. & Hennon, C. (2005). Conceptualizing parental stress with family stress theory. In P. McKenry & S. Price (Eds.), *Families and change: Coping with stressful events and transitions* (3rd ed.) (pp. 25–48). Thousand Oaks, CA: Sage.

Peterson, G. & Hennon, C. (2006). Influencias parentales en la competencia social de los adolescentes en dos culturas: una comparación conceptual entre los Estados Unidos y México [Parental influences on the social competence of adolescent in two cultures: A conceptual comparison between the United States and Mexico]. In R. Esteinou (Ed.), *Fortalezas y desafíos de las familias en dos contextos: Estados Unidos de América y México* (pp. 111–66) [Strengths and challenges of families in two contexts: The USA and Mexico]. México, DF: Centro de Investigaciones y Estudios Superiores en Antropología Social (CIESAS) y Sistema Nacional para el Desarrollo Integral de la Familia (DIF).

Radina, E., Hennon, C., & Gibbons, H. (in press). Divorce and mid and later life families: A phenomenological analysis with implications for family life educators. *Journal of Divorce and Remarriage*, 49(1/2).

Radina, M., Wilson, S., & Hennon, C. (in press). Parental stress among U.S. Mexican heritage parents: Implications for culturally relevant family life education. In R. Dalla, J. Defrain, J. Johnson, & D. Abbott (Eds.), *Strengths and challenges of new immigrant families: Implications for research, policy, education, and service*. Lanham, MD: Lexington Books.

Rank, M. & Hirschl, T. (2002). Welfare use as a life course event: Toward a new understanding of the U.S. safety net. *Social Work, 47*, 237–312.

Sandstrom, K. Martin, D., & Fine, G. (2003). *Symbols, selves, and social reality: A symbolic interactionist approach to social psychology and sociology*. Los Angeles, CA: Roxbury.

Shipler, D. (2004). *The working poor: Invisible in America*. New York: Alfred K. Knopf.

Unger, D., Cuevas, T., & Woolfolk, T. (2007). Human services and cultural diversity: Tenuous relationships, challenges, and opportunities ahead. In B. Trask & R. Hamon (Eds.), *Cultural diversity and families: Expanding perspectives* (pp. 173–93). Thousand Oaks, CA: Sage.

United Nations Development Program. (2001). *Making new technologies work for human development* (Human development report 2001). New York: Author.

United Nations Development Program. (2006). *Beyond scarcity: Power, poverty and the global water crisis* (Human development report 2006). New York: Author.

United Nations Population Fund. (2007). *State of world population 2007: Unleashing the potential of urban growth*. New York: Author.

U.S. Census. (2005). *Poverty status in the past 12 months of families* (S1702). Available HTML: http://factfinder.census.gov/servlet/STTable?geo_id=01000US&ds_name=ACS_2005_EST_G0 0_&qr_name=ACS_2005_EST_G00_S1702 (accessed 19 June 2007).

U.S. Department of Labor. (2002, March). *A profile of the working poor, 2000* (Report 957). Available HTML: http://www.bls.gov/cps/cpswp2000.htm (accessed 22 June 2007).

Voydanoff, P. & Majka, L. (Eds.). (1988). *Families and economic distress: Coping strategies and social policy*. Newbury Park, CA: Sage.

Wagstaff, A. (2002). Poverty and health sector inequalities. *Bulletin of the World Health Organization, 80*(2), 97–105.

Walsh, F. (2002). A family resilience framework: Innovative practice applications. *Family Relations, 51*, 130–7.

Williams, D. & Williams-Morris, R. (2000). Racism and mental health: The African American experience. *Ethnicity and Health, 5*, 243–68.

Wood, D. (2003). Effect of child and family poverty on child health in the U.S. *Pediatrics, 112*, 707–11.

World Health Organization and World Bank. (2002, Jan.). *Dying for change: Poor people's experience of health and ill-health*. Geneva: Author.

Critical Thinking Questions

1   What, in your opinion, are the strengths and/or weaknesses of the MRM model? How might this model be improved?

2   Many students think about family poverty in vary narrow terms. They think mechanically about the family as being above or below some seemingly arbitrary income number. How has this chapter changed your way of thinking about family poverty and family stress?

3   What does "making meaning of social situations" mean to you? Give examples from your own life.

14 Poverty, Policy, and Ideology

Katharine Briar-Lawson and Sandra Austin

The United States is the richest country in the world. It is also a remarkably accomplished nation. In fact, time and again our nation has demonstrated that with resolve, political will and financial investments, major achievements can be accomplished. For example, in 1961, President John F. Kennedy declared the U.S. national space mission to put a "man" on the moon. Subsequently, the U.S. space program was stepped up with large public investments. Public policies supported the trial-and-error approach to launching spacecraft and getting humans into space. By 1969, we eventually reached and walked on the moon. This achievement demonstrates that money, political will, and a trial-and-error approach to reaching desired goals are powerful tools for change.

At the same time as the space program was attracting great attention in public policy circles, a War on Poverty was being launched. This legislative initiative was first introduced by President Lyndon Johnson in 1964, and its goal was to eliminate U.S. poverty through creating equal opportunities for all. Unlike the successful space program, the War on Poverty was deemed a failure (Moynihan, 1969). In fact, the Office of Economic Opportunity, responsible for administering most antipoverty programs, was dismantled by President Richard Nixon in 1973; many of its initiatives did not succeed.

Some people might attribute failure to flawed assumptions undergirding the War on Poverty or to underinvestment in the poor and pathways out of poverty. Regardless of the cause, poverty persists: about 12% of the population is affected at any time. While reduced from the 25% levels before the War on Poverty, in 2004 poverty afflicted 37 million people, including 13 million children and 3.5 million elderly (DeNavas-Walt, Proctor, & Lee, 2006).

Moreover, the United States is faced with some of the greatest income inequities in history. The top fifth of the population now receives 50% of the income and the bottom fifth receives 3.4% (Allegretto, 2006). In the face of such profound wealth, the persistence of family poverty remains a paradox. Furthermore, given huge income disparities, the relative nature of family poverty is vexing. These profound inequalities severely diminish the quality of life and life chances for the poor (deLone, 1979). They lead to reduced longevity as the poor are deprived of adequate health care, and experience poor education that limits employment prospects, and a host of blocked opportunities that affect the quality of their lives (Wilkinson, 2006).

This chapter lays out some of the ideological underpinnings and policy approaches that foster the persistence of family poverty, along with poverty measures and belief systems regarding the causes of poverty. We will discuss the application of century-old principles, such as "less eligibility," in relation to several aid programs, including unemployment benefits, food stamps, housing, and the Earned Income Tax Credit. The chapter focuses also on women and their work roles in the home and in the labor market, and examines the changing ideologies that have governed public assistance approaches to mothers and children. We examine the antipoverty agenda of other nations and raise questions about the absence of attention to poverty in the United States. We conclude with an analysis of the diminishing quality of life among the poor, and increasingly among the middle class, as economic resources are reduced or withdrawn and prospects for the emergence of new twenty-first-century ideologies and social reforms shrink.

Values and the Measurement of Poverty

Poverty measures vary. The standard measures in the United States, growing out of the War on Poverty, involve a "market basket" approach to measuring poverty and counting the poor. Developed by Orshansky (1965), the common measure calculates the poverty index by determining the cost of a minimal food budget and tripling it. As the official U.S. poverty index, this measure also factors in family size and rural versus urban status.

Selective comparisons of this poverty measure indicate that the U.S. approach is flawed. For example, a comparison between the U.S. measure and the United Nations Poverty Index reveals that the UN index uses more discerning variables as yardsticks to calculate poverty numbers. The UN Poverty Index factors in longevity (likelihood of living to the age of 60), functional literacy, long-term unemployment rates, and low to median income. By the UN measure, the United States—the wealthiest nation in the world—ranks 17th (US Department of Human Development, 2003). In other words, while U.S. poverty measures are based on income alone, the UN poverty measures factor in two more variables— quality of life and longevity. These two variables reflect vast differences in the concept of poverty and in values, beliefs, and attitudes toward the poor.

Beliefs, Belief Systems, and the Poor

Values inform public policy. They shape the beliefs that people hold. As noted in Chapter 11, people's beliefs reveal how they think and what actions they take. Beliefs are not only shaped by values but also by experience. They discern which information is screened in or out and which ideas are embraced or rejected. For example, those with an investment in the status quo, in winning power struggles that protect their economic and political interests, will work very hard to discredit anyone who may lay claim to more of their share of the power or income pie. Contenders might argue that the status quo is unconscionable. For example, to have 48 million without health insurance and millions of poor children is a blight on the nation. They would be moved by data about the human costs and the life-scarring effects of such inequities. At the same time, the status quo contingent may believe that the poor have brought poverty upon themselves: that it is not the responsibility of government or taxpayers to subsidize those who are responsible for their plight. Such beliefs de facto reinforce policy inaction and add to the debates about the "worthy" versus "unworthy" poor.

Ideologies are systems of interconnected beliefs that serve as doctrines, shape the views of political systems and lead to the adoption of social policies that determine how government funds programs to serve citizens. Ideologies or doctrines drive public policies regarding the poor and the wealthy. If an ideology states that the cause of poverty is inequality, then poverty is seen as a "systems" or "structural" problem. Wealth redistribution might be a policy response from this ideological perspective. If another doctrine holds that the cause of poverty lies within the individual and can be attributed to certain individual deficits, then the policy response may involve fixing the deficits, or worse, punishment and stigmatization. Public policy informed by the latter doctrine would entail a minimalist approach to helping. If people believe, as do conservative thinkers such as George Gilder (1981) and Charles Murray (1984), that the cause of poverty is public policy that initiates programs to aid the poor, then the policy response might be to alter or eliminate such programs.

Doctrines that hold that the welfare state is bad for the economy and society and that the poor should fend for themselves will reemerge in multiple debates about social welfare policy regardless of the topic (e.g. aging, children, disasters, communities that have lost their tax-base through corporate flight). Such doctrines are so fixed and predicable that they become routinized among those who embrace them and make it possible to anticipate policy responses to issues.

In effect, individuals in power that has been derived primarily from privilege and vast financial resources, shape—even dictate—the terms of public policy debates, as well as the outcomes. Those with an investment in amassing vast wealth will protect their interests with a variety of tactics, including mounting fear campaigns or discrediting anyone who fights to advance better outcomes, especially if it means reducing their power or wealth. Wealth used to enhance privilege and power by demonizing the poor and their advocates is also used to oppress the poor through such mechanisms as discrimination, punishment, marginalization, and exclusion.

Those in power ultimately determine whose doctrines and values rule. Thus public policy is not just the by-product of values, beliefs, and ideologies, but ultimately those with the most political power. Fig. 14.1 depicts how values and ideologies, along with political power, shape policy and services. Later in the chapter, we will see the power dynamic of this values ideology playing out with issues like children's health insurance.

Beliefs and Debates about a "Culture of Poverty"

The implications of some of these ideologies and belief systems are most evident in assertions that there is a "culture of poverty," which leads to castigation of the poor. There is a long U.S. tradition of attributing poverty to cultural deficits seen

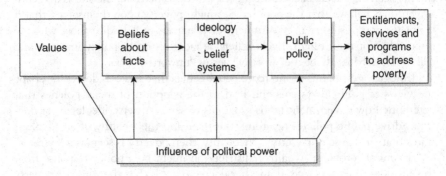

Figure 14.1 Power-Driven Values, Ideology, and Public Policy.

as part of a "culture of poverty." Anthropologists, such as Oscar Lewis (1966), introduced the idea that "cultural variables" (e.g. dependency, apathy, the inability to defer gratification) could explain poverty. These characteristics were seen to set in motion attitudes that impede progress toward self-sufficiency, and in fact create vicious cycles. Furthermore, they believed such cultural values, norms, and beliefs were learned and handed down through generations. "Culture of poverty" writers posit the need to induce new cultural values. In the extreme, Banfield (1970) and others suggested that sterilization would be one mechanism to end the "culture of poverty" and its generational transmission.

The Poor as Surplus Labor

Exclusionary practices involving the poor are well depicted in labor market policy. Some theorists and activists argue that the poor are used as commodities to address labor shortages. Cloward and Piven (1971) and Abramowitz (1996) claim that welfare policies regulate the supply of low-wage workers available for the labor market. They argue that welfare policies are expanded during periods of economic downturn to ensure that the poor and unemployed do not create political problems by protesting their economic condition. During periods of economic upturn, welfare benefits are curtailed to drive low-wage workers into the labor market. In Chapter 3 of this book, Abramowitz argues that patriarchal values and views about the poor, many of whom are women and children, guide public policies. Patriarchal approaches to policy result in strict controls over the allocation and receipt of public funds. Poor single mothers have become scapegoats for the "demise" of the traditional family structure. Increased numbers of single parents among the poor have contributed to increasingly punitive policies toward their receipt of public assistance because they allegedly avoid work in favor of welfare (Haskins, 2006).

Families and Poverty

The U.S. approach to the poor is closely linked to family public policy. Families have no protection or rights because they are seen as independent private social arrangements responsible for the provision of cradle-to-grave supports for members. More importantly, the United States has no comprehensive family policy. While most other western industrialized nations have demogrants, insurance-like programs that provide family or child allowances among other things, the United States has deliberately avoided such investments. The most that is available is the federal Child Tax Credit of $1,000 per child, which allows families to deduct $1,000 from their reported taxable income to receive a reduction in tax liability. While the Child Tax Credit is available to all families, they do not receive the benefit unless they file taxes, or if the credit exceeds their tax liability. In 1994, Garfinkel proposed a modest taxable basic income grant (BIG) that would be given to every adult as a way of equalizing income disparities (Garfinkel, Huan & Naidich, 2006). BIG would eliminate poverty and supplement education, childcare, and health care.

Such proposals do not fare well in the United States. In fact, policy neglect involving income supports creates multiple jeopardies for families. Absent social policy investments in families and their capacity to be economic providers, caregivers, childrearers, and so forth, the effectiveness of this most powerful institution—the family—is impeded. Moreover, families are expected to cope with the vagaries of the labor market; for many, wages dictate whether they have access to housing, health care, food, education, transportation, and subsistence supports. Labor market policies in the United States have never guaranteed full and equitable employment (Briar-Lawson, Lawson, Hennon, & Jones, 2001). If work were equitable, then family work roles would be monetarized. At present, families are not remunerated for caregiving; however, when child or adult care is provided outside the family, such work is monetarized. The irony is that families provide over 90% of all childcare, elder care, counseling, teaching, and socializing. Yet there is no policy investment in their roles or in their success. That family roles are not monetarized depicts another way in which critical functions are excluded from the market. Such marginalization and social exclusion are deliberate by-products of U.S. economic policy.

U.S. capitalism requires that a cushion of surplus workers be maintained as an anti-inflationary strategy. Thus, unemployment rates of at least 4.5% consign millions to joblessness during the year. The rising number of homeless families—many of whom are working—deepens the indelible scar on the nation's policy toward the poor. It is against this backdrop of absence of full and equitable employment policy that we discern some of the thinking and public policy correlates that have adversely affected U.S. poor.

Free market ideologies hold that all working-age adults must earn employment incomes and that those who do not must fend for themselves. Such ideology promotes regulatory practices that force increasing numbers of wage-earners into marginal low-paid jobs. Many poor families work full-time, remain poor, and face increased stress juggling work and family. Absent a car, many parents may have to take several buses to reach their employment. Absent health insurance, they may forgo necessary medical care. Absent a living wage, they are caught in jobs that offer no capacity to support their family beyond mere subsistence living, if that. Such jobs hark back to servitude. Stuck in dead-end jobs, most poor people lack labor union resources and advocacy that might foster more occupational mobility, benefits, wages, and economic power. Jobs and working conditions spawned in a full employment economy would provide workers with economic, employment, and occupational power for advancement.

Increasingly, the current "new economy" consists of low-wage and service sector jobs without benefits or job mobility. This "new economy" has brought pressing economic insecurities to rising numbers of families. Despite changing ideologies about women's work in the home, women are now working full-time while juggling the demands of family caregiving.

Ideology Regarding Women's Work

Family issues are women's issues. Parenting was once seen as valued work for low-income single mothers. When Mothers' Pensions were enacted in the early 1900s in about 26 states, the ideology was that no mother should be forced to work. Mothers' Pensions were seen as the solution to the higher cost of orphanages. They were deemed investments in child welfare because they helped children stay in the home, preventing institutional placement. It should be noted, however, that Mothers' Pensions were racially based allowances; in some states women of color were denied access (Mink, 1996).

When Aid to Dependent Children (ADC) was passed as part of the Social Security Act of 1935, the belief persisted that mothers should not be required to work outside the home and should be subsidized to stay home and care for their children. Later becoming AFDC, ADC was extended to include income-eligible mothers and their children. Until the last nine decades, two-parent families were denied benefits. Such entitlements can be contrasted with the more recent PRWORA and TANF, which require recipients to demonstrate work efforts in exchange for time-limited public assistance. Noncompliance with work requirements results in sanctions and loss of cash benefits.

How is it possible that old belief systems that held that no mother should be expected to parent while working full-time are now replaced with doctrines that require all low-income mothers to work (except the few that may be exempted due to disabilities)? We argue that these changed policies are derived from the changed public attitudes about women's work in the home, the backlash toward dependent poor mothers and children, and the need for more low-wage workers in the new economy. The change toward stay-at-home mothers was fueled by decades of conservative views and rising political power among conservatives with great wealth, who saw welfare rolls to be increasingly inhabited by single Black women and their children, whom they believed received benefits unfairly. The undertone of racism inherent in this assessment was fueled by beliefs that Black women lacked a work ethic, devalued marriage, and sought intergenerational dependence on the state to care for their children. At the same time, sexist attitudes defined single mothers as flawed and unworthy of benefits because they chose not to marry (Abramovitz, 1996). Thus, the demonization and punishment of some of these mothers reflect the intersection of racism, sexism, and classism wielded by those with the political and financial power to shape the debates.

Emblematic of such belief systems are dichotomizing views regarding the "worthy" and the "unworthy" or the deserving and undeserving poor (Trattner, 1999). The "unworthy" poor are seen as the able-bodied who "could" and "should" work. The "worthy" poor are more likely to be absolved of responsibility for their condition. A century ago, poor White single mothers were seen as "worthy" of assistance. They claimed Mothers' Pensions and were expected to stay home and care for their children. Racism and backlash toward growing numbers of ethnic minority single parents who became welfare recipients fueled beliefs that they are "unworthy" of assistance.

Entrenched ideologies about poverty causes and consequences ensure that victim-blaming practices and policies ensue. Instead of those with few financial means being seen as predictable causalities of economic policies linked to free market ideologies, poor families are punished and blamed for conditions over which they may have no control. When their conditions are compounded by racism and sexism, the jeopardy poor families face grows.

Retrenchment in entitlement programs together with the imposition of time limits implemented in TANF, foster care, and some public housing programs further aggravates the harms to poor families. For some families, TANF five-year lifetime limits are compounded by 18-month foster care time limits. Thus, poor women who lose their TANF grants may also be at risk for child neglect charges unless they find a new source of income to support their families. While access to TANF may be the best protective factor leading to child–parent reunification (Wells & Guo 2004), unreasonable time limits drive some poor children into adoption. The rate of U.S. adoptions has doubled in the past decade, with the number of children of color available for adoption growing disproportionately. In some communities, time limits on public housing further compound the risks and profound vulnerabilities that poor families endure.

Children who are raised in poverty, in many instances, are also causalities of the social exclusion that their families and communities face. Thus, the cycle of poverty may continue, not because of values different from those of the mainstream, but because of caste-like conditions and blocked pathways.

Children and Pathways out of Poverty

Instead of guaranteeing equal opportunities and outcomes or sufficient safety nets to help those sliding into or stuck in poverty, U.S. policies marginalize and disenfranchise millions of poor children. In fact, instead of "cradle-to-grave" safety nets for families who are at risk of poverty, the pathway for their children is increasingly a pathway to prison.

In 1978, Ogbu wrote about the induction of children of color into caste-like pathways. He argued that many poor children do not fare well in school because school has not been a pathway to success for their parents or for others in their communities. In fact, the realities they face—their parents' unemployment or poverty-level wages, community disenfranchisement, and marginalization—alienate them from school and from those who argue that hard work in school would pay off. Despite these realities, rugged individualistic U.S. ideologies hold that anyone "can make it from the log cabin to the White House." The belief holds that one must pull oneself up by one's bootstraps and that through rugged individualism one can achieve. This belief system is so entrenched in the United States that data to the contrary do not penetrate policy debates.

Data marshaled by the Children's Defense Fund (CDF) reveal that, for many poor minority children, the pipeline is not one of social mobility and success, but incarceration. For example, CDF data (2007) show that in comparison to Caucasian youth, disproportionate numbers of Black and Latino youth are placed in detention and incarcerated for crimes. Minority youth from low-income families face tremendous obstacles that make their access to jobs and successful futures uncertain. Consequently, for poor minority children, facilitators on this prison pathway include their increased risk of abuse, neglect, poor academic performance, delinquency, and violence. When parents earn insufficient income, it affects their ability to feed their children, support them in their academic achievement, and counter their induction into delinquent activities. Caste-like dynamics shape their trajectory.

Costs of Social Exclusion

In 2003, the cost of U.S. prisons was $40 billion (Kennedy, 2003), exceeding investments in children's schooling. At an earlier time, $40 billion was more than sufficient to eliminate child poverty in the United States. The lack of decent housing and entitlements to cost-effective programs like Head Start, childcare, health care, after-school programs, and jobs for youth reflects ideologies that require that the poor fend for themselves despite the high-cost outcomes. Moreover, public funds flow freely to support rising prison and jail costs, but not to support programs that would deter young people from crime and prison pathways. The political will that prizes investments in deep-end high-cost programs like prisons, rather than prevention and human capital development, derives from deep-seated rugged individualistic and "bootstrap" ideologies regarding an individual's culpability if he or she does not succeed.

Given the horrific human and economic waste as poor children are inducted into prisons rather than jobs, and lives of social marginalization rather than social mobility and inclusion, one would think that antipoverty agendas would be high on the public policy priority list. Racism is tied to exclusionary dynamics, and thus an antipoverty campaign would need to engage race and entitlements issues.

Current policy debates that limit or block aid to immigrants also reflect a growing xenophobia in the United States. This trend, coupled with explicit or veiled racism that often undergirds poverty policy deliberations, suggests that the debates are not just about income support but also about basic human rights.

Less Eligibility and Aid in Wages

Much of the social policy that affects poor families today was developed in 1935 as the federal government's response to the Great Depression. In the early 1900s, ideologies held that government had a limited role in providing supports to families in times of need. Families themselves, religious institutions, and charitable organizations were responsible for providing most of the services for families with social or economic needs.

The Depression changed the way society viewed social welfare and ushered in some human rights in the form of income entitlements. Widespread unemployment and a sense of collective and personal disasters created new ideologies about the necessary role of government in addressing massive economic and social disruption. The ideology underpinning several newly enacted public aid programs was that of less eligibility—stemming from the Poor Laws—in which aid was thought of as undesirable compared to work. Demeaning, meager benefits and in-kind supports were purposely enacted to aid the poor as incentives to seek pathways out of poverty. In addition, aid was often constructed to bolster local and national economic interests (e.g. housing, unemployment benefits, and food stamps).

A major challenge policymakers have faced in recent decades has been upholding the principle of less eligibility, given the package of benefits possible (housing, food, health insurance). For example, TANF and unemployment benefits uphold "less eligibility" to prevent nonworking poor from receiving more than working poor. Passed in 1935 to address the jobless problem during the Depression, unemployment benefits are pegged at a proportion of prior salary; states can also set a maximum allowable benefit. In this way, deriving few income incentives from unemployment benefits, jobless individuals will presumably be incentivized to find work. Moreover, in the United States, unemployment benefits are usually available for up to 26 weeks. When there is a severe downturn in the economy, Congress may vote to extend benefits for up to 52 weeks. Retrenchment in the numbers and types of employees eligible for unemployment benefits in the past two decades has resulted in fewer jobless workers accessing benefits.

The earliest efforts to address the national needs of the poor regarding housing occurred in the 1930s. With a thousand evictions a day, the Depression caused a crisis for many people (Fisher, 1994). Bauer (1934), an early housing advocate, believed that two-thirds of the population should be provided housing by the federal government. Advocates thought that only government could build safe, sanitary housing. Public housing advocates argued for a mix of social classes to foster integration and the "uplifting" of poor residents. However, instead of making public housing a mixed housing strategy for low- and moderate-income persons, public housing policy targeted the very poor who often were in receipt of welfare.

In the 1970s, when Section 8 was introduced as a housing voucher strategy, rent supplements replaced federal investments in building public housing. Despite vast Section 8 housing waiting lists, and with the growing number of homeless families with working parents, housing policy has also been aligned with the doctrine of "less eligibility" (i.e. making it undesirable). Public housing is often stigmatized for its institutionalized and drab look and for the concentration of poor families in one geographic location with limited community resources (i.e. jobs, shopping plazas). Because of this, public housing is linked to a host of social problems for poor families and their communities. In contrast to this housing policy for the poor was the policy adopted for lower- to middle-income families. The 1935 public policy, through the Federal Housing Authority (FHA), fostered low-interest mortgage loans for the middle class while large high-rise buildings were constructed for the poor (Levitan, Mangum, & Mangum, 1998). Only recently have debates shifted in support of home ownership for the poor. The very loans once directed to the middle class are now being expanded to serve selected poor persons who qualify for low-interest mortgage loan assistance. Unfortunately, over the past several years the private market has been increasingly seen as a viable mechanism to address the needs of the poor. Housing in this society is not seen as a right; it is seen as a commodity. Housing is to be sold for profit to people who can secure adequate resources. The recent sub-prime housing crisis is an excellent example of the problems that can arise when the market is relied upon to supply people with what they need. Now, instead of people securing low-interest loans for housing, we have the phenomena of people losing their homes due to unscrupulous lenders taking advantage of the poor eager to attain a house and a piece of the American dream.

Agricultural economic interests are advanced by food stamps. While never providing sufficient funds for food and nutrition, food stamps emerged from the feeding programs of the 1930s. Such programs were as much directed at supporting farmers as they were at aiding the poor (Trattner, 1999). Initially, surplus agricultural and farm products, including cheese, other dairy products and canned goods, were distributed to the poor. In 1964, the Food Stamp Act was passed with the goal of using the nation's food to provide nutritional supports for the poor. The passage of the food stamp bill resulted in a 10-fold increase in food availability (Levitan, Mangum, & Mangum, 1998). The program has the de facto effect of advancing income supports for the working poor. Rather than raising wages, food stamp programs function for the working poor as an "aid in wages." This "aid in wage" practice goes back to early Poor Law days and again focuses on governmental subsidies for impoverished workers rather than their rights to wage increases.

To ensure that the principle of less eligibility was upheld through the centuries, aid in wage programs and policies have been adopted. From the early days of the Speenhamland Act of 1795 in England to current times, efforts to supplement poverty-level wages have necessitated public investments. The EITC program in the United States is the largest antipoverty program and is responsible for lifting as many as four million people out of poverty (Nagle & Johnson, 2006). Initiated in 1975, the EITC is a refundable tax credit to the working poor. It offsets taxes paid by working poor by returning tax funds to them. A family with two or more children received as much as $4,400 in 2005 (Greenstein, 2005). Policy analysts agree that EITC has been the most successful income support program for the poor because it rewards work while providing income subsidies to reduce the number of families living in poverty (Greenstein). Critics of EITC indicate that the refund fails to go far enough in providing ample refunds to families who have more than nine children (Ozawa & Hong, 2003).

While this EITC program helps to offset low wages through public aid in the form of tax credits, it still has the same deterrent effects that were decried in the Speenhamland Act in England. It serves as a deterrent to wage increases and de facto may set a maximum on wages. Like food stamps, TANF, unemployment benefits, and housing support, EITC is not claimed by all who are eligible. GAO (2001) estimated that up to 25% of the working poor do not access the EITC entitlement.

While mechanisms such as EITC in the United States, and Family or Children's Allowances in all other industrialized nations, exist to lift people out of poverty, there are no national campaigns to address U.S. poverty.

Salient Antipoverty Campaigns

The UN has adopted the millennium goals of eliminating extreme poverty by 2015. Progress is charted, and investments are seen as trial-and-error approaches to poverty reduction. The World Bank has adopted poverty-alleviation goals involving extreme deprivation. The UK has adopted a 20-year goal to eliminate child poverty by 2020. The United States, however, has not set any poverty reduction goals. If pressed, the current administration might argue that its healthy marriage and fatherhood initiatives constitute antipoverty programs. In both cases, the goal is to bring men back into single-mother families (HHS, 2007). The purpose is to offset the rise of single-mother households and to increase access to income, which is more likely in two-parent than in one-parent households. What such programmatic strategies often overlook, however, is the fact that domestic violence is a source of grave concern to many low-income women. While public policy may encourage women to marry and may foster more fathers' involvement in the lives of their children, many women work to avoid problematic relationships (NOW Legal Defense and Education Fund, 2006).

While there is no federal antipoverty campaign, local communities may undertake poverty-reduction initiatives. Despite Vice-Presidential hopeful John Edwards' argument that poverty reduction should be a policy goal, most politicians steer away from poverty policy, which has no political cachet. Instead, there is much concern over declining wages and the demise of the middle class. Books popularized by talk show hosts like Dobbs (2006) decry the fact that it takes two family wage-earners to adequately support a family. Plant closures and job losses, disproportionately affecting the poor and minorities, dominate the debates. Thus, the poor are now seen as being under siege only in relation to the job market and as an extension of the middle class (Hartman, 2006).

Economic Insecurity and the American Dream:
New Class Alliances?

The American Dream is a concept that suggests that anyone in this society can reap rewards if they work hard. In a National League of Cities survey (2005, p. 25), the American Dream was defined as "financial security, finding a good job and having access to and obtaining a quality education." The barriers to attaining the American Dream were linked to poor education, low-paying jobs, and concerns about financial security. Many low-income workers strive to achieve the American Dream with the belief that it will result in upward mobility for their children. This survey showed that 72% believed that the government should help families succeed. However, 45% believed that the federal government has done more to hamper than to support their quest for the American Dream (National League of Cities).

Increasingly, the painful uphill struggles and experiences of the working poor, portrayed by authors like DeParle (2004) and Ehrenreich (2001), have struck fear in the middle class. Middle-class workers are increasingly facing economic insecurity as they lack job stability, health care insurance, and wages sufficient to meet basic needs. Economic insecurity unites the working poor with growing numbers of the middle class. Income and economic insecurity are compounded by health insurance deficits.

From 2004 to 2005, an employment-based health insurance decrease (DeNavas-Walt, Proctor, & Lee, 2006) was accompanied by an upward trend in numbers of uninsured persons. They noted that in 2005, 46.6 million people (15.9%) were uninsured compared to 45.3 million (15.6%) in 2004 and 14.6% in 2001.

Until very recently, the minimum wage had not been increased from its 1997 level of $5.15 an hour. Consequently, the economic disparity of low-wage workers has been sustained by the inaction and neglect of policymakers. Some argue that raising the wage threatens low-wage entry-level jobs (Kane, 2005). Others contend that the minimum wage should be indexed to inflation by using the Consumer Price Index to ensure that wages keep pace with inflation and that buying power is not eroded. Linking wage increases to inflation would eliminate the political process of devolving decisions on minimum wage hikes to bodies like Congress, which until very recently, impeded increases. Battles over the minimum wage illustrate the absence of social policy pertaining to economic disparities and income insecurity.

In the new, more service-based economy of the twenty-first century, low- and middle-income workers are experiencing similar losses in opportunities because the economy has not rewarded them. Workers in both classes are struggling. The lower class is trying to acquire some of the symbols of the American Dream. Yet they are employed in jobs that do not provide opportunities to obtain a good wage, benefits, or options for promotion.

At the same time, the middle class is experiencing erosion in their income and employer benefits along with job and livelihood instability and pension plan defaults. "Occupational social welfare," which links employment and private sector policy and benefits, is now undergoing some of the same retrenchment as public social welfare programs (Titmuss, 1966).

In the new economy, globalization has enticed and driven U.S. capital to other parts of the world, resulting in the loss of higher-wage employment at home. However, when concerns are raised about how all of these factors are creating social and economic injustice, especially for the middle class, the arguments are reminiscent of those used to block investments in the poor. Ideologies hold that government should not regulate corporations as they globalize; nor should government impact corporate productivity or interfere with wages, benefits, pensions, or mobility as corporations compete globally.

"Race to the Bottom" Welfare State Cutbacks: Tipping Points and Opportunities

The belief that investments in the economy and wealth creation are the solution to economic security and poverty elimination has dominated arguments for dismantling welfare state programs and imposing time limits on eligibility programs. As disinvestments in safety net programs continue to drive public policy, and arguments for tax cuts for the rich and for corporations succeed, the trajectory for the welfare state could be "a race to the bottom." This means that retrenchments in welfare state programs are promulgated as good for the economy and the long-term economic well-being of individuals and families. Thus instead of building and fine-tuning welfare state programs to offset economic casualties of the new economy, the economic trickle-down doctrine, with its presumed benefits for all, continues to dominate policy decision-making.

As the middle class feels increasingly threatened by private sector cutbacks in occupational social welfare such as health benefits and pension plans, and public aid programs such as unemployment benefits, they may be less likely to support further retrenchment in universal programs such as Social Security. In fact, despite proposals to privatize Social Security, the public policy debate has been laced with fears about risks in dismantling safety nets.

Is it possible that the tipping point has been reached and that the combined effects of income inequalities, economic insecurity, and low-wage jobs in the new economy mitigate against more safety net losses? Actually, as middle-class workers feel pressed by the changes in the economy and see little to support them in an economic slide downward, there may be a countervailing momentum afoot. This downward trend combined with the potential for low- and middle-income workers to unite around job and benefit losses in the workplace might spark new discourses about entitlements and universal services.

A preview of future social policy deliberations is epitomized in recent Congressional debates about reauthorizing the 1997 State Children's Health Insurance Program (SCHIP). SCHIP is a child health insurance program for families who have incomes too high for Medicaid eligibility and too low for private insurance. Debates have focused on worthy and unworthy families with low and middle incomes. Since its passage, SCHIP has been expanded for families so that 23 states allow middle-income families with incomes at 200% above the poverty level to acquire SCHIP for their children. Despite SCHIP popularity, ideologies and values drive the predictable debates.

One doctrine involves beliefs and values that hold that SCHIP creates disincentives for middle-income families to purchase private health insurance. The values inherent in this debate center on the ideology that government (and ultimately taxpayers) should not undermine the market economy by offering any subsidy that would supplant private health insurance. There is also fear that this new legislation would drive up the per child cost of health insurance while reducing the overall availability of private health insurance. When data to the contrary are presented, they are discredited as "media myths." Instead what is proposed is a redesigned program linked to a tax incentive to encourage middle-class families' to participate in private insurance and to minimize reliance on SCHIP.

This debate highlights values that privilege the market economy over government subsidies to shape public policy. Ultimately those with the most political power have the votes in Congress to influence the outcome.

Public discourse about the importance of quality health care is increasingly surfacing as an issue that citizens expect Congress will address. Eventually Congress will enact some legislation on more health insurance guarantees that will represent a hybrid model, with as little government subsidy as possible and as many supports as feasible for private sector insurance and health care providers.

Regardless of power differentials, doctrines about protecting the free market at the expense of the poor and increasingly economically vulnerable middle-income individuals and families will dominate the policy choices and potential outcomes. Protecting the market is a central component of U.S. capitalist values and ideologies. Some argue that the stakes are very high. These debates are not just about the fears and threats engulfing the poor and the middle class, they are ultimately about threats to our democracy (Hartman, 2006).

Many of the middle class, now fearing the demise of the safety net, may have once supported the dismantling of welfare and other welfare state programs. Some might have scapegoated welfare recipients because of their own fears about their growing economic vulnerability. New unity might emerge between the classes as they face the prospect of further degradation of both the welfare state and the economy in terms of wages, benefits, and economic security. This may lead to new opportunities for forging improved social and economic justice in the twenty-first century.

Together families in both classes face the absence of a comprehensive social policy that would support successful outcomes for their members. Human capital development requires investments in families, not "race to the bottom" cuts in benefits and supports. Given globalization and its impact on the economic and social well-being of families and communities, it is essential that welfare state policies reverse the minimalist approaches that have been shaping life chances for many in our society. Demands by those threatened with losses of livelihoods, incomes, and services for their families in middle-income brackets may help usher in more empathy and protection. Such demands may also compel more supports, services, and entitlements for those who are at rock bottom.

For the most part, European models of social insurance are not means-tested and set aside just for the poor. Housing, health, and family income support schemes are more universal in scope. Thus, middle-income beneficiaries will, more often than not, fight to protect what they have had as threats increase to their welfare state benefits. In the United States, the job that lies ahead is one of convincing middle-income families that they have rights and opportunities to demand more supports and entitlements to offset the rollercoaster effects of job and livelihood loss, health and pension benefit loss, along with nonmonetarized family caregiving demands and crises that take them out of the labor market.

The most obvious next step is to institute full and equitable employment, demograms such as BIG or family allowances together with other entitlements that ensure a more robust welfare state. To attend to the needs of very poor families requires intensive investments to eliminate poverty.

Reprogramming dollars spent on incarceration into antipoverty agendas may demonstrate that the investments made in the poor help not only conserve the human capital of a nation, but also demonstrate a more humane return on investments than current approaches to the poor offer. Instead of being marginalized as surplus labor and then castigated for their plight, the poor represent high-promise and high-impact investments for the twenty-first century.

It took a major Depression with cataclysmic consequences for thousands of families to usher in the modern welfare state of the last century. While mass effects of Depression-like consequences are now "managed" by governmental interventions, case by case casualties in the current economy of uncertainty and instability are every bit as compelling. Movements to unite around entitlements and benefits have yet to fully emerge. These might be led increasingly by working poor and middle-income families who recognize that the free market doctrine cannot replace their rights to more stabilized work and income supports.

Advocates for families and family support can begin to lay the foundation for a more family-centered social and economic justice movement as destabilized workers affect entire families and communities. A family-centered social and economic justice movement may be a stepping-stone to investments and more universal supports for economically vulnerable individuals and families in our society.

References

Abramovitz, M. (1996). *Regulating the lives of women.* Boston: South End Press.

Allegretto, S. (2006). *Wealth inequality is vast and growing.* Economic Policy Institute. Available HTML: http://www.epi.org/content.cfm/webfeatures_snapshots_20060823 (accessed 1 December 2007).

Banfield, E. (1970). *Unheavenly city: The nature and future of our urban crisis.* Boston: Little Brown.

Bauer, C. (1934). *Modern housing.* Boston: Houghton Mifflin.

Briar-Lawson, K., Lawson, H., Hennon, C., & Jones, A. (2001). *Family centered policies and practices: International implications.* New York: Columbia University Press.

Children's Defense Fund. (2007). *America's cradle to prison pipeline* (CDF Report). Washington, DC: Author.

Cloward, R. & Piven, F. (1971). *Regulating the poor: The functions of public welfare.* New York: Vintage Books.

deLone, R. (1979). *Small futures: Children's inequality and the limits of liberal reform.* New York: Harcourt Brace Jovanovich.

DeNavas-Walt C., Proctor, B., & Lee, C. (2006). The income, poverty, and health insurance coverage in the United States: 2005. In U.S. Census Bureau, *Current Population Reports* (pp. 60–231). Washington, DC: Government Printing Office.

DeParle, J. (2004). *American dream: Three women, ten kids, and a national drive to end welfare.* New York: Viking.

Dobbs, L. (2006). *War on the middle class: How the government, big business, and special interest groups are waging war on the American dream and how to fight back.* New York: Viking.

Ehrenreich, B. (2001). *Nickel and dimed: On (not) getting by in America*. New York: Metropolitan Books.

Fisher, R. (1994). *Let the people decide: Neighborhood organizing in America*. New York: Twayne.

Garfinkel, I., Huang, C., & Naidich, W. (2006). The effects of a basic income guarantee on poverty and income distribution. In B. Ackerman, A. Alstott, & P. Van Parijs (Eds.), *Redesigning distribution: Basic income and stakeholder grants as cornerstones of a more egalitarian capitalism* (pp. 143–74). New York: Verso.

Gilder, G. (1981). *Wealth and poverty*. New York: Basic Books.

Greenstein, R. (2005). *The earned income tax credit: Boosting employment, aiding the working poor*. Center on Budget and Policy Priorities. Available HTML: http://www.cbpp.org/7-19-05eic.pdf (accessed 7 July 2006).

Hartman, T. (2006). *Screwed: The undeclared war against the middle class—and what we can do about it*. San Francisco: Berrett-Koehler.

Haskins, R. (2006). *Poverty and income in 2006: A look at the new census data and what the numbers mean for children and families*. Washington, DC: Brookings Institute.

Kane, T. (2005). *Minimizing economic opportunity by raising the minimum wage*. The Heritage Foundation. Available HTML: http://www.heritage.org/Research/Economy/wm676.cfm (accessed 1 January 2007).

Kennedy, A. (2003, 9 August). Speech at the American Bar Association annual meeting. Anthony M. Kennedy, Associate Justice Supreme Court of the United States.

Levitan, A., Mangum, L., & Mangum, L. (1998). *Programs in aid of the poor* (7th ed.). Baltimore, MD: Johns Hopkins University Press.

Lewis, O. (1966). *Children of Sanchez*. New York: Random House.

Mink, G. (1996). *The wages of motherhood: Inequality in the welfare state, 1917–1942*. New York: Cornell University Press.

Moynihan, D. (1969). *Maximum feasible misunderstanding*. New York: Free Press.

Murray, C. (1984). *Losing ground: American social policy 1950–1980*. New York: Basic Books.

Nagle, A. & Johnson, N. (2006). *A hand up: How state earned income tax credits help working families escape poverty in 2006*. Available HTML: http://www.cbpp.org/38-06sfp.htm (accessed 27 September).

National League of Cities. (2005). *The American Dream in 2004: A survey of the American people*. Washington, DC: Author.

NOW Legal Defense and Education Fund (2006). *Why NOW legal defense opposes federal marriage promotion in TANF reauthorization*. Available HTML: www.nowldef.org/html/issues/wel/marriage backgrounder.pdf (accessed 20 September 2006).

Ogbu, J. (1978). *Minority education and caste: The American system in cross-cultural perspective*. New York: Academic Press.

Orshansky, M. (1965). Counting the poor: Another look at the poverty profile. *Social Security Bulletin*, 28, 3–29.

Ozawa, M. & Hong, B. (2003). The effects of EITC and children's allowances on the economic well-being of children. *Social Work Research*, 27, 1.

Titmuss, R. (1966). *Essays on "the welfare state"* (2nd ed.). London: Allen and Unwin.

Trattner, W. (1999). *From poor law to welfare state* (6th ed.). New York: Free Press.

U.S. Bureau of the Census. (2006). *Current population survey*. Washington, DC: U.S. Government Printing Office.

U.S. Congress. (1996). Personal Responsibilities and Work Opportunities Reconciliation Act of 1996. 104 Congress. 2nd Session.

U.S. Department of Health and Human Services. Administration for Children and Families (2007). *The healthy families initiatives*. Available HTML: http://www.acf.hhs.gov/healthymarriage/about/mission.html#ms (accessed 29 September).

U.S. Department of Human Development. (2003). *Report 2003: Millennium development goals compact among nations to end human poverty*. Available HTML: http://hdr.undp.org/reports/global/2003/indicator/indic_27_1_1 (accessed 1 December 2006).

U.S. General Accounting Office. (2001). *Earned income tax credit eligibility and participation* (Letter Report GAO-02-290R). Washington, DC: Author.

Wells, K. & Guo, S. (2004). Reunification of foster children before and after welfare reform. *Social Service Review*, 78, 74–95.

Wilkinson, R. (2006). *The impact of inequality: How to make sick societies healthier*. New York: Routledge.

Critical Thinking Questions

1 What can one person, such as yourself, do to improve the plight of poor families? Does your solution address the structural level or the individual level?

2 How are poverty and "social exclusion" addressed in western Europe? What appeals to you about some of their policies? Why? Could their policies work in the United States? Why, or why not?

3 Think about what happens when class and gender intersect. Search online for statistics on gender and income disparities. Develop a chart that shows comparisons between the earnings of men and women, in general. How about income disparities between divorced men and women? Are there differences in your field? Do you think this will change on its own in the future? If not, what can you do to move the United States toward income equity?

Index

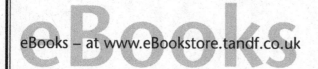

eBooks – at www.eBookstore.tandf.co.uk

A library at your fingertips!

eBooks are electronic versions of printed books. You can store them on your PC/laptop or browse them online.

They have advantages for anyone needing rapid access to a wide variety of published, copyright information.

eBooks can help your research by enabling you to bookmark chapters, annotate text and use instant searches to find specific words or phrases. Several eBook files would fit on even a small laptop or PDA.

NEW: Save money by eSubscribing: cheap, online access to any eBook for as long as you need it.

Annual subscription packages

We now offer special low-cost bulk subscriptions to packages of eBooks in certain subject areas. These are available to libraries or to individuals.

For more information please contact
webmaster.ebooks@tandf.co.uk

We're continually developing the eBook concept, so keep up to date by visiting the website.

www.eBookstore.tandf.co.uk

Printed in the United States
by Baker & Taylor Publisher Services